Nutrition and Sensation

Nutrition and Sensation

Alan R. Hirsch, MD

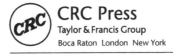

CRC Press
Taylor & Francis Group
Boca Raton London New York

CRC Press is an imprint of the
Taylor & Francis Group, an **informa** business

CRC Press
Taylor & Francis Group
6000 Broken Sound Parkway NW, Suite 300
Boca Raton, FL 33487-2742

First issued in paperback 2021

© 2015 by Taylor & Francis Group, LLC
CRC Press is an imprint of Taylor & Francis Group, an Informa business

No claim to original U.S. Government works

Version Date: 20150330

ISBN 13: 978-1-03-209878-4 (pbk)
ISBN 13: 978-1-4665-6907-2 (hbk)

Library of Congress Cataloging-in-Publication Data

Nutrition and sensation / [edited by] Alan R. Hirsch.
    p. ; cm.
    Includes bibliographical references and index.
    ISBN 978-1-4665-6907-2 (hardcover : alk. paper)
    I. Hirsch, Alan R., editor, contributor.
    [DNLM: 1. Nutritional Physiological Phenomena. 2. Sensation. QU 145]

RA784
613.2--dc23   2015011629

Visit the Taylor & Francis Web site at
http://www.taylorandfrancis.com

and the CRC Press Web site at
http://www.crcpress.com

Contents

Preface..vii

Acknowledgments..ix

Editor xi

Contributors xiii

Chapter 1 Tasting History 1

Gabriella Petrick

Chapter 2 Chemosensory Disorders: Emerging Roles in Food Selection,
Nutrient Inadequacies, and Digestive Dysfunction............................25

Carl M. Wahlstrom, Jr., Alan R. Hirsch, and Bradley W. Whitman

Chapter 3 Retronasal Olfaction..65

Jason J. Gruss and Alan R. Hirsch

Chapter 4 Taste and Food Choice 81

Thomas R. Scott

Chapter 5 Psychophysical Measurement of Human Oral Experience 103

Derek J. Snyder and Linda M. Bartoshuk

Chapter 6 Color Correspondences in Chemosensation: The Case of Food
and Drinks... 139

Betina Piqueras-Fiszman and Charles Spence

Chapter 7 Effect of Visual Cues on Sensory and Hedonic Evaluation of Food...159

Debra A. Zellner

Chapter 8 Chemesthesis, Thermogenesis, and Nutrition 175

Hilton M. Hudson, Mary Beth Gallant-Shean, and Alan R. Hirsch

Chapter 9 The Look and Feel of Food.. 193

Sanford S. Sherman, Mary Beth Gallant-Shean, and Alan R. Hirsch

Chapter 10 Auditory System and Nutrition 203

Alan R. Hirsch

Chapter 11 Sensory-Specific Satiety and Nutrition 209

Alan R. Hirsch

Chapter 12 Chemosensory Influences on Eating and Drinking, and Their
Cognitive Mediation 221

David A. Booth

Chapter 13 Review of Chemosensation for Weight Loss 295

Darin D. Dougherty

Chapter 14 Chemosensation to Enhance Nutritional Intake in Cancer Patients 309

Cheryl A. Bacon and Veronica Sanchez Varela

Index 323

Preface

Of the estimated 130 million books published in the last two millennia, nutrition has maintained a preeminent position. While mostly about weight reduction diets, topics have spanned the spectrum ranging from anthropological to zoological nutrition. What has been missing has been a book solely devoted to the effect of the senses on nutrition. Clearly, the sensory influence on food choice is ubiquitous. It is trite to highlight that if a food does not look, taste, or smell good, then it will not readily be eaten. However, there are exceptions: the ugly fruit or capsaicin-induced trigeminal pain. Part of hedonics, and thus consumption of foods, is based on past experience and expectation. When indigenous cultures cannibalize the captivated warriors' brains, they are dapatical; raw, poisonous puffer fish sushi is a delicacy in Japan; and scrotum is treasured to many as an Asian gourmet.

Such expectations are grounded in the sensory properties of the consumable. Whether it be the color of soda; the creaminess of ice cream, the astringency of wine, the viscosity of maple syrup, the bitterness of coffee, or the aroma of chocolate, the sensory experience is the fuel of the locomotion of the hedonics of consumption.

Ultimately, behavior results from integration and higher cognitive interpretation of the sensory experience of eating. Sensory components of consumption are integrated in the posterior insular cortex (for taste) and orbitofrontal cortex (for smell) (Rolls 2006). The behavioral response to such sensations is directed through these and the anterior cingulate cortex to control behavior, and it is these behaviors that ultimately act to regulate nutrition (Benarroch 2010).

REFERENCES

Benarroch, E.E. 2010. Neural control of feeding behavior. Overview and clinical correlations. *Neurology* 74:1643–1650.

Rolls, E.T. 2006. Neural mechanisms of taste, smell, and flavour. *Chemical Senses* 31:E38–E39.

Alan R. Hirsch, M.D.
Smell & Taste Treatment and Research Foundation
Chicago, IL

Acknowledgments

With this in mind this text has been created. Thanks to the many without whose help this project would not have come to fruition. To each of the chapter authors who have devoted so much uncompensated time in this effort, to Denise Fahey for her administrative and organizational assistance, and to Jill Jurgensen and Randy Brehm at CRC Press for their motivation and foresight, I thank you all.

Editor

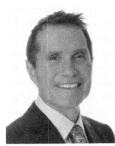

Alan R. Hirsch, M.D., F.A.C.P., a neurologist and psychiatrist who specializes in the treatment of smell and taste loss, is the neurological director of the Smell & Taste Treatment and Research Foundation in Chicago. He is a faculty member in the Department of Medicine at Mercy Hospital and Medical Center.

Dr. Hirsch is board-certified by the American Board of Neurology and Psychiatry in neurology, psychiatry, pain medicine, geriatric psychiatry, and addiction psychiatry. Dr. Hirsch has served as an expert on smell and taste disorders for many local governmental agencies, the Environmental Protection Agency (EPA), and many State's Attorney offices and the US Attorney General.

Dr. Hirsch earned both his medical and BA degrees from the University of Michigan.

He has also authored *Dr. Hirsch's Guide to Scentsational Weight Loss* (Element Books, 1997), *Scentsational Sex* (Element Books, 1998), *What Flavor is Your Personality?* (Source Books, 2001), *Life's a Smelling Success* (Authors of Unity Publishing, 2003), *What Your Doctor May Not Tell You about Sinusitis* (Hachette Book Group, 2004), *What's Your Food Sign?* (Stewart, Tabori and Chang, 2006), and *How to Tell if Your Teenager is Lying: and What to Do about It* (Hilton Publishing, 2010).

Contributors

Cheryl A. Bacon
Ingalls Memorial Hospital
Harvey, Illinois

Linda M. Bartoshuk
Center for Smell and Taste
University of Florida
Gainesville, Florida

David A. Booth
Food Quality Research Group
School of Psychology
College of Life and Environmental
    Sciences
University of Birmingham
Edgbaston, Birmingham,
    United Kingdom

and

School of Psychology
University of Sussex
Falmer, Brighton, United Kingdom

Darin D. Dougherty
Division of Neurotherapeutics
Department of Psychiatry
Massachusetts General Hospital and
    Harvard Medical School
Boston, Massachusetts

Mary Beth Gallant-Shean
Smell & Taste Treatment and Research
    Foundation
Chicago, Illinois

Jason J. Gruss
Smell & Taste Treatment and Research
    Foundation
Chicago, Illinois

Alan R. Hirsch
Smell & Taste Treatment and Research
    Foundation
Chicago, Illinois

Hilton M. Hudson
Smell & Taste Treatment and Research
    Foundation
Chicago, Illinois

Gabriella Petrick
College of Health & Human Services
George Mason University
Fairfax, Virginia

Betina Piqueras-Fiszman
Marketing and Consumer Behaviour
    Group
Wageningen University
Wageningen, Netherlands

Thomas R. Scott
Department of Psychology
San Diego State University
San Diego, California

Sanford S. Sherman
Northwest Neurology
Lake Barrington, Illinois

Derek J. Snyder
Division of Occupational Science &
   Occupational Therapy
University of Southern California
Los Angeles, California

Charles Spence
Crossmodal Research Laboratory
Department of Experimental Psychology
University of Oxford
Oxford, United Kingdom

Veronica Sanchez Varela
High Custody Intermediate Treatment
   Center
Department of State Hospitals-Vacaville
Vacaville, California

Carl M. Wahlstrom, Jr.
Smell & Taste Treatment and Research
   Foundation
Chicago, Illinois

Bradley W. Whitman
Sensory Neuroscience
Weston, Florida

Debra A. Zellner
Department of Psychology
Montclair State University
Montclair, New Jersey

1 Tasting History

Gabriella Petrick

CONTENTS

1.1 Galen's Bitter World 3
1.2 Tasting the Future: Umami.. 10
1.3 Conclusion: Much Too Sweet—The Late Twentieth-Century Diet and
    Obesity..20
References...22

People do not eat nutrition nor do they eat nutrients. People eat food but not just any food. They eat food that tastes good to them. Yet, what tastes *good* varies across time and space and, of course, has serious implications for health. Although nutrition is a young science, barely a century old, the impact of chemosenses on health dates to Galen's observations on diet and likely well before that. But the relationship between chemosenses and health has resonated today as our population ages, drugs change perceptions of taste and flavor, and global obesity becomes a worrying trend. Yet, as a scientific field, taste is understudied, and its effect on health is only now becoming an important field of medical and scientific inquiry, as I am sure others in this volume elucidate much more elegantly.

Anthropologists have been writing for decades about how food and culture are intertwined, which at some level is also about the taste of foods. Here, I think of the work of Claude Levi-Strauss, Mary Douglas, and Sidney Mintz, among others. Yet, there is little historical literature that helps us to better understand the taste preferences, priorities, and landscapes of past generations or how these fit into particular social, political, economic, and cultural patterns, let alone their impact on health. For the most part, historians of food and foodways take a cultural tack that interrogates the relationship between food and identity or the globalization of particular ethnic or regional foods (Pilcher 2012). That is, how did particular foods come to be associated with different ethnic, religious, or national groups? There is also a significant literature on the Columbian Exchange and the flow of particular commodities from one part of the world to another. The sensory aspects of these foods rarely if ever come into play, although the existence of particular taste or flavor preferences is a recurring subtext in many of these studies.

The biological aspects of taste also complicate its cultural dimensions. There is no denying that humans are biologically *hardwired* to eat what tastes good. As a species, we have long preferred sweet to bitter, salty, and sour in measured quantities. Humans also have a strong preference for umami, which is the most recently *discovered* basic taste. But these are only the most fundamental *tastes* and have nothing to do with flavor, which is much more complex and combines the basic tastes with visual, olfactory, tactile, and auditory stimuli. In fact, some taste combinations like sweet and salty are complementary. A bit of salt in a cake tames the sugar and produces a more unctuous and balanced flavor. A bit of sugar in salty products cuts the bite of the salt rounding out the savory components. Yet, there is equally no doubt that this combination of salt and sweet is a product of global trade and industrial production and is far more common in the United States and Western Europe than in East Asia, the Middle East, or many traditional cultures in Latin America, Polynesia, or Africa. This illustrates how flavor distorts the cultural and historical boundaries of *scientific taste*.

To further complicate our understanding of human taste preferences, the idea of what is sweet versus what is saccharine varies not only within geographic regions but also within cultures. For example, consumption of soda pop was much more prevalent in the American south before and shortly after World War II than it was in New England or the Midwest, with Georgians drinking the most soda pop per capita in the nation (Petrick 2007). In thinking about why Southerners, or Georgians, drank three times more soda than New Englanders, historians are confronted with how and why sweetness pervaded Southern foodways. The large amount of sweet beverages, including both soda pop and sweet tea, that Southerners consumed points to the need to interrogate localized taste preferences and the larger effects that these preferences had on the region and the people living there. That molasses, cane syrup, and sorghum syrup were daily fare in many Southern households, particularly in African-American households, helped entrench not only sweet tastes but also overly sweet tastes as part of a Southern palate. These sweeteners added flavor to cornbread, hoecake, or Johnny bread and tamed the saltiness of cured pork (Opie 2008). In investigating the sensory aspects of taste that lay beyond the scientific, we can start to appreciate how the flavor and taste of food circulate and permeate everyday life and, in fact, how they shape people, communities, nations, and, increasingly, the world.

Popular understandings of taste suggest that there are four basic tastes consisting of sweet, sour, salty, and bitter. For more than a century, millions of American children took for granted that the tongue is segregated into taste zones with sweet at the tip of their tongue, sour on the sides, salty midtongue, and bitter at the back. In classrooms across the country, schoolchildren even did experiments to confirm that their tongues had these zones, putting sugar, salt, vinegar, and caffeine on the appropriate taste zones (Bartoshuk 1993). This, however, is not at all the way taste is perceived on the tongue. Any taste bud can detect any basic taste. Yet, generations of Americans misunderstood how taste worked based on the mistranslation of a scientific paper (Bartoshuk 1993). The recent *discovery* of umami challenged popular understandings of the basic tastes as well as helped to discredit the taste map, since the flawed map could not account for more than four basic tastes. This example illustrates how a quirk of history actually constrained how a culture and society thought about taste for generations.

Many sensory researchers emphasize that basic taste reception (sweet, sour, salty, bitter, umami) is only a small part of how food is perceived. Smell, sight, feel, and even auditory stimuli affect taste. So rather than thinking about taste in isolation from the other senses, taste perception must be viewed holistically, especially since food tastes even more delicious when we are hungry and nauseating when we are full. Additionally, psychologists have found that emotions cannot be divorced from the taste of foods (Rozin 2002). While the biology of taste is important, it is also based on social relationships and ritual eating whether around a dinner table, at the county fair, or in a church. The taste, flavor, and context of food all contribute to the importance of taste in history.

Without a doubt, understanding the biological aspects of taste is important. And yet, no one eats just sweet or sour or bitter or salty or umami. Taste in the biological sense of only five basic tastes does not exist in the taste landscape. Food is a complex combination of different flavors. Both lime and lemon are clearly sour, but each has a flavor that makes it distinctive and sometimes iconic. For example, tea and lemon go together but not tea and lime. Likewise, the citrusy acid paired with tequila in either shots or margaritas is lime but not lemon. To bite a lemon after downing a shot of tequila would be odd, inauthentic, or simply wrong. Thus, in approaching the lifestyle and health consequences of taste, the biological cannot outweigh the cultural, as ingrained cultural tastes can take a toll, such as diabetes or cardiovascular disease; but they can also bring joy, conviviality, and pleasure.

This chapter argues that at particular historical moments, not only did taste matter but also it was important to everyday life, and the choices individuals made, based on what was available, reshaped human bodies as well as cultures and societies. In it, I will begin with Galen's humoral concepts of bitterness and then jump more than two millennia to think about umami and the sensory world of the twenty-first century to suggest how the chemosenses have influenced and continue to influence what tastes *good* at any given moment. This, of course, is woven into broader social, cultural, economic, political, and health agendas.

1.1   GALEN'S BITTER WORLD

Even the earliest physicians, like Hippocrates, recognized that mixtures that helped heal the body routinely tasted bitter and unpleasant and distorted the palate so that everything tasted bitter. Thinking about bitterness and its relationship to health not only sheds new light on taste and medicine but also helps us think about how central taste was to early physicians. With the rise of Galenic rational and humoral medicine in the second century CE, health became inseparable from diet. The dominance of humoral medicine from early Rome to the Enlightenment placed bitterness at the center of medical discourse and made bitter foods into tools for healing or corrupting the body.

Arguably the most influential advocate for humoral medicine was Galen. Through his prolific writing, he prescribed and promulgated a distinctive approach to diet and health. As a result, his work on food as medicine provides a window into how taste informed ancient life. Born in the Eastern Roman Empire in September 129 CE, Galen lived a life of privilege (Grant 2000). Although he started his medical education in Pergamum, Galen traveled widely to enhance his career. Galen began his medical practice by attending to Pergamum's gladiators. This was an unusual job for him given his family's high social status. However, caring for these men gave Galen invaluable insights into the human anatomy, and according to one historian,

"Working with gladiators also allowed Galen to experiment with regulating the diet for healing and building strength" (Grant 2000, p. 2). Regulating the gladiators' diets gave Galen firsthand knowledge of food's impact on the body. He also gleaned how the taste of a variety of foods healed or corrupted these active bodies. This experience certainly influenced his later writing on diet and use of bitter foods and medicine to restore humoral balance.

Although many of Galen's works are lost to history, his books on diet are particularly important for understanding the place of taste and, more importantly, bitterness in humoral medicine and everyday life. His major writings on diet, nutrition, and health include *On the Power of Foods*, *On Barley Soup*, *On the Cause of Disease*, *On the Humors*, and *On Black Bile*. Taken together, they help scholars understand not only how taste and disease were intertwined but also the dietary habits of Imperial Rome. Or, as Grant (2000, p. 10) suggests, "what makes the dietetic treatises so important" is that "they are both a record of medical practice and a contemporary commentary on the social mores of the Roman empire."

Galen's writings on diet were wide-ranging. Because he traveled so extensively, he recorded what starving peasants ate as well as the sumptuous meals of Rome's elites. He frequently contrasted country and city life through the lens of food (Grant 2000). Many scholars argue that in describing what common laborers and peasants ate as well as the exotic fare of those who lived outside the Greco–Roman world, Galen is describing the boundaries of the human diet, that is, what is fit for man and what is fit for animals. Equally, by excluding foods eaten by the wealthy, particularly fish, he emphasizes the medicinal rather than the gustatory aspect of food (Grocock and Grainger 2006; Wilkins and Hill 2006). It appears that Galen left the pleasures of the table to cooks like those who created the *Apicius* cookbook. The tension between what was healthy and what tasted good was no less contentious in Galen's time than it is in our own.

Galen believed that only when an individual's four humors were evenly balanced could they be truly healthy. He explained, "The human body has in itself blood, phlegm, yellow bile, and black bile; these make up the nature of the body, and through these pains are felt or health enjoyed. The most perfect health is enjoyed when these humours are in correct proportion with each other—that is in compound, power or quantity—and when they are properly mixed" (Grant 2000, p. 25). Food was the lynchpin of this humoral balance. On his essay "On Humors," Grant (2000, p. 15) wrote, "When we make proper use of foods in recipes, the attendant humours follow." In *On Black Bile*, he went into much greater detail on how the qualities inherent in foods were mirrored in the body. He explained, "I have shown that the humour which is called phlegm stems from phlegmatic foods during the initial stages of digestion in the stomach, just as whatever is full of yellow bile or black bile arises in the liver" (Grant 2000, p. 33).

Just as the four humors composed the human body, according to Galen and other like-minded doctors, they also reflected a quadripartite approach to the world encompassing both its temporal and spatial dynamics. Conventional wisdom across the empire asserted that the elements air, fire, water, and earth combined to create the world. Likewise, the four seasons—spring, summer, winter, and autumn—marked the passing of time. Each humor was also either moist or dry and cold or hot (Grant

2000). Just as humors were hot, cold, wet, or dry, they also had a corresponding taste, which also ordered the universe quadratically. According to Galen, "Blood is sweet to the taste; yellow bile is bitter; black bile is sharp; phlegm is ordinarily neutral, but it can also be salty, sharp and frequently sweet" (Grant 2000, p. 6). That blood tasted sweet is surprising to us. If we taste blood, we might call it metallic, minerally, or perhaps even salty, but never sweet. Yet, because blood nourished the body and kept it in good working order, it was logical for Galen to associate it with sweet tastes such as those found in fruits, grains, and honey. Sweetness did not have the same intensity for Galen and his contemporaries as it did by the twentieth century. Galen also told his readers that the most dangerous humors—yellow and black bile—had the harshest and most intense flavors: bitterness in the case of yellow bile and sharpness, intense sourness, and astringency in the case of black bile. As a result, it became very important for physicians to study the properties of foods in order to learn their taste, consistency, and temperature. Without this knowledge, doctors could do great harm to their patients.

In an effort to educate others, Galen inventoried a wide range of foods commonly eaten across the Roman Empire. His compendium *On Food*, which was laid out in three books, inventoried the physical and medical properties of a wide variety of foods. The first book illustrated how the taste of food depended on its natural properties. He explained, "Not only the principal and primary temperament of each food must be known, as has been shown in my work *On Drugs*, but also the temperaments that stem from them. Essentially many of the useful temperaments, if not all, happen to reside in the juices, but some are also in the smell. For from the blending of so much heat, cold, dryness and wetness come their sweetness, bitterness, saltiness, astringency, harshness or sharpness" (Grant 2000, p. 6). Equally, these tastes translated into nourishment. He told readers, "You should bear in mind a factor common to all foods: that whatever is sour and bitter furnishes little nourishment for the body, whilst whatever is flavourless, and even more so whatever is sweet, provides a lot of nourishment. This is still more pronounced if the foods have a compact substance, and are neither moist, thick nor spongy in their consistency" (Grant 2000, p. 149). His distinction between taste and nourishment ultimately separated food from drugs. In Galen's pantheon, bitter-tasting foods were, in fact, drugs. I will return to this in much greater detail in Section 1.2, but suffice it to say that Galen repeatedly expounded on the medicinal properties of bitter foods. While sour, salty, and sweet tastes appear throughout his writing on food, bitterness and its association with healing became central to his medical philosophy and by far the most important of all the tastes.

In an extremely graphic example of how bad taste caused illness, Galen tells the story of how a wet nurse caused a baby's suffering through her diet of bitter wild foods.

Milk which does not taste good is of no help to a healthy state of the humours, with the result that it makes those who use it full of bad juices. This is clear from a baby who, after its first wet-nurse had died, was covered all over its body with sores because another wet-nurse provided it with milk containing bad juices. This second wet-nurse lived on a diet of wild vegetables from the countryside, for it was springtime and a food shortage was pressing. So she was also full of these sores, as were some other people in the same area who were living on a similar diet. I noticed this with lots of other women who were feeding their babies at that same time. (Grant 2000, pp. 164–165)

This effect was not limited to breast-feeding women, but any animal eating bitter grasses such as *scammony* or *spurge* transferred yellow bile to whoever drank their milk, causing dysentery-like symptoms as the bile loosened the bowels (Grant 2000).

In Galen's humoral world, bitterness became an extremely powerful tool. Because it was believed that phlegm was frequently responsible for disease, since its viscosity blocked the stomach, liver, or spleen, it was thought that ingesting bitter compounds, whether foods or drugs, cut through the mass relieving the patient of their pain and discomfort. Additionally, combining bitter foods such as garlic and onion with thick foods like beef allowed for nourishment without fear of blocking digestion or causing constipation. By way of anecdote, Galen told the readers,

I personally know of someone who complained about the area that is around the mouth of the stomach, and I reckoned from his description that phlegm had collected at this point, and so I advised him to eat his food with mustard, leeks and beets, since phlegm is cut by these foods. He excreted a great deal of phlegm from his stomach and was completely cured of his complaints. But then conversely he suffered from indigestion after eating biting foods and felt biting pains in his stomach. He had eaten mustard with beet, and not only was he taken unawares by the biting, but also was made considerably worse. He was of course amazed that he should be hurt so much by what had before been so beneficial, and he came to me to find out the reason. (Grant 2000, p. 75)

Because the patient did not understand that both yellow and black bile were extremely caustic, in eating mustard greens with beets, both bitter foods, he caused his own illness. In expounding on the biting effects of yellow and black bile if eaten immoderately, Galen wrote, "it is in fact possible to recognize [that] both yellow and black bile clearly appear to gnaw at one intestine or the other, wherever in fact they are particularly lodged, and they render dysentery completely incurable. ... Therefore just as an intestine is incurably ulcerated by black bile, and ulcerated by yellow bile in a way that is difficult to cure" (Grant 2000, p. 25).

Yet, it was not so simple to prescribe a diet by simply ensuring that the humors were equally proportional. Galen's model required that the physician know if his patient was naturally more phlegmy or full of yellow bile so that he could prescribe foods to restore the patient's natural state. In other words, humoral balance was based on an individual's tendency toward a predominant humor rather than simply balancing the four humors. In *On Black Bile*, he commented on variations in the natural humoral state. Galen wrote, "But it can be seen that some people, however they live, collect a lot of fluid that is either full of yellow bile, black bile or phlegm" (Grant 2000, p. 17). He also observed "some people who have a constitution that is hot without being moist, and a rather bad temperament that is dry and fiery. For these people rot whatever in others is easily transformed and digestible, and a belching occurs which is completely greasy" (Grant 2000, p. 114).

This variation required a good doctor to know how each food affected his patient. Perhaps that is why Galen quipped that good doctors also needed to be good cooks (Grant 2000). To illustrate his deep knowledge of the body and how food could nourish it, he gave an example of how cooking could transform a dangerous food into a wholesome one. He wrote, "Wild leeks differ from cultivated leeks in the same way as all similar species of wild plants are different from their cultivated types. Some people store them in vinegar for a whole year, just like onions. You can do the same for wild leeks, and this improves them as a food ..." (Grant 2000, p. 152). Yet, even though boiling the bitter wild foods "removes some bad juices," people who are full of yellow bile should "... avoid continual use of all bitter foods, especially when the person eating them is by nature rather bilious. For such foods are suitable only for those who collect either phlegmatic juice or juice that is raw, thick and viscous" (Grant 2000, p. 153).

Because the body is ever-changing, an optimal humoral state was constantly in flux. An individual's life stage also affected the concentration of humors. In describing how the humors shifted over the life course, Galen argued,

> The blood increases at puberty; hence teenagers are cheerful and enthusiastically disposed to games. But the yellow bile in adolescents makes for anger, sexual drive and bullying early in this stage of life; whilst later there is a surge of black bile, the worst sort of humour, since wherever it rushes it is hard to resist or divert, thus making this stage of life devious, revengeful and stubborn. In old age there is phlegm, when there reigns sluggishness, loss of memory and lethargy. This is because old age is moist and cold, just as the prime of life is dry and cold. Puberty is hot and moist, whilst adolescence belongs to an analogous and superior humour. (Grant 2000, p. 15)

In a more personal example, Galen described how lettuce restored his humoral balance as an adolescent and as an older man. He explained, "When I was young I used to use lettuce to refresh my upper bowel which was constantly filled with bile, but when I reached middle age this vegetable provided me with relief from insomnia, since I then yearned for sleep in contrast to when I was in my teens" (Grant 2000, pp. 138–139). Here is an example in which a single food, lettuce, could be used for different purposes as the body's humoral balance naturally shifted across the life course.

Throughout the ancient world, a humorally balanced diet was essential to a healthy body. Galen, like other empirical physicians, believed that food had power through its natural properties to modify an individual's humoral state. Despite the well-documented dietary excesses of Rome's elite, most people across the empire ate a simple grain-based diet made more flavorful by a simple side dish of vegetables or legumes. These flavorful and frequently bitter accompaniments were called *opsa* (Wilkins and Hill 2006). Much like today, many Romans believed that individuals controlled what they ate, and therefore, they were responsible for their own health, giving food a moral dimension espoused by Galen and many of his contemporaries. In other words, immoderate patients, especially those who banqueted frequently, caused their own illness by eating too much of the wrong foods and throwing their humors out of balance (Grant 2000). To illustrate how wealth and access to food got corrupted, Galen wrote in *On Uneven Bad Temperament*, "Bad temperament is unequal [for] ... those who shiver ... For it [shivering] to come about, one must lead a life of idleness, or eat large quantities of food over a long period, the result of which is the slow, cold, raw and phlegmatic humour which Praxagoras considered to be vitreous. Long ago, so it seems, no one suffered like this, because to live with such ease and abundance was unheard of ..." (Grant 2000, p. 44). Thus, according to Galen, a pursuit of sensual pleasure necessarily led to physical and moral decay, resulting in gluttony. According to historian Mark Grant, "Moderation and balance were essential in the pursuit of truth and the ultimate good. Diet was therefore raised from mere eating for the sustenance of the body to a higher philosophical plane that bolstered its importance within medicine as a whole" (Grant 2000, p. 7).

Depending on how a particular foodstuff affected the body, it could either be a food or a drug. In his first book of *On the Power of Foods*, Galen explained the medicinal aspects of food: "Everything that sheds its bitterness when cooked becomes like those foods which have no effect on the senses. It is logical, therefore, that such foods are not serviceable when it comes to evacuation or to the checking of stomach flux ... Such qualities belong to them not when they act as foods, but as medicines" (Grant 2000, pp. 100–101).

In a similar vein, he argued,

Some foods, as I said a little before, exhibit no distinct quality regarding smell or taste; they are in fact called inert and watery. But other foods have a very obvious astringency, innate sweetness or bitterness, just as indeed some appear rather salty and others have a clear element of bitterness. It is obvious that such foods have in them the same power as medicines, which they resemble in flavor. (Grant 2000, p. 76)

Foods seem to have a swift or slow passage through the body depending on the constitution of the stomach at the outset, or a condition that is acquired. I am talking of what is eaten and drunk, since some of these things are moist, others dry, some slippery, others friable and easily broken down, some containing an element of pungency, others sharpness, bitterness, sweetness, saltiness, harshness, astringency or, beyond these properties, some medicinal power with the general character of a purgative drug. (Grant 2000, p. 72)

Where I live cows eat vetch, whilst elsewhere people eat vetch that have been sweetened beforehand. But you should really leave off this seed, for it is unpleasant and contains bad juices. However in a famine, as Hippocrates remarked, they come into their own out of necessity. If you prepare them first, you can use them like lupins with honey as a medicine for purging the thick humours in the chest and lungs. Among the vetches, the white variety is less medicinal than those which have a hint of yellow or cream. When boiled twice and sweetened in water their unpleasantness is removed, but in this unpleasantness is held their purgative and cutting power, so that of their general substance only the earthy part is left behind, and this is a drying food without any distinct bitterness. (Grant 2000, p. 105)

As these examples illustrate, to Galen's palate, medicinal foods were overwhelmingly but not exclusively bitter. In another example relating to the taste of beef, he noted, "In cows, however, the spleen is by nature darker, and as they grow older the spleen gradually becomes even darker. The taste too of this offal, even when it is cooked, seems to hold some bitterness and never becomes like the liver" (Grant 2000, p. 28). Apparently, as the liver was cooked, its bitterness dissipated and turned foods sweet, while the spleen, which stored bitter compounds, never completely shed its bitter taste—a taste that became more pronounced as the animal aged.

Just as a cook manipulates the flavor of food to satiate a hungry body, Galen sought to alter the taste of foods to promote health or healing. For example, Galen describes how boiling transferred bitterness and thus a food's medicinal properties to the water. To tame the bitterness of cabbage, he endorsed the following technique: "... boil the cabbage in water, carefully drain off all this water from the pan, add more hot water, boil the cabbage a second time ... to ensure that if any of its own moistness is retained after the first boiling, it will be removed. Everything boiled in water experiences a shift of its own power and also a transfer of the power belonging to itself and the water" (Grant 2000, p. 71). He went on to explain that it was not just food that is boiled in water that transferred the taste and therefore the humoral aspects of food. He told his readers, "It is essential for you to realize that this occurs every day with things that are cooked in sauces, whether some pulses are being boiled, or part of an animal or a vegetable. Whatever has been boiled reveals through its taste and smell the quality and power of the sauce, whilst the sauce discloses the quality and power of what has been boiled in it" (Grant 2000, p. 71). This shift of flavors between the solids and the liquid allowed physicians to feed their patients with either tamed solid foods or flavorful sauces to restore their health. In the second book of *On the Power of Foods*, he reiterated how cooking could neutralize the bitter, medicinal components of food. He reminded his reader, "It is a trait common to all foods with a marked medicinal quality that ... they lose this power through boiling, baking or soaking ... The same thing happens with onions and leeks" (Grant 2000, p. 124). Again, in the third book of *On the Power of Foods*, Galen repeats how flavor was transferred through boiling. He explained, "... a solid body, when boiled in water, releases into it that quality it had at the start, so that after a while it becomes inert (so to speak) and watery, exhibiting neither any saltiness, bitterness, sharpness or astringency. You can see how true this is more clearly if you boil whatever you want after changing the water, for you will find that whatever is being boiled has lost its particular quality since the water has absorbed it" (Grant 2000, p. 183). In this passage, he went on to explain how reducing a flavorful liquid could induce bitterness and therefore become dangerous as yellow bile accumulates. He warned, "when most things are reduced (or if you wish when everything is reduced), the longer they are boiled, the saltier they always become, then a little later, as they themselves want, they also turn bitter" (Grant 2000, p. 183).

Although Galen continually expounds on the dangers of bitter foods, the empirical evidence suggested otherwise. In an effort to explain why most Romans, who largely subsisted on bitter-tasting vegetables, remained healthy, he wrote in his essay "Mixtures,"

The reason that all substances [such as mustard, pickles, garlic, and onion] which cause injury externally do not do so when taken internally are: that they are changed and transformed by digestion in the stomach and the blood-making process in the veins; that they do not remain in one place, but are divided into small parts which are carried in all different directions; that they are mixed with many humours, as well as with other foods taken at the same time as themselves; that their digestion and excretion are carried out quickly, by which process that in them with is proper to the nature of the animal is assimilated while the excess sharpness is excreted by stomach, urine, and sweat. (Wilkins and Hill 2006, p. 227)

This passage is one of the few instances in which bitter foods did no damage to the body or health; thus, even Galen acknowledges the limits of his observations and proscriptions of bitter foods.

Galen's taste world was colored by his medical thinking. As a physician who wanted to heal sick patients, bitter tastes perhaps overshadowed others as medicines, and medicinal foods tended to be bitter. Throughout his writing, he spends very little time on sweetness or saltiness but continually speaks about sharp and astringent tastes, which are also cast in medical language. While we might not consider garlic, onions, or leeks bitter, in Galen's medical lexicon, the fact that they helped with constipation made them bitter. Yet, Galen's world was also a place with virtually no sweetness or salinity, as only the wealthiest Roman had regular access to honey or salt. Vinegar was ever present as was fish sauce, the first being sour and the second umami. Olive oil was ubiquitous and can also taste bitter, astringent, or rancid. As most Romans ate very little meat and some fish, bread and simple vegetable accompaniments sustained most people on a daily basis. Although these might be seasoned with vinegar, wine, fish sauce, or olive oil, the natural taste of vegetables tends to be bitter even when combined with other tastes. This is certainly not to say that the food was so bitter that it was unpalatable; in fact, herbs, greens, and vegetables made bread more palatable. But far more than in our contemporary world, bitter tastes and flavors formed the foundation of the Roman palate.

1.2 TASTING THE FUTURE: UMAMI

In early September 1912, University of Tokyo chemist Kikunae Ikeda stood before an audience in Washington, DC, and announced his exciting discovery to the International Congress of Applied Chemistry. He told his audience, "... there is still another quality, which is quite distinct from all these, and *must be considered primary* [emphasis added], because it cannot be produced by any combination of other [taste] qualities" (Nakamura 2011). In an effort to convey to listeners where they might experience this new taste, he suggested, "An attentive taster will find ... something common in the complicated taste of asparagus, tomato, cheese, and meat, which is quite peculiar and cannot be classified under any of the above mentioned qualities [sweet, sour, bitter, or briny]. It is usually so faint and overshadowed by other stronger tastes, that it is often difficult to recognize it unless the attention is specially directed towards it" (Nakamura 2011). In this talk, he called this new taste *glutamic taste*. But in an earlier paper in *Nippon kagaku zasshi* (*Journal of the Tokyo Chemical Society*) in 1909, he referred to this new taste as *umami* (Ikeda 2002). In order to better explain this subtle taste, Ikeda attempted to describe the difference between umami as it is found in food and its pure form. By way of analogy, he explained, "Had we nothing sweeter than carrots or milk, our idea of the quality of 'sweet' would be just as indistinct as it is in the case of this peculiar quality. Just as honey and sugar gave us so clear a notion of what sweet is, the salts of glutamic acid are destined to give us an equally definite idea of this peculiar taste quality" (Ikeda 2002, p. 847). It was through pure monosodium glutamate (MSG) that scientists could fully experience the taste of umami.

The existence of umami as a basic taste like sweet, sour, salty, or bitter seems *new* to the American palate. Although the other four basic tastes have been identified in the West since well before the Enlightenment, the number of basic tastes has varied widely from region to region and from epoch to epoch. Aristotle identified only two tastes, whereas Qing commentators noted as few as six and as many as nine. Based on the amino acids glutamic acid and the 5′-ribonucleotides guanosine monophosphate (GMP) and inosine monophosphate (IMP), umami has a distinctly East Asian pedigree as many of the foods eaten throughout the region combine these amino acids in much larger quantities than in European or American diets. In other words, Ikeda's and the Japanese palate were trained to experience umami unlike citizens or researchers in either Europe or the United States.

In 1909, Ikeda published the first of his papers arguing that there was a new fifth basic taste produced by glutamic acid. His essay, "New Seasonings," postulated that there were not five but six tastes. In the Japanese taste landscape, at the time, there were four basic Western tastes in addition to the taste of capsicum and other chemicals that give foods their hot and spicy flavors. However, Ikeda did not consider hot a basic taste. He explained, "a hot sensation is just a skin mechanical sensation," and scientists did not consider it a basic taste (Ikeda 2002, p. 847). In differentiating basic tastes from other flavor perceptions, Ikeda eliminated *metallic*, *alkaline*, and *astringent* tastes because "they cannot be tastes (at least not pure tastes), because they cannot be separated from the sensation accompanied by tissue damages" (Ikeda 2002, p. 847). Yet, based on over 2 years of research, he was convinced that another—*new*—basic taste existed. He found umami in "fish, meat and so forth" or in foods with high protein content (Ikeda 2002, p. 847).

Ikeda's *discovery* of umami was based as much on his mastery of physical chemistry as it was on his own taste experiences and the flavors endemic to Japanese foods. Japanese cuisine, more than European and Eurocentric cuisines, is centered on umami as a foundational element and is a key taste in the Japanese palate. The two foods Ikeda focused on to extract glutamic acid were *konbu* and *bonito*, which are the key elements in dashi—a savory broth ubiquitous throughout Japanese cooking. As it happens, both *konbu* (dried brown kelp) and *katsuobushi* (bonito or skipjack tuna that is fermented, dried, smoked, and flaked) contain large amounts of glutamate. In fact, miso soup, a twice-daily habit in most Japanese households even today, is a combination of two strong umami flavors: dashi and miso (a fermented soy paste). Miso soup also generally has a few strands of green seaweed (*wakame*) and a few cubes of soft bean curd (*tofu*) (Cwiertka 2005). Ikeda also singled out soy sauce as a food that amplifies umami. In particular, soy sauce, with its high salt and glutamic acid content, was an excellent example of how salt intensified the taste of umami (Ikeda 2002). Given the complementarity between salt and umami, Ikeda began developing salt-based glutamate compounds. He explained that the taste of his early glutamate salts were "so great that two or three grams dissolved in one liter of water impart to it a very agreeable taste. It is especially palatable in combination with common salt [sodium rather than potassium or magnesium chloride]. Thus we see that sodium glutamate is an almost ideal flavoring substance for the glutamic acid" (Nakamura 2011).

By the time Ikeda gave his paper to the International Congress of Applied Chemistry in Washington, DC, in September 1912, he believed that umami was a central taste in both Chinese and Japanese food culture. He stated, "In Japan and China a large quantity of *Laminaria japonica*, a sort of brown sea-weed, is consumed as food. Its decoction is much employed to impart an agreeable taste to soup and other articles of food. It is briny on account of … common salt, it is sweet as a large quantity of mannite is present, but what makes it valuable is its strong glutamic taste" (Nakamura 2011). He went on to describe the long history of strong umami foods in Japan: "Impure flavoring substances for the glutamic taste were known of old. In this country, besides *Laminary japonica* dried, prepared fishes were used for this purpose in ancient times" (Nakamura 2011). Here, Ikeda is referring to the importance of both *konbu* and *katsuobushi* in the development of Japanese cuisine and a unique Japanese palate.

While China and Japan might have highly concentrated umami foods and dishes, Ikeda also noted that European cuisines also had foods that are high in umami. He explained, "In Europe and America, Liebig's meat-extract and allied preparations are essentially flavorings of the same category" (Nakamura 2011).* Leibig's meat extract was essentially veal stock that was reduced until it was thick and gelatinous. In French cuisine, this type of stock reduction is called an essence. The expense of producing an essence (it took 34 lb. of meat to produce 1 lb. of meat extract) made these rare flavors for the average European or American. These were certainly not working- or middle-class foods until the second half of the twentieth century, when cheap, industrial beef extracts laced with glutamates, like Maggi or Bovril, became common (Parren 2006). Unlike *dashi*, umami tastes in Europe and the United States were not everyday affairs.

Further, Ikeda based his claim for umami as a basic taste on human evolution. He commented, "Taste sensations must have been developed as a guide to food choice" (Nakamura 2011). He went on to explain that humans avoid bitterness because many bitter substances induce a spectrum of unpleasant sensations from an upset stomach or indigestion on the mild side to death on the most extreme. He reasoned that humans like "briny taste[s]" because of our natural need for sodium chloride in many biological processes. He further contended that sweet foods provide the calories to fuel our bodies. As for glutamic acid, he concluded, "The reason why we find glutamic taste so pleasant must be sought in the fact that glutamates are often present in minute quantities in nutritious matter of albuminous nature and mostly of animal origin. Hence, the appetite for these three taste qualities are [*sic*] quite normal" (Nakamura 2011). He continued, "Since many generations, pure salt and pure sugar are the flavoring substances for the first two qualities [saltiness and sweetness], and in the future a pure glutamate must form the principle flavoring substance for the third, [umami]" (Nakamura 2011). In other words, as saltiness helps regulate

---

* Ikeda would have known about Liebig's work on human nutrition and proteins not only from Liebig's fame as a chemist but also from Ikeda's time in Germany.

electrolytes and sweetness helps regulate caloric intake, umami would regulate protein consumption.

Building on Ikeda's discovery, many of his students continued to research the characteristics of umami. The first researcher to identify inosinic acid, another umami-inducing compound, was Ikeda's student Shintaro Koadamada in 1913. Building on Ikeda's research on bonito and *katsuobushi*, he discovered that a histidine salt found in inosinic acid also produced an umami taste. While it was actually the inosinic acid (IMP) that produced umami, it would take another 40 years for Japanese researchers to start to put the pieces together on the chemicals that produced umami.

Yet, all of the compounds found by early Japanese umami researchers were already known to Western scientists. In fact, research on glutamic acid in wheat proteins dates to 1866, inosinic acid in beef broth to 1847, and guanylic acid in pancreatic juices to 1898. Yamaguchi and Ninomiya (1998, p. 124) in their review of umami research noted, "the taste of these substances went unnoticed for decades." They further observed that one German scientist found that "glutamic acid had a peculiar insipid [or] (weak) acid taste" (Yamaguchi and Ninomiya 1998, p. 124). Even Ikeda found that glutamic acid was subtle and rather nondescript in its natural form. Perhaps its subtlety was one of the reasons scientists in both Europe and the United States rejected umami as a basic taste.

Yet, Ikeda's own research raised additional scientific questions about umami as a basic taste. For one, the fact that salt enhanced the flavor certainly suggested to many American researchers that it was a salt or a combination of the other three basic tastes that made umami a flavor enhancer rather than a basic taste. With a strong predisposition to only four tastes, American scientists concluded that if glutamate amplified the taste of various salts, then it must be a variant of saltiness and not a new taste. Additionally, early in his research, Ikeda found that acids neutralized the taste of umami. Again, because umami essentially disappeared with acids (Ikeda speculated that it bonded with free hydrogen), then how could it be a *true* basic taste? Despite resistance to embracing umami as a new taste, Ikeda hoped that because "the taste imparting power of glutamate is so great, it is to be expected that the glutamic taste will be found in [a] great many articles of food, even where analytical chemistry cannot demonstrate its existence" (Nakamura 2011).

Ikeda rightly predicted the power of glutamate but not quite in the way that he imagined. While the search for glutamate in a wide array of foods did not occupy the emerging field of food science, the commercialization of MSG based on Ikeda's work did. In another more prescient prediction, Ikeda remarked that MSG "will develop into a great industry in the future" (Nakamura 2011). And indeed it did. After patenting his process for making MSG, Ikeda partnered with one of the most prominent iodine producers in Japan. He and Saburosuke Suzuki founded the Suzuki Seiyakusho Co. and trademarked their MSG seasoning called Ajinomoto or quintessence in Japanese. By 1912, the company was manufacturing 25 tons of MSG largely for domestic consumption. Very quickly, the company was selling Ajinomoto across East Asia and before the end of World War I in the United States. By mid-century, Suzuki Seiyakusho, now renamed Da-Nippon Chemical, dominated the global market for MSG. At the turn of the twenty-first century, glutamate production for seasoning and flavor enhancement exceeded 2 million tons, with 89% being consumed in Asia in 2009. On a global scale, the United States consumes relatively little even though domestic consumption in the postwar period has increased (Sano 2009).

Even as American researchers saw the value in MSG from a commercial and sensory perspective, they clung to their traditional construction of taste as having only four components: sweet, sour, salty, and bitter. From the Depression to the fall of the Berlin Wall, American researchers in government, industry, and universities sought to discredit the idea that MSG had a taste and that it was anything more than an echo chamber amplifying the four tastes that constructed the American palate. The most prominent flavor scientist of his generation, E.C. Crocker, a research scientist at the most important food laboratory in the United States, A.D. Little Inc., which was located just a few steps off of Massachusetts Institute of Technology (MIT)'s campus, seemed quite hostile to the idea that umami existed. Early in his research career, Crocker set out to interrogate whether glutamate had a taste as Japanese scientists, Japanese and Chinese producers, and some American consumers argued.

Crocker's critique of glutamic taste is a direct response to Han's article, which, being an industrial chemist, Crocker no doubt read. Crocker (1948, p. 26) began by explaining that "Monosodium glutamate appears to be entirely without odor when pure." And since his earlier research found that "meat flavor is predominantly odor, and pure monosodium glutamate is odorless, that meaty flavor cannot be due to, or be reproducible by, monosodium glutamate" (Crocker 1948, p. 26). He further asserted, "Pure glutamate has taste but essentially no odors [and because meat flavor is derived from odor] it cannot substitute for meat. It is not meaty, or chicken(y), and the reason for its successful use in food must be sought in some other direction" (Croker 1948, p. 30).

But Crocker went even further in his critique of glutamic taste. In this case, building on Han's description as well as his own and other Americans' research, Croker (1948, p. 26) found that "The taste of those [glutamates] in the neutral range of pH seems always to be sweet but usually somewhat bitter. Saltiness and sourness, which characterizes glutamic acid and its sodium salt [MSG], are exceptional tastes among the amino acids." He continued, "The taste of glutamic acid is reminiscent of that of sodium glutamate, but much sourer. ... As an acid it is about as sour as the same concentration of tartaric or citric acid" (Crocker 1948, p. 29). While to Crocker MSG seemed to only be salty or sweet, in the solution, he found sweet, sour, salty, and bitter. He concluded that glutamate was a combination of "all four components: sweetness, saltiness, sourness and bitterness" (Crocker 1948, p. 29). So, rather than a new taste centered on meatiness, glutamates simply embodied the four tastes that already made up the American diet. But Crocker (1948, p. 29) was left with a puzzle that he ultimately ignored. His research indicated, "Due to the buffering action of the saliva and of the tissues of the tongue, we get the glutamate taste whether glutamic acid or its monosodium salt is applied to the taste buds ..."

Crocker with his colleague L.F. Henderson sought to reproduce the taste of glutamate by combining other tastes. Crocker (1948, p. 28) said, "We made up solutions of sugar, salt, tartaric acid and caffeine and combined these in various ways in an attempt to match the taste of sodium glutamate." He continued, "At the time, we felt well enough satisfied with this match that the glutamic was considered as operating only through the usual four kinds of taste buds" (Crocker 1948, p. 28). With subsequent

research, Crocker found additional complexities in umami. He noted that MSG produced a "tingling feeling" and a persistent taste sensation or what he described as "a
feeling of satisfaction" or fullness (Crocker 1948, p. 28). Beyond taste, umami created
a multisensorial experience for the taster. Not only did the mouth tingle but glutamates
also actually made people feel full. No other taste had these qualities. In the course of
these investigations, he asked an extremely interesting question that in some ways suggests that umami was a basic taste. He posed, "What can be the cause of this glutamic
effect, which is apparently independent of true taste, but which adds psychologically to
the flavor or whatever has been eaten" (Crocker 1948, p. 28). He concluded that MSG
stimulated the nerves that innervate the tongue, which then send stronger taste signals
to the brain. Another way to think about Crocker's explanation is that MSG served
as a taste amplifier or enhancer. That MSG and glutamates enhanced taste and flavor
framed the conversation around umami until the twenty-first century.

Yet, in the United States, taste researchers regularly described MSG as a combination of the other four primary tastes with *salty-sweet* being a not uncommon
description until the 1970s (O'Mahony and Ishii 1986). The reluctance to classify
umami as a new taste could in part be because the strongest umami flavors were
endemic to the Japanese palate but largely anathema to American and European
food cultures. Chemist Sanishiro Mizushima implied as much in his 1972 essay on
the history of physical chemistry in Japan. He argued that Japan's attention to subtle
tastes and flavors not only inspired Ikeda but also led him to discover umami. He
further argued that Western scientists interested in sensory experiences would have
chosen to study vision or hearing because "frequencies … are common to every-
body," and given these objective data, studying these senses was more empirical and
less impressionistic than taste (Mizushima 1972). Rather than following research that
broke away from Japan's long tradition of valuing simplicity and understatement in
aesthetics, including their culinary traditions, Mizushima suggests that Ikeda, in his
taste research, actually bridged Japanese aesthetics with Western science in a way that
was not accessible to either European or American researchers. In a way, Mizushima
suggests that Japanese taste researchers had an artistic approach to science that predisposed them to investigate taste and find what Western researchers could not.

While American researchers did not think that glutamic acid was a new taste,
they did know that it changed the perception of food by enhancing its flavor. It did
not strike many as odd that Japanese researchers found these compounds. American
researchers continually emphasized the long history of eating foods high in glutamates across East Asia as the reason that glutamates were discovered. For example,
Joseph A. Maga, a food scientist at Colorado State University, observed, "For centu-
ries Oriental cultures have used naturally occurring sources of flavor potentiators in
their food preparations" (Maga 1983, p. 231). He continued, "Thus the … major flavor
potentiators in commercial use today … were identified in naturally occurring products that historically have been used … in Japanese food preparations" (Maga 1983,
p. 232). That glutamates were already familiar to Ikeda and other Japanese researchers
predisposed them to finding them, or so American scientists contended into the 1980s.

It would take until after the end of the U.S. occupation of Japan in the early 1950s
for Japanese researchers to further advance umami research and once again argue
that it is a new basic taste. By far, the most important new contribution to umami

research in the second half of the twentieth century was the discovery that umami was far more complex than any of the other basic tastes. The first major breakthrough on umami research was that glutamic acid was not the only compound that produced umami. Akira Kuninaka, working as a researcher at Japan's oldest and most renowned soy sauce producer, the Yamasa Shoyu Company in Choshi, Japan, identified guanylic acid (GMP) as an umami-inducing compound. Rather than marine products, Kuninaka found that a broth made from dried black shitake mushrooms, also a common ingredient in many Japanese dishes, produced umami (Yamaguchi and Ninomiya 1998). Building on his discovery of GMP, Kuninaka realized that not only GMP produced the taste of umami, but also when he combined it with MSG, the umami became 30 times stronger. While both MSG and GMP are subtle on their own, in combination, a truly recognizable and distinct taste developed. That is, while both MSG and ribonucleotides each produce distinct umami flavors, when they are combined, the perception of umami is more than the sum of its parts. No other basic taste has this capability to ratchet up taste perception. This was certainly a profitable discovery to many food processors who, by the 1960s, began using GMP and IMP in a variety of industrial foods. The usual combination of MSG to GMP or IMP was 95:5 resulting in a sixfold flavor increase (Kuninaka 1964, 1966). MSG remained the dominant umami compound because it was far less expensive to produce than either IMP or GMP. Yet, by adding a small amount of these new amino acids, processers could dramatically improve the flavor of their goods. Canned and dehydrated soups and a wide variety of other products were greatly improved with glutamates (Maga 1983).

Scientific research into taste as a sensory experience has always been a much smaller subfield within sensory sciences. Like sensory history, we know far more about vision and visuality and hearing and aurality from both a cultural and a scientific perspective than we do about taste. Yet, by the mid-1970s, a small group of researchers interested in the physiology of taste and the neurotransmission of taste sensation to the brain reinvigorated taste research with a less industrial or applied approach by focusing on the biological mechanisms of taste and not the sensory experience of it. This shift refocused the conversation about umami in the United States, and the question of whether or not it was a primary taste was reconsidered (Yamaguchi and Ninomiya 1998).

One of the most important new developments in the field of taste science was debunking a myth. Linda Bartoshuk was and still is one of the most important scientists in taste research. In her 1993 paper titled "The Biological Basis of Food Perception and Acceptance," in *Food Quality and Preference*, Bartoshuk explains that our understanding of how the tongue processes taste is wrong. She explains,

One of the most widespread 'facts' about taste concerns the distribution of sensitivity to the other 4 basic tastes. This 'fact' was reexamined by Collings (1974). The tongue map with 'sweet' on the tip, 'bitter' on the back, etc., dates back to the PhD thesis of Hänig, which was published in *Philosophie Studien* in 1901. Hänig wanted to measure taste thresholds around the perimeter of the tongue where the taste papillae are most densely distributed. He believed that if the thresholds for his four stimuli (sucrose, salt, quinine sulfate, and hydrochloric acid) could be shown to vary differently around the perimeter of the tongue, then this would support the argument that these four tastes had distinctly physiological mechanisms. (Bartoshuk 1993, p. 22)

In 1942, Edwin Boring, a historian of psychology at Harvard University, transformed Hänig's observations into a graph that located taste sensitivity along the contours of the tongue. While Boring did not create the taste map per se, his interpretation of Hänig's work led to the taste map, which related specific tastes to specific regions of the tongue. As Bartoshuk (1993, p. 23) notes, "much of the time, maps that appear in modern texts ... do not cite any source for the map. That map has become an enduring scientific myth." Yet, even in this paper, in which Bartoshuk explains that the Americans' general understanding of the physiology of taste is wrong, she only invokes the four Western tastes of sweet, sour, salty, and bitter. Umami is not yet in the pantheon of basic tastes, but her biological approach helps open the door.

In addition to challenging the taste map, Bartoshuk is well known for her work on supertasters. Through her work on bitterness, using 6-n-propyl-thiouracil (PROP), she found that not all people perceive taste with the same intensity. She concluded that roughly 25% of the population cannot taste PROP (nontasters); 50% of the population taste PROP (tasters); and 25% of the population taste PROP intensely (supertasters) (Bartoshuk 1991, 2000).* Based on her early research on supertasters, Bartoshuk found that supertasters have more taste buds per surface area than either tasters or nontasters. The effects of enhanced taste perception actually made eating a less pleasant experience and, in certain instances, even painful for her subjects (Karrer and Bartoshuk 1991). Bartoshuk (2000, pp. 456–457) observed that "both female and male supertasters were thinner among subjects with normal body weight." Additionally, supertasters experience even sweet and fatty sensations more powerfully than the rest of the population. It seems that supertasters are less interested in food because it is too intense and it does not taste particularly good to them. Supertasters appear to eat to live and not live to eat. Perhaps what is most interesting in Bartoshuk's review essay is that she concedes that taste is far more complex than genetic or biological disposition would indicate. As different cultures favor a wide variety of flavors that reflect ethnic, regional, or national palates, which are based on long-held flavor preferences and food availability, a purely scientific or biological approach to food choice does not fully explain what is eaten or, more importantly, what is tasted.

In conjunction with Bartoshuk's work on taste receptors, the use of the term *umami* gained acceptance within the scientific community. The movement to use umami to refer to glutamic compounds began in earnest in Japan with the founding of the Umami Research Association in 1982. In an effort to expand research on umami, the Umami Research Association reached out to other scientific communities to organize symposia. This effort led the American Chemical Society to partner with the Chemical Society of Japan to launch umami into the American

---

* PROP, a bitter compound, is perceived at varying degrees based on an individual's genetic sensitivity to taste. Through her PROP experiments, Bartoshuk coined the term *supertaster*. Supertasters are highly sensitive to strong flavors and tend not to like highly flavored foods. Rather than enjoying food more, supertasters tend to dislike and avoid intensely flavored foods because they find them so unpleasant.

lexicon of tastes (Kurihara 2009). While the focus of the conference was taste chemistry, umami was presented as both a concept and a scientific term. In 1985, the first symposium on umami was held in Hawaii characterizing MSG, GMP, and IMP as imparting a unique taste or umami. The pace of umami research accelerated with the discovery of supertasters, the debunking of the taste map, and a new interest in physiology taste.

With this new biologically based interest in taste, researchers working on perception increasingly used a wide array of new tools to evaluate basic tastes. Additionally, the case for umami grew stronger as researchers in various fields, including physiology, neuroscience, psychology, and statistical modeling, among others, became interested in it. The case for umami as a new basic taste began to build steadily from the mid-1980s and accelerated throughout the last decade of the twentieth century. In further support of the existence of umami, Japanese scientists at Tokyo University worked to counter Crocker's and other American researchers' assertion that umami was simply a combination of the four basic Western tastes. In 1987, Shizuko Yamaguchi found that umami did not fit a pattern that allowed it to be made up of the other tastes. Based on new statistical tools, Yamaguchi (1987) found that individuals given sweet, sour, salty, bitter, and umami compounds could distinguish umami from the other four. This work firmly put to rest Crocker and other researchers' claim that umami was derived from the other four tastes (de Araujo et al. 2003). While not all taste scientists were yet convinced that umami was a new taste, they certainly began looking more earnestly for what it was. Yamaguchi's work was a watershed moment that increasingly pointed to Ikeda's research 8 years earlier.

Another crucial piece of the umami puzzle was solved in 2000 when Nirupa Chaudhari at the University of Miami found that, just like the other four tastes, taste buds have unique receptors that only respond to umami compounds. These receptors convert chemical stimuli into neural impulses. That there are taste receptors unique to glutamates seemingly redefined umami as a basic taste (Chaudhari et al. 2000; Lindemann 2000). But given that there are many different forms of glutamate that produce an umami taste, it also became clear "that umami is much more complex than just the taste of MSG" or, for that matter, IMP or GMP, each of which seems to have its own unique receptors (Chaudhari et al. 2009, p. 738S).

By the 1990s, functional magnetic resonance imaging (fMRI) provided researchers with the ability to map the brain, including taste. By giving a research subject sugar water while hooked up to an fMRI, researchers could see, in real time, how the brain recognized sweetness. Interested in how different sensory stimuli were interpreted in the brain, British psychologist and neuroscientist Edmond T. Rolls began work with collaborators in the United States that explored how vision, taste, and odor converged in the brain. His early research in primates used electrodes that recorded brain activity, and he and Leslie L. Baylis at the University of San Diego began studying umami in primates (Rolls and Baylis 1994). By the turn of the twenty-first century, Rolls began using a human subject to explore umami. In a jointly authored paper, Rolls and his colleagues explained, "Nothing is known ... about the cortical responses to umami substances and their interaction in the human brain" (de Araujo et al. 2003, p. 313). Knowing the brain map for sweet, sour, salty, and bitter, Rolls and his colleagues attempted to see if umami is mapped onto the brain in a similar way. They found that when subjects were fed an umami solution, there was brain activity in the taste and vision areas of the brain, and that when MSG was combined with IMP, the taste of umami was amplified. It was as if the brain not only tasted a substance but also visualized its flavor. They concluded, "umami works in generally the same way as other tastants and is consistent with umami being considered as a 'fifth taste'" (de Araujo et al. 2003, pp. 315, 317). By the first decade of the twenty-first century, researchers had confirmed what Ikeda found a century earlier. The combination of different fields—psychophysiology, neuroscience, and biophysiology, among others—each builds a case for umami that began after World War II but gained steam in the closing decades of the twentieth century. Because it is impossible to study a phenomenon that you do not believe exists, it took a shift away from Crocker's model of umami to one based on Ikeda. This was one of the cultural aspects of scientific research on umami throughout the twentieth century. It is striking that Japanese scientists continued to probe the existence of umami by identifying those chemical compounds that to their palate produced the taste of umami, whereas American scientists ignored it. It was only after the seminars sponsored by both the American Chemical Society and the Japanese Chemical Society (and publication of Japanese research in English) that umami began to be thought of as, at first, a taste enhancer and subsequently as a unique taste and finally, by 2000, a new basic taste.

Yet, we should take sensory scientist Jennine Delwiche's caution that "the concept of four basic tastes can become somewhat of a self-fulfilling prophecy" (Delwiche 1996, p. 422). The way in which culture shapes our beliefs about what we do and do not taste, I believe, played an important part in shifting research toward discovering umami as a basic taste. That both American and Japanese researchers found what they were looking for when trying to understand taste reinforces that the palate of a nation encompasses far more than a biological predisposition.

Perhaps what is most interesting about the controversy surrounding the existence of umami is the vastly different flavor profiles that exist in both Japan and the United States. While umami flavors certainly exist in American food culture, they are not profound. Umami flavors like tomato paste, Parmesano Reggiano cheese, and deeply cooked mushrooms frequently made it onto American dinner tables. Yet, these flavors were supplements rather than staples in the American diet. Moreover, both Parmesan cheese and tomato paste are imported from Southern Italy and only became a ubiquitous part of the American diet as Italian Americans became integrated into the American society rather than lived in ethnic and cultural enclaves as they did before World War II.

In an example of sensory struggle and the foreignness of umami, historian Connie Chiang (2008, p. 406) argues that "the social and material dimensions of order became inseparable ... To exercise power over the natural world was also to exercise power over other people." She further explained, "... people can project their fears, desires, and prejudices on to smell. ... Radical and ethnic minorities and the working class often suffered the most from the negative connotation associated with the smell ..." (Chiang 2008, p. 405–406). Chiang's observations related to smell are equally true for taste when they are associated with marginalized groups and Asian foodways. Chiang (2008) noted that Chinese fishermen air-dried squid, which is high in umami, and that residents and tourists found the smell *abominable*. She further explained the cultural dissonance between those who ate the squid and those who merely smelled it. According to Chiang (2008, p. 411), "Since they [residents and hotel promoters] did not eat dried squid, the odor was all the more foreign and objectionable." One can imagine that those unfamiliar with eating dried squid would be equally repelled by the flavor of umami for all the same reasons. Chiang (2008, p. 411) explained, "Thus, the Chinese produced a completely alien stench," unlike the alien taste of umami in Japanese and other East Asian foods.

Just as Chiang makes clear that the materiality of objects affects the perceptions of smell, so too the perceptions of taste shift over time. In the case of umami, the assimilation of glutamic tastes helped shift the American palate and diet and allowed Americans to *discover* a fifth taste. The subtle taste of umami, while obvious to Kikunae Ikeda, was much less so to E.C. Crocker largely because, as an American entrenched in a quartet of tastes, he literally could not taste it. He and many other sensory researchers before the last few decades of the twentieth century were taste-blind to umami.

The path to umami becoming a new taste or its rediscovery was based not just on scientific debates over meatiness or flavor enhancement but also about the place of Asian immigrants in American society. Umami became a taste just as Chinese- and Japanese-Americans were becoming more integrated into American society, and a new wave of immigrants were allowed to emigrate to the United States due to immigration reform that favored Asians. While Chinese restaurants exploded in the postwar period and became an essential part of our restaurant culture, Joyce Chen taught cooks how to make *real* Chinese food at home. Favorable trade policies to stem the spread of communism across Asia also brought more expatriate Japanese businessmen and their families to the United States. Immigrants who were once confined to Chinatowns and Little Tokyos were now moving to suburbia and taking their taste and foodways with them.

1.3 CONCLUSION: MUCH TOO SWEET—THE LATE TWENTIETH-CENTURY DIET AND OBESITY

"There are glimmers of good news," the *New York Times* editorial board wrote on February 27, 2014 (*New York Times* Editorial Board 2014). The Board was referring to new data from the Centers for Disease Control and Prevention that obesity rates in children between two and five dropped 43% between 2003 and 2013. The Board continued, "There is little hard proof, but there are many theories about the factors that might have driven down obesity rates in young children" (*New York Times* Editorial Board 2014). Chief among them is a reduction in sugary beverages that children, and in fact most Americans, are drinking. Beginning in the early 1980s, both soda pop consumption and obesity began to increase dramatically. Although Americans had been drinking ever more carbonated beverages since the end of World War II, the increases between 1980 and 1998, when consumption peaked, were exponentially greater than previous increases (Associated Press 2013). Both sugar and salt consumptions have been grist for the mill of the obesity debate. The weight that Americans have put on since the 1980s when the *epidemic* first began is largely blamed on Americans' collective sweet tooth and the central place of sugar in the

American diet. As more highly processed foods including soda pop, snack foods, frozen meals, and fast food became a daily habit rather than a treat, Americans ate more sugar, even if the foods were savory. Because highly processed foods require large amounts of salt to both preserve them and make them palatable, they tend to be overly salty. By adding some sugar, perceptions of salt were mitigated making the food more palatable, and hence more highly processed, resulting in more salt and sugar consumption. The sugar in processed foods is commonly referred to as hidden sugar because consumers frequently do not even know that it is there.

According to cultural critics like Michael Pollan, Alice Waters, Michael Moss, Frank Bruni, and Mark Bittman, among many others, industrial foods are largely to blame. If there was a villain in their stories, it is food companies that substituted the cheaper and more industrially friendly high-fructose corn syrup for sucrose beginning in the early 1970s. While some nutrition advocates (Science in the Public Interest, Marion Nestle, and Kelly Brownell being some of the most vocal) condemn high-fructose corn syrup, the scientific data are far more suggestive on these matters than they are conclusive. Yet, there is no doubt that Americans have enormously increased the amount of sugar that they eat, most frequently in the form of soda and highly processed foods (Kaplan 2014). Sugar became so vilified within the health community that in August 2012, a nursing organization equated sugar with cocaine (Walton 2012). Sugar was no longer a benign food but rather an addictive drug or a toxin. This vitriolic and shrill debate surrounding sweetness, high-fructose corn syrup, and obesity suggests two major shifts in the American palate. First is that sweetness has lost its cultural power. Eating or drinking lots of sugar has now become a stigma, and being obese has taken on moralistic underpinnings that are associated with lack of control or discipline despite the scientific evidence that obesity is not simply caused by diet. Obese people are perceived as simply eating too many processed foods and drinking too many sugar-rich soft drinks, thus causing their own health problems. Second, both the economics and politics of industrial foods are changing. In an effort to respond to consumers' fears of high-fructose corn syrup and sugar more generally, food companies like H.J. Heinz have also reduced the amount of sugar in their products, eliminating high-fructose corn syrup (Heinz 2014). Even Coca-Cola and PepsiCo are trying to reduce the sugar in their iconic beverages (Schultz 2013). Because consumers are demanding less sugar, industry leaders who want to retain their market share are being forced to reengineer their products while simultaneously not changing the taste of their products. It is not yet clear if sweetness or just sugar is being eliminated from industrial and highly processed foods. Beyond rhetoric, the 2014 Farm Bill makes progress on moving Americans away from subsidized corn and toward fresh fruits and vegetables. For the first time, the federal government is rewarding those on Supplemental Nutrition and Assistance Plan (SNAP, formerly Food Stamps) who choose to purchase fresh fruits and vegetables by doubling their produce dollars (Steinhauer 2014). New Food and Drug Administration policies on labeling will highlight the amount of sugar in products trying to help consumers consume less sugar (and salt and fat). The culture, economics, and politics of sweetness at the dawn of the twenty-first century are an inversion of those same forces a century ago, illustrating that tastes really do change dramatically.

Taste in its most basic form is a chemical reaction in the mouth in which an individual perceives sweetness, sourness, saltiness, bitterness, and umami. Yet, I have argued that taste and taste perceptions are far from simply a chemical reaction. Beyond the science of taste that includes olfaction, or even ideas of flavor that are created through sight, hearing, and touch in addition to taste and smell, our sense of taste shapes not just what is good to eat but also a wide array of other economic, political, social, and cultural institutions that are historically contingent. Rather than being a strictly biological function that is hardwired, our sense of taste changes over time and space.

REFERENCES

Associated Press. 2013. Water becomes America's favorite drink again. *USA Today*, March 11, 2013. Available at http://www.usatoday.com/story/news/nation/2013/03/11/water -americas-favorite-drink/1978959/ (accessed March 3, 2014).

Bartoshuk, L.M. 1991. Sweetness: History, preference and genetic variability. *Food Technology* 45:108–113.

Bartoshuk, L.M. 1993. The biological basis of food perception and acceptance. *Food Quality and Preference* 4:21–32.

Bartoshuk, L.M. 2000. Comparing sensory experiences across individuals: Recent psychophysical advances illuminate genetic variations in taste perception. *Chemical Senses* 25:447–460.

Chaudhari, N., A.M. Landin, and S.D. Roper. 2000. A metabotropic glutamate receptor variant functions as a taste receptor. *Nature Neuroscience* 3:113–119.

Chaudhari, N., E. Pereira, and S.D. Roper. 2009. Taste receptors for umami: The case for multiple receptors. *American Journal of Clinical Nutrition* 90:738S–742S.

Chiang, C.Y. 2008. The nose knows: The sense of smell in American history. *The Journal of American History* 95:2:405–416.

Crocker, E.C. 1948. Meat flavor and observations on glutamate and other amino acids. In *Monosodium Glutamate—A Symposium*. Chicago: Quartermaster Food and Container Institute for the Armed Forces.

Cwiertka, K.J. 2005. *Modern Japanese Cuisine: Food, Power, and National Identity*. London: Reaktion Books.

de Araujo, I.E.T., M.L. Kringelbach, E.T. Rolls, and P. Hobden. 2003. Representation of umami taste in the human brain. *Journal of Neurophysiology* 90:313–319.

Delwiche, J. 1996. Are there 'basic' tastes? *Trends in Food Science & Technology* 7:411–415.

Grant, M. 2000. *Galen on Food and Diet*. New York: Routledge.

Grocock, C., and S. Grainger. 2006. *Apicius: A Critical Edition*. Devon, England: Prospect Books.

H.J. Heinz Company, L.P. 2014. Product Gallery 2014. Available at http://www.heinzketchup .com/Products.aspx (accessed March 4, 2014).

Ikeda, K. 1912. On the taste of the salt of glutamic acid. *Proceedings of the 8th International Congress of Applied Chemistry* 38:147.

Ikeda, K. 2002. New seasoning. (Trans.) *Chemical Senses* 27:847–849.

Kaplan, K. 2014. Americans consume too much added sugars, study says, and it's killing us. *Los Angeles Times*, February 3, 2014. Available at http://articles.latimes.com/2014/feb /03/science/la-sci-sn-added-sugars-death-risk-heart-disease-20140203 (accessed March 4, 2014).

Karrer, T., and L.M. Bartoshuk. 1991. Capsaicin desensitization and recovery on the human tongue. *Physiology & Behavior* 49:757–764.

Kuninaka, A. 1964. Symposium of flavor potentiation. In *Flavor Chemistry and Technology*, Second Edition, ed. G. Reineccius. Cambridge, MA: Arthur D. Little.

Kuninaka, A. 1966. Recent studies of 5′-nucleotides as new flavor enhancers. In *Flavor Chemistry* Advances in Chemistry Series, Vol. 56, ed. R.F. Gould, 261–274. Washington D.C.: American Chemical Society.

Kurihara, K. 2009. Glutamate: From discovery as a food flavor to role as a basic taste. *American Journal of Clinical Nutrition* 90:3:719S–722S.

Lindemann, B. 2000. A taste for umami. *Nature America* 3:99–100.

Maga, J.A. 1983. Flavor potentiators. *CRC Critical Reviews in Food Science and Nutrition* 18:231–312.

Mizushima, S. 1972. A history of physical chemistry in Japan. *Annual Reviews in Physical Chemistry* 23:3–22.

Nakamura, E. 2011. One hundred years since the discovery of the 'umami' taste from seaweed broth by Kikunae Ikeda, who transcended his time. *Chemistry: An Asian Journal* 6:7:1659–1663.

New York Times Editorial Board. 2014. Driving down childhood obesity. *New York Times*, February 27, 2014. Available at http://www.nytimes.com/2014/02/28/opinion/driving -down-childhood-obesity.html?action=click&module=Search&region=searchResults% 230&version=&url=http%3A%2F%2Fquery.nytimes.com%2Fsearch%2Fsitesearch% 2F%23%2Fobesity%2F7days%2F (accessed March 3, 2014).

O'Mahony, M., and R. Ishii. 1986. A comparison of English and Japanese taste languages: Taste descriptive methodology, codability and the umami taste. *British Journal of Psychology* 77:161–174.

Opie, F.D. 2008. *Hog and Hominy: Soul Food from Africa to America.* New York: Columbia University Press.

Parren, R. 2006. *Taste, Trade and Technology: The Development of the International Meat Industry since 1940.* Aldershot, England: Ashgate Publishing.

Petrick, G.M. 2007. *The Arbiters of Taste: Producers, Consumers, and the Industrialization of Taste in America, 1900–1960.* PhD dissertation, University of Delaware.

Pilcher, J. 2012. *Plant Taco: A Global History of Mexican Food.* New York: Oxford University Press.

Rolls, E.T., and L.L. Baylis. 1994. Gustatory, olfactory, and visual convergence within the primate orbitofrontal cortex. *The Journal of Neuroscience* 14:5437–5452.

Rozin, P. 2002. Human food intake and choice: Biological, psychological, and cultural perspectives. In *Food Selection: From Genes to Culture*, eds. H. Anderson, J. Blundell, and M. Chiva, 7–24. Paris: Danone Institute.

Sano, C. 2009. History of glutamate production. *American Journal of Clinical Nutrition* 90:3:728S–732S.

Schultz, E.J. 2013. How PepsiCo and Coca-Cola Are Creating the Cola of the Future. *AdAge*, December 3, 2013. Available at http://adage.com/article/news/pepsico-coca-cola-creating -cola-future/245457/ (accessed March 4, 2014).

Steinhauer, J. 2014. Farm bill reflects shifting American menu and a senator's persistent tilling. *New York Times*, March 8, 2014. Available at http://www.nytimes.com/2014/03/09 /us/politics/farm-bill-reflects-shifting-american-menu-and-a-senators-persistent-tilling .html?hp (accessed March 9, 2014).

Walton, A.G. 2012. How much sugar are Americans eating? *Forbes*, August 12, 2012. Available at http://www.forbes.com/sites/alicegwalton/2012/08/30/how-much-sugar-are-americans -eating-infographic/ (accessed March 6, 2014).

Wilkins, J.M., and S. Hill. 2006. *Food in the Ancient World.* Malden, MA: Blackwell Publishing.

Yamaguchi, S. 1987. Fundamental properties of umami in human taste sensation. In *Umami: A Basic Taste*, eds. Y. Kawamura and M.R. Kare, 41–73. New York: Marcel Dekker.

Yamaguchi, S., and K. Ninomiya. 1998. What is umami? *Food Reviews International* 14: 123–138.

2 Chemosensory Disorders
Emerging Roles in Food Selection, Nutrient Inadequacies, and Digestive Dysfunction

Carl M. Wahlstrom, Jr., Alan R. Hirsch, and Bradley W. Whitman

CONTENTS

2.1 Introduction 26
2.2 Epidemiology...26
2.3 Anatomy and Pathophysiology 27
    2.3.1 Anatomy of Smell...27
    2.3.2 Neurotransmitters That Mediate Smell 29
    2.3.3 Physiology of Taste 30
    2.3.4 Etiologies of Chemosensory Disorders....................................30
        2.3.4.1 Aging..30
        2.3.4.2 Nasal Obstruction 36
        2.3.4.3 Viral 36
        2.3.4.4 Endocrine Disorders 36
        2.3.4.5 Meningiomas 37
        2.3.4.6 Temporal Lobe Lesions 37
        2.3.4.7 Thalamic and Hypothalamic Lesions.........................38
        2.3.4.8 Parkinson's Disease 38
        2.3.4.9 Alzheimer's Disease 39
        2.3.4.10 Toxic Agents 40
        2.3.4.11 Trauma 41
        2.3.4.12 Nutritional Deficiencies 41
        2.3.4.13 Diagnoses Associated with Olfactory Impairment..............42
2.4 Patient Evaluation 43
    2.4.1 Assessing Olfaction 44
2.5 Treatment..46
    2.5.1 Phosphatidylcholine..46
    2.5.2 Thiamine...47
    2.5.3 Vitamin A 47

2.5.4   Caffeine 47
2.5.5   Zinc 47
2.5.6   Pentoxifylline 48
2.5.7   Intranasal Calcium Inhibitors 48
2.5.8   Theophylline 49
2.5.9   Prednisone 49
2.5.10 Sniff Therapy 49
2.5.11 Chiropractic Manipulation 50
2.5.12 Increasing Patients' Awareness of Altered Eating Habits 50
2.6   Summary 52
References 52

2.1   INTRODUCTION

Exploration of the myriad pathophysiological states with co-occurrence of chemosensory and nutritional dysfunction may help to clarify the nature of such an association.

Since the experience of prandial consumption engages multisensory integration, including smells, tastes, somatosensation, and viscosity, it cannot truly be isolated. This is illustrated in the paradigm of gustatory synesthesia of retronasal smell (Small 2009). For purposes of organization in this chapter, however, sensations of smell and taste will be segregated and individually delineated.

Nutrition regulates the chemosenses, and reciprocally, taste and smell greatly influence food selection, satiety, digestion, dietary patterns, and nutrient intake. While the name *gustation* suggests the link between the sense of taste and food, the sense of olfaction is linked in a variety of complex ways. The quintessential position of smell in the chemosensory hierarchy is epitomized by the human's ability to discriminate over 1 trillion unique olfactory stimuli as opposed to only four or five different tastes (Keller et al. 2014). Approximately 90% of *taste* or flavor is actually smell (Hirsch 1992a). It is a nonpathological form of synesthesia wherein orthonasal smell is perceived as aroma, and retronasal smell, from the posterior of the mouth, through the oropharynx, is construed as taste (Murphy and Cain 1980; Bingham et al. 1990). Olfaction begins exerting its effects when stimuli are remote, and its potential roles in nutritional assessments are an area of ongoing research (Griep et al. 1999). Attributes of nutritional metabolism and physiology are both enmeshed in this nexus and serve as a powerful milieu regulating disparate chemosensory forces that powerfully come together and impact one another to yield relevant changes in the human sensory response and behavioral outcomes, and finally in resulting in impact upon human health.

Approaching olfaction in a balladromic fashion, subdivision into a physiological and pathophysiological condition may be useful.

2.2   EPIDEMIOLOGY

Chemosensory dysfunction is endemic. It has been estimated that approximately 15 million Americans 55 years of age or older have olfactory abnormalities, and more than 200,000 individuals seek the medical advice of general practitioners and specialists each year because of complaints regarding smell or taste (Murphy et al. 2002). More recent studies suggest that chemosensory loss is an even more ubiquitous condition, with an overall prevalence of smell dysfunction in 23% of the general population or more than 75 million in the United States alone (Rawal et al. 2014). The causes of chemosensory dysfunction are myriad, and the underlying disorders are often associated with nutritional dysfunction (Estrem and Renner 1987).

2.3 ANATOMY AND PATHOPHYSIOLOGY

Smell is the only sensation to reach the cortex before reaching the thalamus. Furthermore, it is the only sensory system that is primarily ipsilateral in its projection to the cortex. In the future, neuroimaging techniques will help to expand the understanding of this evolutionarily precortical limbic system sense.

2.3.1 ANATOMY OF SMELL

Dirhinous inhalation occurs asymmetrically due to the olfactory cycle, which alternates open nostrils every 40 min to 4 h (Eccles 1978). Parenthetically, olfaction demonstrates the greatest sensitivity ipsilateral to the restricted nostril, as a result of eddy currents created by the smaller aperture. These vertiginous gusts of odorant, like rhinal tornadoes, stochastically distribute odorants with greater concentration reaching the olfactory epithelium at the top of the nose, as opposed to bypassing this area in favor of the bronchi and lungs (Frye 2003). For a putative olfactory substrate to be processed, it needs to be solubilized in mucus. If through suboptimal alterations in nutritional metabolism, a disturbance in mucus production arises, it is possible that subsequent olfaction might be adversely affected. Increased nasal mucus production in the setting of the biology of a hyperimmune state might yield a disturbance in olfaction. Features of these conditions such as nasal polyps may also separately engender problems with taste and smell (Smith et al. 1987).

Once an odor passes through the olfactory epithelium, it must stimulate the olfactory nerve, which consists of unmyelinated olfactory fila. The olfactory nerve has virtually the slowest conduction rate of any nerve in the body (Wolfe 2006). The olfactory fila pass through the cribriform plate of the ethmoid bone and enter the olfactory bulb. Different odors localize in specific areas of the olfactory bulb (Kratskin and Belluzzi 2003). During trauma, damage often occurs in this bulb, resulting in greater impact in identification than threshold (Hirsch and Wyse 1993; see Figure 2.1).

Inside the olfactory bulb is a conglomeration of neuropil called glomeruli. Approximately 2000 glomeruli reside in the olfactory bulb. Four different cell types make up the glomeruli: processes of receptor cell axons, mitral cells, tufted cells, and second-order neurons, which give off collaterals to the granule cells and to cells in the periglomerular and external plexiform layers. The mitral and tufted cells form the lateral olfactory tract and establish a reverberating circuit with the granule cells. The mitral cells stimulate firing of the granule cells, which in turn inhibit firing of the mitral cells (Brodal 1969).

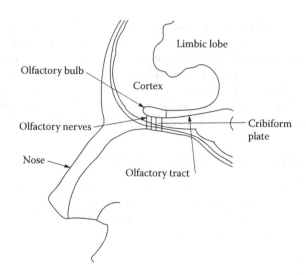

FIGURE 2.1   Cross-sectional anatomy of the nose and cranial nerve I.

A reciprocal inhibition exists between the mitral and tufted cells, which results in a sharpening of olfactory acuity. The olfactory bulb receives several afferent projections, which include the primary olfactory fibers, the contralateral olfactory bulb, the anterior nucleus, the inhibitory prepiriform cortex, the diagonal band of Broca (with the neurotransmitters acetylcholine and gamma-aminobutyric acid [GABA]), the locus coeruleus, the dorsal raphe, and the tuberomammillary nucleus of the hypothalamus.

The olfactory bulb's efferent fibers project into the olfactory tract, which divides at the olfactory trigone into the medial and lateral olfactory striae. The striae project to the anterior olfactory nucleus, the olfactory tubercle, the amygdaloid nucleus (which in turn projects to the ventral medial nucleus of the hypothalamus, a feeding center), the cortex of the piriform lobe, the septal nuclei, and the hypothalamus, especially the anterolateral regions of the hypothalamus, which are involved in reproduction, which may partially explain the significance of olfactory stimuli in the reproduction process (Hirsch 1998).

The anterior olfactory nucleus receives afferent fibers from the olfactory tract and projects efferent fibers, which decussate in the anterior commissure and synapse in the contralateral olfactory bulb. Some of the efferent projections from the anterior olfactory nucleus remain ipsilateral and synapse on internal granular cells of the ipsilateral olfactory bulb.

The olfactory tubercle receives afferent fibers from the olfactory bulb and the anterior olfactory nucleus. Efferent fibers from the olfactory tubercle project to the nucleus accumbens as well as the striatum. Prominent neurotransmitters of the olfactory tubercle include acetylcholine and dopamine (Kratskin and Belluzzi 2003).

The area on the cortex where olfaction is localized, that is, the primary olfactory cortex, includes the prepiriform area, the periamygdaloid area, and the entorhinal area. The piriform cortex and the amygdala are the primary olfactory cortex, whereas the insula and orbitofrontal cortex are the secondary olfactory cortex association areas (Doty et al. 1997). Afferent projections to the primary olfactory cortex include the mitral cells, which enter the lateral olfactory tract and synapse in the prepiriform cortex (lateral olfactory gyrus) and the corticomedial part of the amygdala. Efferent projections from the primary olfactory cortex extend to the entorhinal cortex, the basal and lateral amygdaloid nuclei, the lateral preoptic area of the hypothalamus, the nucleus of the diagonal band of Broca, the medial forebrain bundle, the dorsal medial nucleus and submedial nucleus of the thalamus, and the nucleus accumbens.

It should be noted that the entorhinal cortex is both a primary and secondary olfactory cortical area. Efferent fibers project via the uncinate fasciculus to the hippocampus, the anterior insular cortex next to the gustatory cortical area, and the frontal cortex. This may explain why temporal lobe epilepsy that involves the uncinate often produces parageusias of burning rubber, sometimes referred to as *uncinate fits* (Acharya et al. 1996).

Some of the efferent projections of the mitral and tufted cells decussate in the anterior commissure and form the medial olfactory tract. They then synapse in the contralateral parolfactory area and the contralateral subcallosal gyrus. The exact function of the medial olfactory stria and the tract is not clear. The accessory olfactory bulb receives afferent fibers from the bed nucleus of the accessory olfactory tract and the medial and posterior corticoamygdaloid nuclei. Efferent fibers from the accessory olfactory bulb project through the accessory olfactory tract to the same afferent areas. The medial and posterior corticoamygdaloid nuclei project secondary fibers to the anterior and medial hypothalamus, the areas associated with reproduction. Therefore, the accessory olfactory bulb in humans may be a mediator for human pheromones (Hirsch 1998a). The microneuroanatomy of these structures and other cortical projections may be adversely impacted by certain forms of poor nutrition.

2.3.2 NEUROTRANSMITTERS THAT MEDIATE SMELL

Neurotransmitters of the olfactory cortex are myriad, including glutamate, aspartate, cholecystokinin, luteinizing hormone-releasing hormone, and somatostatin. Furthermore, odor perception causes modulation of olfactory neurotransmitters within the olfactory bulb and the limbic system. Virtually, all known neurotransmitters are present in the olfactory bulb. Thus, odorant modulation of neurotransmitter levels in the olfactory bulb, tract, and limbic system intended for transmission of sensory information may have unintended secondary effects on a variety of different behaviors and disease states that are regulated by the same neurotransmitters. For instance, it is possible that the odorant modulation of dopamine in the olfactory bulb/limbic system may affect the manifestations of Parkinson's disease. Mesolimbic override of aspects of Parkinson's disease has been documented in response to motoric activation associated with emotional distress and fear of injury in a fire (Thierry et al. 1976; Javoy-Agid and Agid 1980).

2.3.3 Physiology of Taste

True tastes—salt, sweet, sour, bitter, umami, and possibly lipids—are mediated through taste receptors on taste buds located primarily in the fungiform and circumvallate papillae (Witt et al. 2003). The fungiform papillae have the lowest threshold to salt and sweet, whereas the circumvallate papillae are more sensitive to sweet stimuli (Jeppson 1969; Smith 1986). Cranial nerves VII, IX, and X, mediating the gustatory stimuli, enter the pons at the pontomedullary junction, ascending and descending through the tractus solitarius and finally terminating topographically on the ipsilateral nucleus of the tractus solitarius. Cranial nerve VII chorda tympani fibers synapse rostrally, whereas glossopharyngeal fibers synapse caudally. Second-order taste neurons progress through the parabrachial pontine nuclei where they diverge. Some of these synapse in the thalamus with tertiary-order neurons, which progress to the primary gustatory cortex in the insula. The others bypass the thalamus and project diffusely to the ventral forebrain with widespread limbic system connections.

Gustatory perception fluctuates between individuals, and such variability is partially genetically determined. Such differences influence consumption patterns and gastrointestinal physiology, thereby influencing metabolic and health outcomes more broadly. The implication of this individual variability may be significant for certain individuals inasmuch as it may impact the degree to which food is optimally digested and assimilated and thus overall heath. Chemosensory stimulation promotes gastric acid production and influences nutrient absorption, food allergenicity, and autonomic responses to food (Rolls 2010).

2.3.4 Etiologies of Chemosensory Disorders

2.3.4.1 Aging

The most common cause of smell loss in the United States is precipitated by aging itself (Kalogiera and Dzepina 2012). But by miraculous juvenescence of a *Ponce de Leon and His Fountain of Youth*, the march of time with the vicissitudes of aging proceeded unabatedly. From birth onward, olfactory bulb neurons are lost at a rate of 1% per year (Meisami et al. 1998). Clinically declining olfactory function can be demonstrated starting at the age of 36 years (Hawkes et al. 2005). Over time, olfactory ability vitiates, atrophying to such an extent that one-half of those over 65 and three-fourths of those over 80 have an impaired olfactory ability (Doty et al. 1984b). Odor sensitivity, in terms of both absolute threshold and odor identification, is reduced with age. Twenty-five percent of those over the age of 75 years are anosmic. These effects of aging parallel those found in other senses (Table 2.1).

Many possible mechanisms have been postulated for age-induced olfactory defects (Doty 1991). One theory posits that degenerative processes caused by toxins and viruses produce a cumulative effect on the olfactory epithelium. A second theory suggests that age-related immunocompromise predisposes people to upper respiratory infections, which may be followed by postviral upper respiratory infection-induced anosmia. The premise of a third hypothesis suggests that in the elderly, the central neural pathway degenerates with concomitant reduction in noradrenergic synesthesia. A fourth theory postulates the ossification of the foramina of the cribriform plate

TABLE 2.1
Pathologic Conditions

Conduction defects:

Airway:

Nasal Polyposis (Scott et al. 1989)

Symptoms: Hyposmia, olfactory windows, subjective hypogeusia

Treatment: Steroids (local/systemic), surgery, systemic steroids followed by nasal steroids, surgery followed by nasal steroids, surgery followed by systemic steroids (Scott 1989a)

Mucus:

Allergic Rhinitis

Symptoms: Hyposmia, olfactory windows, subjective hypogeusia

Mechanisms: Histamine release → change in mucus → decreased ability for the odorant molecule to dissolve in the mucus → blocked olfactory experience prior to reaching the olfactory nerve (Mott and Leopold 1991)

Treatment: Local or if ineffective, systemic steroids, (1) Flunesolide two puffs inhaled per nostril b.i.d. in head-down position (Scott et al. 1988); (2) Prednisone 50 mg PO q/day for five days (Apter et al. 1992)

Cranial Nerve I Disorder (1° neuron)

Olfactory Receptor Damage:

Postviral Infection

Symptoms: Hyposmia, dysosmia, no olfactory windows, subjective hypogeusia

Treatment: None. Zinc, no effect in double-blind, placebo-controlled study (Henkin et al. 1976)

Olfactory Nerve (Receptor Damage?)

Atmospheric pressure-sensitive paroxysmal unilateral phantosmia (Hirsch et al. 1992)

Symptoms: Phantosmia, hyposmia, olfactory windows

Mechanisms: Virus causes receptor damage → partial denervation occurs → in response to denervation, there is sprouting of new receptor sites that are sensitive to touch (trigeminal neuralgia model of synesthesia with perception of temperature or touch as pain)

Treatment: (1) Mechanical obstruction; (2) Valproic acid; (3) Tegretol; (4) Mysoline

Olfactory Nerve Axon at the Cribriform Plate

Head trauma (Hirsch and Wyse 1993)

Symptoms: Subjective hypogeusia, no olfactory windows, anosmia, hyposmia, phantosmia, dysosmia

Mechanisms: *Shearing of olfactory nerve* 40% of the time damage rostral to cranial nerve I *central hyposmia*

Treatment: For central hyposmia: (1) thiamine 100 mg PO q. d., (2) phosphatidylcholine 9 gm q. d.

For peripheral anosmia: None

Olfactory Nerve (at the axon hillock)

Toxins (Amoore 1986; Doty et al. 1986): Trichloroethylene (Hirsch 1995b), cigarettes (Frye et al. 1990), nitrogen tetroxide (Hirsch 1995c), pyrethroid insecticides (Hirsch 1997), hydrogen sulfide (Hirsch 1996), lead, methyl ethyl ketone (Hirsch 1997), aluminosilicates (Roberts 1986), mercury (Furuta et al. 1994), solvents (Schwartz et al. 1990), chlorine (Hirsch 1995a)

Symptoms: Hyposmia, anosmia, subjective hypogeusia, no olfactory windows, phantosmia

Mechanisms: With no blood–brain barrier, toxins overwhelm the nasal xenobiotic mechanism, inducing olfactory nerve cell death. Aluminosilicates, in addition, are transported transaxonally causing continued rostral destruction (a postulated mechanism for the pathogenesis of senile dementia of the Alzheimer's type)

(Continued)

TABLE 2.1 (CONTINUED)
Pathologic Conditions

Central Pathway Dysfunction

Olfactory bulb and tract: Olfactory groove meningioma (Jafek and Hill 1989)

    Symptoms: Phantosmia, hyposmia, subjective hypogeusia

    Treatment: Surgical intervention

Hippocampi: Wernicke–Korsakoff syndrome (Potter and Butters 1980)

    Symptoms: Anosmia

    Treatment: Thiamine

Temporal Lobe: Complex partial seizures (Acharya et al. 1996)

    Symptoms: Anosmia ipsilateral to the seizure focus, hyposmia contralateral to the seizure focus, *uncinate fits*, phantosmia, foul burning rubber, metallic phantageusia, not well localized

    Mechanism: Spontaneous olfactory cortex discharge possibly ipsilaterally mediated

Frontal Lobe: Pick's disease

Anterior Olfactory Nucleus: Parkinson–dementia complex of Guam (Doty et al. 1991)

    Symptoms: Hyposmia

Limbic Lobe: Dysthymia, generalized anxiety disorder (Hirsch and Trannel 1996), schizophrenia (Serby et al. 1990)

    Symptoms: Hyposmia, subjective hypogeusia, phantosmia

    Mechanism: Neighborhood effect; reaction to narcissistic insult: the greater the duration of the schizophrenia, the greater the olfactory loss (Moberg et al. 1997)

    Treatment: Amitriptyline, group therapy

Schizophrenia (Rubert et al. 1961; Meats 1988) olfactory hallucination—prevalence: acute schizophrenia 79%, chronic schizophrenia (hospitalized) 92%

Olfactory dysmorphophobia (Hirsch 1990a): Olfactory reference syndrome

    Symptoms: Self-perception of cacosmia

    Treatment: Haloperidol, MAOI

Diffuse Brain Dysfunction

Senile dementia of the Alzheimer's Type

    Symptoms: Anomic anosmia, subjective hypogeusia

    Mechanism: Decreased choline acetyltransferase in the basal nucleus of Meynart—questionable decreased acetylcholine in the olfactory bulb, tract, and cortex—pathology in the anterior olfactory nucleus, uncus, and medial amygdaloid nuclei olfactory vector hypothesis allows toxin or virus to penetrate transaxonally (Pearson et al. 1985) deep into the brain where it causes selective damage based on susceptibility of specific neurons (Doty 1997)

    Treatment: Phosphatidylcholine 9 gm q. d.

Olfactory Dysfunction in Other Neurologic Diseases

Movement Disorders

Parkinson's disease (Markopoulou et al. 1977):

    Symptoms: Hyposmia, subjective hypogeusia

    Mechanism: Question if due to depletion of dopamine in the olfactory bulb (not seen in MPTP-induced Parkinsonism) (Doty et al. 1992a)

    Treatment: Unresponsive to L-DOPA (Doty et al. 1992b)

Huntington's chorea

    Symptoms: Hyposmia of threshold and identification

    Mechanism: Not a presymptomatic indicator of disease—appears coincidentally with motor findings (Moberg and Doty 1997)

TABLE 2.1 (CONTINUED)
Pathologic Conditions

Progressive supranuclear palsy (Doty 1995): None

Essential tremor (Busenbark et al. 1992): None

Multiple sclerosis:

> Symptoms: Hyposmia in 23% (Doty et al. 1984b)

> Mechanism: Olfactory ability correlated with the number of plaques in temporal lobes and frontal cortex (Doty et al. 1997)

Amyotrophic lateral sclerosis:

> Symptoms: Hyposmia in 64%, anosmia in 11% (Sajjadian et al. 1994)

Headache

Sinusitis (Apter et al. 1992):

> Symptoms: Hyposmia, foul phantosmia, dysosmia, subjective hypogeusia, olfactory windows

> Mechanism: Prevents odorant molecule from getting to or dissolving in the mucus

> Treatment: Antibiotics

Migraine (Hirsch 1992):

> Symptoms: Subclinical hyposmia in 17%

> Mechanism:

> 1. Migraine may induce olfactory dysfunction

>> —Recurrent small vascular insults may induce a persistent neurologic deficit (as in complicated migraine) affecting the olfactory system

>> —Lacrimation and rhinorrhea may engorge the nasal passages to such a degree as to totally obstruct air flow to the olfactory epithelium

>> —A learned response to *tune out* environmental odorant triggers

> 2. Olfactory loss may predispose to the development of migraines

>> —Decreased olfactory ability → increased likelihood of exposure to environmental chemical inducers of headache

>> —Olfactory sensory deprivation → compensatory psychological response → headache

> 3. Unified limbic system theory

>> —A single pathogen induces both migraine and olfactory deficit concurrently (due to neighborhood effect?)

> 4. Genetics

> 5. Medication effect

> Treatment: Multipronged and may respond to specific antimigraine agents

Cluster headaches (Hirsch and Thakkar 1995):

Symptoms: Transient hyperosmia concurrent with and ipsilateral to the hemicephalgia

Mechanism:

> —Transient cortical deficiency (physiologic Addisonian state)

> —Transient hypothalamic/pituitary axis dysregulation

> —Increased substance P: (an excitatory olfactory neurotransmitter?)

> —Change in 5HT (olfactory bulb neurotransmitter)

> —Change in ACH (olfactory bulb neurotransmitter)

> —Increased DA (olfactory bulb neurotransmitter)

> —Increased NE (locus coeruleus projects to the olfactory bulb): NE → granule cell discharge → GABA → mitral cell discharge → increased olfaction

> —Increased gastrin (olfactory bulb neurotransmitter)

(Continued)

TABLE 2.1 (CONTINUED)
Pathologic Conditions

—Beta endorphin (olfactory bulb neurotransmitter)

—Decreased met-enkephalin (inhibitory olfactory bulb neurotransmitter)

—RAS activation

—Generalized limbic/anterior hypothalamic discharge (neighborhood effect)

—Partial nasal congestion → eddy currents

—Nasal engorgement → increase in air temperature

—Nasal secretions → wet mucosal membrane → better dissolution of odorant

—Change in estrogen/testosterone balances (estrogen changes mucosal composition → increased odorant absorption; testosterone changes mucosal composition → decreased odorant absorption)

—Cyclic limbic/hypothalamic instability → activation of the olfactory component of the limbic system → cyclic hyperosmia → detection of otherwise subthreshold ambient irritants

→ trigeminal nerve activation → substance P release → cluster headache

—1° hyperosmia (odor-induced limbic dysregulation; odor-induced changes in CNS electrical activity)

Columella variant of glossopharyngeal neuralgia (Bruyn 1986):

Symptoms: Unilateral or bilateral burning tongue, mouth grittiness, pain, dyesthesias, hyperpathia

Mechanism: virus-induced deinervation with reinnervation hypersensitivity? reinnervation synesthesia?

Treatment: Tegretol, Dilantin, valproic acid, Neurontin

Features Common to Many Neurologic Diseases:

Medication effect (Scott 1989b):

Symptoms: Hyposmia, anosmia

Mechanism: possibly inhibits olfactory nerve regeneration from stem cell

Treatment: Discontinue the medication, zinc sulfate

Senescence (Venstrom and Amoore 1968):

Symptom: Subclinical hyposmia

Mechanism: Generalized reduction in neurotransmitters, cumulative effect of recurrent mild head trauma or recurrent viral infection-induced olfactory nerve destruction, medication effect, presence of other neurologic disease (i.e., senile dementia of the Alzheimer's type, multi-infarct dementia), cumulative effect of exposure to exogenous toxins (cigarette smoke), nutritional deficiency state

Treatment: Thiamine 100 mg q. d., phosphatidylcholine 9 g q. d.; amantadine not effective; aminophylline not effective, amitriptyline not effective

Malingering:

Symptoms: Anosmia with loss of trigeminal preceptor as well; after head trauma or toxic exposure; no olfactory windows

Mechanism: U.S. Armed Forces recognize anosmia as a 10% total body disability, awards in California exceeding $3,000,000 for smell loss

Acute alcohol intoxication:

Symptom: Subclinical hyposmia

Mechanism: possibly transiently anesthetizes olfactory nerve cells; inhibits the reticular activating system thus reducing attention to external stimuli

Treatment: Routine breathalyzer testing

Individual variation:

Symptoms: Subjective hyposmia (Hirsch 1995d)

Subclinical hyposmia—four-star chefs (Hirsch 1990)

TABLE 2.1 (CONTINUED)
Pathologic Conditions

General Treatment Approaches:

Remove gas from house; gas detector, smoke detector. Food taster; date all food. Hygienic checker—smell buddy. Group therapy (Hirsch et al. 1992)

Flavor enhancers (Schiffman and Warwick 1988)

Modify foods: Horseradish, black pepper, cayenne pepper, hot pepper, fresh mint texture, colorful visual displays (Duffy and Ferris 1989) capsaicin, mustard, ginger, clove, cinnamon, peppermint, spearmint, and pimiento (Davidson et al. 1987)

Stop smoking

For idiopathic or not surgically correctable anosmia or hyposmia; from Z to A (Hirsch et al. 1996):

Zinc sulfate (Davidson et al. 1987) (no better than placebo) (Henkin et al. 1976)

Vitamin B_1 (Goodspeed et al. 1987)

Vitamin A (Snow, Jr. and Martin 1994) 100,000 IU IM q wk for 6 weeks, followed by 50,000 I.U. POqd for 12 weeks

Strychnine (CNS stimulant) (Estrem and Renner 1987)

Prednisone 40 mg, taper by 5 mg/day (Knight 1988)

Phosphatidylcholine (Hirsch 1990; Hirsch and Dougherty 1992)

L-cysteine ethylester hydrochloride (topical) ± topical steroids (Takagi 1984)

Alcohol

Amantadine (Hirsch and Aranda 1992)

Aminophylline 500 mg—1 gm q day (Henkin et al. 1981)

Amitriptyline (Hirsch and Vanderbilt 1992)

Amphetamine (methylphenidate) (Wysocki et al. 1989)

For smell blindness:

Sniff therapy—3 min tid for 6 weeks (Hummel et al. 2005)

Unusual Treatment Approaches of Questionable Validity:

Chiropractic manipulation

Intranasal steroid injection

Acupuncture

Homeopathic

with secondary occlusion and compression of the olfactory fila. These hypotheses are not mutually exclusive.

The implications of olfactory deficits among the aged are important, particularly regarding the detection of gas used for heating and cooking (Croy et al. 2014). Elderly persons succumb to accidental injury from leaking gas at a much higher rate than do younger people; 75% of such deaths were among persons over 60 years of age. Among persons over 65 years old, 30% could not smell town gas in concentrations below 50 parts per 10,000 if they could smell it at all. Among those under age 65, in comparison, 95% could smell town gas in concentrations below 20 parts per 10,000 (Stevens et al. 1987). Half of the people over age 60 could not detect the odor of gas at the maximum concentration allowed by the Department of Transportation. One-seventh of persons 70 to 85 years of age could not detect the odor of gas at explosive concentrations (Stevens et al. 1987).

In reference to ethyl mercaptan, the agent that is added to propane gas to give it a noxious odor; persons 70 to 85 years of age have a threshold 10 times higher than that of persons under age 70 (Stevens et al. 1987).

The impaired olfactory abilities among the elderly imply impaired flavor abilities since odor forms a large component of the sense of *taste*. This may explain why the elderly consume an unbalanced diet such as one lacking in vegetables. Green peppers, for instance, have a bitter taste and a pleasant odor, but to the elderly, they merely taste bitter, making it unlikely that elderly people would eat them. The same is true with other green, leafy vegetables leading to avoidance of their food with a secondary effect of vitamin deficiency state and constipation.

Among the aged, retronasal odor perception (odor perceived while chewing and swallowing) is also reduced (Stevens and Cain 1986). Despite this, elderly persons rarely complain of food lacking taste, possibly because of the slow, gradual loss of smell whose decline is unrecognizable to the person.

True gustatory ability also worsens with age. The majority of 60-year-olds have lost 50% of their taste buds, with a concordant reduction in taste, initially to sweet and salty followed by loss of sour and bitter (Zegeer 1986).

Coincident with this chemosensory loss, weight shows a reciprocal elevation with age. Excluding the extreme elderly, from the age of approximately 20 onward, the average American gains approximately 1 lb./year (Lewis et al. 2000). This chemosensory loss may be part of the cause of age-associated weight gain, which is partly due to reduced effectiveness of sensory-specific satiety (Chapter 11 of this book). Cooks preparing food for the elderly should use higher concentrations of odorants compared with those preparing food for the young. The elderly, because of their deficits, prefer foods with enhanced flavor.

2.3.4.2 Nasal Obstruction

Decreased ability to detect odors can occur secondary to nasal obstruction from adenoid hypertrophy. Adenoidectomy causes a recovery of the threshold of odor detection. Steroid-dependent anosmia is a syndrome whose triad includes inhalant allergy, nasal polyps, and steroid reversal anosmia (Jefek et al. 1987). Its pathology is that of polyps, which cause a mechanical obstruction causing a conduction effect preventing odorants from reaching the olfactory epithelium.

2.3.4.3 Viral

Acute viral hepatitis causes a reduction in olfactory sensitivity with dysgeusia and associated anorexia, which improve as the illness improves (Deems et al. 1991b). Olfactory sensitivity in acute viral hepatitis is inversely proportional to the plasma bilirubin and directly proportional to the plasma retinal binding protein level (Deems et al. 1991b). The function of these and other signaling molecules in connection with food choice-related chemosensory variability will become increasingly pertinent in the epidemiology of obesity and metabolic disturbance.

2.3.4.4 Endocrine Disorders

Several endocrine disorders are associated with anosmia. In hypothyroidism, 39% of afflicted individuals are aware of an alteration of sense of taste, 17% have dysosmia or distortion in sense of smell, and 39% have dysgeusia (Mackay-Sim 1991). Thyroid replacement reverses these problems. Individuals with both olfactory or gustatory problems and hypothyroidism have low parotid zinc levels (Mackay-Sim 1991).

Pseudohypoparathyroidism is a syndrome that includes a short stature, a rounded face, mental retardation, brachymetacarpia, brachymetatarsia, hypocalcemia, hyperphosphatemia, and resistance to parathyroid hormone (Mackay-Sim 1991). Hyposmia and hypogeusia are also seen in pseudohypoparathyroidism. With onset at birth, patients are usually unaware of their hyposmia and are unresponsive to hormones. In this condition, hyposmia has been localized to an X-linked dominant chromosome.

Turner's syndrome, or chromatin-negative gonadal dysgenesis, is characterized by a short stature, cubitus valgus, a webbed neck, a shield-like thorax, and an XO-chromosome pattern. Though patients are almost always unaware of olfactory defects, they are found to have both hyposmia and hypogeusia (Henkin 1967).

Olfactory sensitivity of patients with adrenal cortical insufficiency is increased approximately 100,000 fold over that of unaffected individuals (Mackay-Sim 1991). Treatment with carbohydrate-active steroids such as prednisone 20 mg/day reduces olfactory sensitivity toward normal within 1 day. Since the olfactory response occurs prior to any change in electrolytes or body weight, one can postulate that endogenous CNS carbohydrate-active steroids normally inhibit olfaction.

Congenital adrenal hyperplasia is a nonhypertensive, virilizing illness. In the nonsalt-losing variant, the classic treatment with steroids reduces the sometimes associated olfactory and gustatory hypersensitivity to normal in 8 to 14 days. Since 17-ketosteroids and pregnanetriol return to normal before the normalization of olfactory and gustatory sensitivity, it is unlikely that the reduction in olfactory sensitivity is due to carbohydrate-active steroids alone.

Kallmann syndrome involves a deficiency of gonadotrophin-associated hypogonadism and impaired olfactory acuity. Clomiphene induces luteinizing hormone and follicle-stimulating hormone release, which causes an increase in both gonadotrophin and testosterone. The olfactory deficit does not respond to clomiphene (Hawkes and Doty 2009).

2.3.4.5   Meningiomas

Olfactory meningiomas are classically described as causing loss of ability to detect odors. These meningiomas, which occur along the olfactory groove, account for less than 10% of all intracranial meningiomas (Murphy et al. 2003). They usually develop in middle-aged patients, with hyposmia as the first and only symptom, years before the meningioma would enlarge, causing dementia and impaired vision.

2.3.4.6   Temporal Lobe Lesions

The temporal lobe also has an important influence on olfaction. One patient, H.M., was studied for his olfactory sensitivity after undergoing bilateral resection of the medial temporal lobe that involved the amygdala, the uncus, the anterior two-thirds of the hippocampus, and the parahippocampal gyrus. Although he could detect odors, he could not identify them, and when given two odors, he could not distinguish whether they were the same or different. This suggests that the medial temporal lobe is critical for the perception of odor quality (Eichenbaum et al. 1983). Temporal lobectomy patients demonstrate a mild, bilateral reduction in absolute olfactory sensitivity. In the ipsilateral nostril, odor perception is reduced as is odor identification. Patients with temporal lobe epilepsy who have had no surgery display a bilateral reduction in odor identification. Of patients with temporal lobe tumors, 20% have an olfactory disturbance (Eskenazi et al. 1986). Speculated to be secondary to temporal lobe infarction, coronary artery bypass surgery can cause both dysosmia and cacosmia, whereby odors are distorted and previously hedonically pleasant aromas postoperatively are perceived as unpleasant (Mohr 1986).

2.3.4.7   Thalamic and Hypothalamic Lesions

Patients with estrogen receptor-positive breast cancer have been found to have hyposmia, possibly secondary to hypothalamic lesions (Lehrer et al. 1985). Hypothalamic lesions produce an increase in the incidence of spontaneous mammary tumors in female rats. This suggests that a hypothalamic lesion may be the primary defect in both estrogen receptor-positive breast carcinoma and associated hyposmia.

Korsakoff's psychosis is associated with an anatomic lesion of the dorsal medial nucleus of the thalamus and with impairment in odor perception corresponding to reduction in cerebrospinal fluid 3-methoxy-4-hydroxy-phenylethylene glycol (MHPG), which is a norephinephrine metabolite (Mair et al. 1986). MHPG is reduced in Parkinson's disease and in senile dementia of the Alzheimer's type, and these patients also display an impaired ability to identify odors (Potter and Butters 1980; Ward et al. 1983). Related studies suggest that norephinephrine is important for olfaction and that a drug to increase norephinephrine could potentially restore olfactory ability in some patients.

One such drug is D-amphetamine. This D2 dopamine receptor agonist increased olfactory detection in rats given 0.2 mg/kg body weight. With much higher doses, i.e., 1.6 mg/kg, the rats' ability to detect odors was reduced (Doty and Ferguson-Segall 1987; Doty et al. 1988b). The mechanism whereby it increases odor detection ability is unknown. D-amphetamine may act as a reticular activity system stimulator. It may also act by increasing catecholamine levels in the olfactory tubercle, anterior olfactory nucleus, amygdala, and entorhinal cortex. It may stimulate the locus coeruleus to release norephinephrine, which projects to the lateral olfactory tract. The lateral olfactory tract then would act to inhibit granule cell discharge, causing a reduction in the inhibition of mitral cell discharge. The disinhibited mitral cells would thus be allowed to fire, causing an increase in olfactory acuity. The latter mechanism is probably not applicable to D-amphetamine, however, because in experiments with rats, norephinephrine depletion of the olfactory bulb had no effect on odor detection ability, implying that D-amphetamine operates on a central basis.

2.3.4.8   Parkinson's Disease

Parkinsonism is associated with a decrease in odor sensitivity in 75% of cases and a reduced ability to identify odors in 90% of cases (Hawkes 2006). These olfactory deficits occur independently of age, gender, stage, and duration of the disease. Before they were tested, 72% of Parkinson's disease patients were unaware of their deficits in olfaction, which tend to occur early in the disease process in both demented and nondemented patients and do not worsen with time (Doty et al.

1988a). In monozygotic twins who both suffer from Parkinson's disease, olfactory impairment has a low concordance rate, indicating that this aspect of the disease is probably not inherited (Doty et al. 1989). Phantosmia has also been described in this setting (Hirsch 2009).

Myriad mechanisms have been postulated for the olfactory defects associated with Parkinson's disease. The same environmental agent that caused Parkinson's disease may have also damaged the olfactory pathway. The olfactory receptor cells may actively transport viruses, proteins, and environmental toxins, bypassing the blood–brain barrier directly infiltrating the central nervous system. The substance so transported could damage the olfactory epithelium and olfactory system before invading the substantia nigra to cause Parkinson's disease. The underlying Parkinson's disease could also reduce the olfactory system's resistance to viral or environmental toxins, which then could destroy olfactory pathways. Alternately, the degenerative process of Parkinson's disease may favor destruction of the olfactory pathways as it affects the substantia nigra. Moreover, a reduction in CNS neurotransmitters can impair olfaction. The absence of effect of levodopa/carbidopa on olfaction in Parkinson's disease argues against this hypothesis. In its favor is the fact that d2 dopamine receptor agonist d-amphetamine increases olfaction in rats, as previously mentioned.

2.3.4.9 Alzheimer's Disease

Patients with Alzheimer's disease (AD) are usually unaware of their olfactory deficits (Doty et al. 1987). The reduced odor threshold and identification ability found in this disorder may be secondary to reduced acetylcholine in the olfactory system (Serby et al. 1985). Acetylcholine has been found to be low in the olfactory tubercle in patients with AD. Arguing in favor of this hypothesis is the effect of the application of nasal acetylcholine producing an increase in olfactory sensitivity.

Alternatively, the decrease in olfactory sensitivity in AD could be secondary to temporal lobe dysfunction (Koss et al. 1988). As mentioned, olfactory defects are found in individuals with temporal lobectomies, and the same mechanism may operate in AD. The olfactory pathway has been suggested to be the initial site of involvement in both AD and Pick's disease (Pearson et al. 1985).

In AD, neuritic plaque and neurofibrillary tangles form in the olfactory bulb, olfactory tract, anterior olfactory nucleus, prepyriform cortex, uncus, and the corticomedial part of the amygdaloid nucleus (Serby et al. 1992). In normal anatomy, the anterior olfactory nucleus, the uncus, and the corticomedial part of the amygdaloid nucleus all receive afferent input from the olfactory bulb. In the entorhinal cortex, layer II stellate cells, which are the end point for the lateral olfactory tract, are lost. This is clinically relevant since secondary connections of the olfactory cortex are involved with memory and cognition, including the amygdala, the dorsal medial nucleus of the thalamus, and the hippocampus.

A unified theory that could possibly explain the occurrence of both olfactory deficits in AD is a variant of the theory described for Parkinson's disease: viruses may enter the olfactory pathway via the olfactory epithelium, thereby bypassing the blood–brain barrier (Monath et al. 1983). Once inside the olfactory pathway, the viruses can spread into the secondary connections of the limbic system. This route of infection is known to operate in the case of St. Louis encephalitis and amoebiasis and may explain some of the features of Parkinsonism, including catatonia, facial hypokinesia, and Parkinsonian tremor, which have occurred in rare arborvirus-induced cases such as St. Louis encephalitis.

Roberts' theory is that AD begins in the nose and is caused by aluminosilicates (Roberts 1986). Labeled glucose placed into the oropharynx is rapidly transported transneuronally to the glomeruli in the olfactory bulb. From there, it spreads into the olfactory projections, i.e., the basal nucleus of Meynert, the locus coeruleus, and the brainstem raphe nuclei. Aluminum and silicon are found to increase in the brain with aging (Schwartz et al. 1988). Widely dispersed in the environment, aluminosilicates can be found in diverse products including talc, deionizers, antacids, underarm spray, dental powder, cat litter, cigar ash, and cigarette ash. Roberts strongly recommends reducing exposure to these aerosolized toxins.

2.3.4.10   Toxic Agents

In addition to aluminum and silicon mentioned above as the possible causes of AD, other more classic toxic agents, notably lead and arsenic, are well known to affect olfaction (Cometto-Muniz and Cain 1991). Perfume workers, varnish workers, and those exposed to cadmium dust also experience a marked reduction in olfactory abilities (Cometto-Muniz and Cain 1991; Schwartz 1991). Other environmental toxins demonstrated to be olfactotoxins include pyrethroid insecticides, chlordane/heptachlor hermaticides, nitrogen tetroxide, chlorine, and hydrogen sulfide (Hirsch 1995a, 1998b, 2002a,b, 2003).

Over 20% of the adult population in the United States smoke, and thus this pathologic action may be the primary cause of smell loss seen today (CDC 2014).

In a Texas petrochemical plant, workers who smoked cigarettes showed reduced olfactory sensitivity; the diminished acuity directly correlated with the amount that they smoked (Frye et al. 1990). Another aspect of cigarette smoking concerns its effect on the trigeminally mediated reflex transitory apnea (the *took-my-breath-away* reflex). Cigarette smoking raised the threshold of the reflex by 67% (Cain and Cometto-Muniz 1982). The mechanism is probably secondary to smoke-induced ciliostasis, which causes a mucostasis that induces viscid, static mucus. The viscid mucus impairs the transfer of odor molecules from the air to free nerve endings. Secondhand smoke may thus act through a similar mechanism to raise both olfactory and trigeminal thresholds.

Such secondhand smoke may further promote obesity. Adult women and men who before 10 years of age were raised by parents, both of whom smoked and were exposed to two or more smokers in their household, respectively, have an elevated body mass index (BMI) (Snyder et al. 2005). The mechanism for such an effect may revolve around the influence of secondhand smoke not on the nose but rather the ear. The smoke promotes childhood otitis media. Such infection damages the chorda tympani. This increases the palatability of energy-dense foods and thus the propensity to adult onset obesity (Bartoshuk et al. 2007).

Another common toxin that adversely impacts upon olfaction is that of alcohol, which with both acute and chronic use reduces olfactory ability (Hirsch and Bissell 1998).

2.3.4.11 Trauma

Head injury is a common cause of olfactory defects and can occur from trauma as minimal as *heading* a soccer ball (Custer et al. 2014). Many possible mechanisms have been suggested (Hirsch and Wyse 1993). One is that acceleration injury produces shearing forces on the olfactory nerves as they pass through the cribriform plate of the ethmoid bone. Fracture of the cribriform plate may compress the olfactory nerves, or a hematoma may compress them, thereby impairing olfaction. Another theory suggests that the primary insult in trauma is the destruction of pathways of central connection of olfaction (Levin et al. 1985). After trauma, surgical intervention with subfrontal exploration of the anterior fossa can stretch or tear the olfactory nerves. Surgical repair of a dural tear with grafts covering the cribriform plate can block regenerating stem cells.

Assessing the results of many studies of olfaction in head injury victims, roughly 5% of them are described to possess olfactory disorders. No correlation has been observed between the loss of olfaction and the age of the victim at the time of the accident or the category of the accident.

The incidence of olfactory disorder is proportional to the severity of the injury, but even a trivial injury can induce anosmia. In trauma severe enough to induce amnesia, occipital trauma is five times as likely to produce anosmia as is trauma to the forehead (Costanzo et al. 1992).

Usually, any olfactory loss occurs shortly after the trauma, but sometimes, anosmia or hyposmia may not be noted until several months later. Recovery from olfactory defects usually begins during the first few weeks after head trauma, but it can be delayed until as long as 5 years later.

Half of the individuals with anosmia secondary to head trauma experience distorted smell in response to odorants. Costanzo reported on 77 persons with anosmia due to head injury: 33% recovered, 27% worsened, and 40% remained unchanged (Costanzo and Becker 1986). Costanzo and Becker (1986) reported on a sample of 1167 patients: 50% recovered except for cases where injury was so severe as to cause amnesia of more than 24 h. In these cases, fewer than 10% recovered.

Temporary anosmia of short duration, often found after trauma, could be due to mechanical blockage of airways, nasal hemorrhaging, inflammation, cerebrospinal fluid rhinorrhea, or an increase in intracranial pressure. Increased intracranial pressure may reduce blood circulation to the olfactory bulbs, causing secondary infarctions with associated anosmia.

The trauma may be so severe as to cause both olfactory and trigeminal system dysfunction with the trigeminal dysfunction of variable degrees with or without loss of trigeminally induced lacrimation (Hirsch et al. 2014).

2.3.4.12 Nutritional Deficiencies

Some primary nutritional deficiency states have also been associated with chemosensory pathology. Hypovitaminosis A induces both hyposmia and hypogeusia, which usually resolves within 2 months with vitamin A replacement (Sauberlich 1975). The mechanism of the deficit may be a result of epithelial proliferation and drying, which forms a physical barrier preventing odorants and tastants from reaching their respective receptors (Friedman and Mattes 1991).

Chemosensory dysfunction has been reported in those deficient in B complex vitamins (Green 1971). Hyposmia is found in Wernicke–Korsakoff syndrome, a disorder usually seen in chronic alcoholism associated with thiamine deficiency (Mair et al. 1986). Dysosmia and dysgeusia are seen in those with reduced vitamin B_{12} levels and pernicious anemia (Green 1971; Smith 1983).

Both zinc and copper status have also been implicated as being relevant to olfactory function. Hypocupria (which often occurs coincidentally with zinc deficiency) causes a reversible hypogeusia and is responsive to both copper sulfate and zinc sulfate (Schechter et al. 1972; Smith and Seiden 1995). Patients with anosmia induced by head trauma have been found to have reduced total serum zinc and increased total serum copper. This same chemical imbalance is found in the syndrome of idiopathic hypogeusia with dysgeusia, hyposmia, and dysosmia. The importance of zinc is further demonstrated in patients treated with L-histidine, which induces zincuria, causing a secondary hypozincemia and reduced total body zinc. This, in turn, causes hypogeusia, hyposmia, anorexia, dysgeusia, and dysosmia. All these symptoms are corrected with zinc. Improvement occurs even when the patient is still receiving L-histidine (Weismann et al. 1979). Further discussion of zinc is found in Section 2.5.5.

2.3.4.13   Diagnoses Associated with Olfactory Impairment

The absence of olfactory data on a patient may impair diagnostic accuracy. For example, Post's pseudodementia, which does not involve olfactory impairment, is sometimes misdiagnosed as AD, which does involve olfactory impairment (Post 1975). Olfactory testing can aid in distinguishing these disorders (Solomon et al. 1998). In parallel fashion, olfactory deficits are seen in idiopathic Parkinson's disease but not in 1-methyl-4-phenyl-1,2,3,6-tetrahydropyridine (MPTP) induced Parkinson's disease, progressive supranuclear palsy, or essential tremor (Busenbark et al. 1992; Doty et al. 1992a; Sajjadian et al. 1994). Olfactory deficits are seen in a substantial proportion of those with sinusitis or migraines but not in those with cluster headaches (Loury and Kennedy 1991; Hirsch 1992b; Hirsch and Thakkar 1995).

Olfactory deficits may be the first manifestation of an underlying disease state. Without olfactory data, vitamin B_{12} deficiency and olfactory groove meningiomas, which display olfactory dysfunction early on, may remain undetected until more serious neurological deficits occur (Estrem and Renner 1987; Hirsch 1995b; Hafek and Hill 1989). General anxiety disorder and sexual dysfunction are associated with olfactory dysfunction; thus, the detection of olfactory deficits may facilitate the diagnosis and treatment of these disorders (Hirsch and Trannel 1996; Hirsch 1998a).

The converse chemosensory ability in the obese or tabescent may also be revealing. Consistent with the suggestion that impaired olfactory ability reduces sensory-specific satiety, inhibiting post-ingestion appetite suppression and thus increasing consumption and weight gain, reduced olfactory ability has been found in the obese as compared to the non-obese (Fox 1966). Over half a century ago, such has been demonstrated in adults and in children, where impaired odor detection thresholds were found to exist (Guild 1956; Obrebowski et al. 2000).

In obesity, chemosensory dysfunction is not limited to the olfactory sphere. Also, in obesity, there are normal sweet taste thresholds and normal sweet suprathreshold intensity judgments (Grinker 1978; Witherly et al. 1980; Fritjers et al.

1982; Drewnowski 1987). In regard to sweet hedonics, studies are inconclusive with results suggesting more, same, or less sweet preference (Rodin et al. 1976; Spitzer and Rodin 1981; Fritjers and Rusmussen-Conrad 1982; Drewnowski 1987). While high-fat, low-sugar mixtures appear to be preferred in the obese, not all studies confirm this preference (Pangborn et al. 1985; Warwick et al. 1990; Drewnowski 1991). Diverse results from studies suggest that presently unidentified subgroups of taste response exist among those with obesity and chemosensory disorders.

Taste blindness to the intensely bitter substance 6-n-propylthiouracil (PROP) is a genetic trait that correlates with obesity and increased BMI (Tepper et al. 2005). This connection may relate to hedonic effects occurring due to the inability to detect the bitter taste of PROP, allowing consumption of a greater number of foods leading to a greater BMI. Such pathophysiology might explain the PROP–obesity association, since PROP nontasters are more likely than tasters to have a larger waist circumference (Hutchins et al. 2002). However, PROP bitterness did not correlate with vegetable and fruit food hedonics, bringing this mechanism into question (Minski et al. 2010).

Those PROP-impaired subjects did, however, demonstrate greater hedonics toward high-fat foods (Duffy et al. 2006). Such a PROP impairment–obesity connection is further muddied, since greater spicy food preferences (in theory, which may be seen with PROP taste deficiency) are associated with lower adiposity rather than obesity (Sullivan et al. 2007).

Furthermore, PROP nontasters have more difficulty detecting free fatty acids and thus may require more fats to induce sensory-specific satiety, allowing greater consumption before satiation and thus a higher BMI (Sollai et al. 2014).

Among the morbidly obese (BMI > 45), there is greater olfactory impairment than even among the moderately obese (BMI < 45) (Richardson et al. 2004). The reduced olfactory acuity in the obese is even further diminished after eating, suggesting that the olfactory component of sensory-specific satiety may be impaired in the obese, thus inhibiting further appetite suppression and predisposing to greater consumption and obesity (Stafford and Welbeck 2010, 2011). Altered brain response to chemosensory stimuli, as documented by functional magnetic resonance image (fMRI), has been postulated as one of the underlying mechanisms for obesity in metabolic syndrome (Murphy et al. 2014).

Among patients with anorexia, there is an elevation in sour and bitter recognition thresholds, but there is no abnormality in sweet or salty taste detection thresholds. Neither are there abnormal sweet superthreshold intensity judgments nor detection threshold in anorexic or bulimic patients (Lacey et al. 1977; Casper et al. 1980; Sunday and Halmi 1990). Furthermore, anorexic patients demonstrate an aversion to high-fat foods, but this may be due to food texture rather than taste (Mela 1988).

2.4 PATIENT EVALUATION

When chemosensory disorders are associated with some of the underlying conditions mentioned above, it is important to diagnose the treatable medical conditions. This assessment is particularly relevant among hospitalized persons where the incidence of olfactory impairment is probably greater than among the general population (Public Health Service 1979; Ackerman and Kasbekar 1997).

Standard medical and neurological text indicates that assessment of the olfactory nerve, the cranial nerve I (CNI), is an essential part of a complete neurological examination (Bates 1974; Parsons 1983; Haerer 1992; Fuller 1993). Given the likelihood of olfactory dysfunction among hospitalized patients, particularly those with neurological disorders, olfactory testing should be routinely performed.

Assessment of CNI allows the detection of hyposmia and anosmia regardless of the origin. Patients may then receive medications, vitamins, food supplements, or special treatment to correct the underlying pathology, such as polypectomy for nasal polyps and steroids for allergic rhinitis (Davidson et al. 1987; Scott et al. 1988, 1989). Appropriate counseling can be life-saving prevention. Risks to personal safety such as inadvertent consumption of spoiled or oversalted food or fire injury can be averted with use of food tasters and gas detectors (Chalke and Dewhurst 1957; Costanzo and Zasler 1991).

2.4.1 Assessing Olfaction

Limiting testing to those who complain of chemosensory problems would leave many cases of smell loss undetected. Self-recognition of olfactory deficits is poor across affected groups. Half of anosmic workers exposed to cadmium and 100% of hyposmic chefs were unaware of any deficits (Adams and Crabtree 1961). Moreover, among working Chicago firefighters, 87.5% of whom were either hyposmic or anosmic, none were aware of their deficits (Hirsch and Colavincenzo 2000a). Geriatric patients and those with neurodegenerative disorders tend to be unaware of their olfactory losses (Nordin et al. 1995). Of those with Parkinson's disease, fewer than 15% recognize their olfactory deficits (Doty et al. 1988a).

In clinical practice, CNI is rarely tested (Fuller 1993). To demonstrate this, histories and physical examinations in 90 patients' charts at a Chicago teaching hospital were evaluated (Hirsch and Colavincenzo 1999). Charts were selected from all adult patients admitted to this hospital over 6 months who met the following criteria: a neurologic diagnosis upon discharge; ability to follow directions and respond verbally; and not intubated, comatose, or admitted to an intensive care unit. None of the 94 physical exams performed by attending-level internists and neurologists indicated that CNI was tested. While four charts (4.2%) note *cranial nerves intact* or *neuro exam grossly normal*, the implication is that olfactory testing may actually not have been performed at all.

Resources for testing have historically been limited and may account for part of the olfactory-testing lacunae. There is a lack of standardization among the traditional test of asking patients to identify readily available fragrant substances such as coffee, almond, lemon, tobacco, anise, oil of clove, toothpaste, eucalyptus, vanilla, peppermint, camphor, rosewater, and soap (Bates 1974; Parsons 1983; Adams and Victor 1989; Haerer 1992; Fuller 1993). Difficulties with standardized tests prevent their widespread use. The Chicago Smell Test is not widely available (Hirsch and Gotway 1993; Hirsch et al. 1993). Individual odor olfactory threshold tests from Olfacto Labs require several bulky bottles and hence are not practical for the clinician (Bakay and Cares 1973; Amoore and Ollman 1983; Gent et al. 1986). The University of Pennsylvania Smell Identification Test (UPSIT), a 40-question scratch-and-sniff test, adjusted for age and sex requires a substantial amount of time to administer, and patients with cognitive dysfunction may have difficulty completing it (Doty et al. 1985).

A simple standardized test is available. The Alcohol Sniff Test (AST) is standardized and can easily be performed at the bedside, even in children and those with cognitive impairment (Davidson and Murphy 1997; Davidson et al. 1998; Freed et al. 1998; Middleton et al. 1998; Schlotfeld et al. 1998). The AST is rapid and cost-effective and requires only a tape measure and an alcohol pad (Figure 2.2). Olfactory ability is quantitatively determined by placing the centimeter (cm) marker of the tape measure at the philtrum (the medial cleft extending from the upper lip to the nose). With the patient's eyes closed, an alcohol pad, one-quarter exposed, is placed at the 40-cm marker and gradually moved inward on inhalation at 1 cm/s until detected. This is repeated four times, waiting 45 s between each test, and the results are averaged. If detection is greater than or equal to 17 cm, it indicates normosmia; detection between 8 and 17 cm indicates hyposmia; and detection at less than 8 cm suggests anosmia.

The AST has been validated in comparison to threshold testing, and threshold testing correlates with the UPSIT (Doty et al. 1984a; Davidson and Murphy 1997). A statistically significant correlation exists between the UPSIT and the AST (Hirsch and Colavincenzo 2000b). UPSIT scores, in addition, can be used to discriminate among anosmic, hyposmic, normosmic, and malingering patients, although its validity in malingering has been questioned (Hirsch and Gruss 1998).

In time-constrained situations, olfaction by the AST can grossly be interpreted as normal if alcohol can be detected beyond the chin. The number of centimeters on

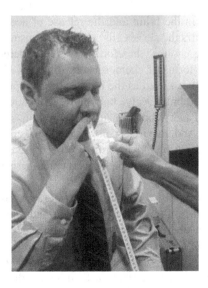

FIGURE 2.2   Demonstrating the AST, a standardized bedside clinical exam of olfaction.

AST can thus be recorded sequentially in office visits, analogous to office testing of visual acuity on the Snellen Acuity Test. More detailed testing such as the UPSIT, PEA threshold, olfactory butanol threshold, and fMRI can then be performed on those with an abnormal AST.

Retronasal smell can also be assessed looking at differences in flavor perception of a cappuccino jelly bean with and without nose clips (Hirsch et al. 2013; Chapter 3 of this book).

2.5 TREATMENT

There are currently no medications labeled specifically for the treatment of chemosensory dysfunction. However, chemosensory disorders have been shown as responsive to several nutritional approaches. Individual nutrient repletion and some medication and other forms of treatment are presented here.

2.5.1 PHOSPHATIDYLCHOLINE

Acetylcholine is important in olfaction as evidenced by the observation that normosmic subjects' olfactory sense is impaired by taking scopolamine, which decreases the effect of acetylcholine (Serby et al. 1989). We cannot ascribe this impairment to drying of the nasal mucus since drying actually improves olfaction (Serby 1987). Rather, it may be due to a decrease in acetylcholine. As further evidence of the importance of acetylcholine in olfaction, patients with senile dementia of the Alzheimer's type lose their ability to detect and identify odors relatively early; in this disease, reduced choline acetyltransferase causes a reduction of acetylcholine in the basal nucleus of Meynert (Adams and Victor 1989). Phosphatidylcholine is converted via choline acetyltransferase into acetylcholine. Thus, choline provides the essential precursor (Wurtman 1979). The amount of choline circulating in the body affects its content in the brain and the release of acetylcholine in the CNS. Insufficient choline impairs the nerve cells' ability to transmit messages across synapses. By supplementing choline, therefore, it was considered possible to amplify these messages in some forms of chemosensory disorders (Wurtman et al. 1981). Phosphatidylcholine has been used as the most optimal approach to increase blood choline, brain choline, and brain acetylcholine levels in patients with brain diseases associated with impaired acetylcholine neurotransmission, such as tardive dyskinesia (Jackson et al. 1979). And, due to its central role in the composition and function of neuronal membranes, phosphatidylcholine has been used for patients with brain diseases associated with dissolution of neuronal membranes such as AD (Little et al. 1985).

In an open label, followed by a double-blind trial of phosphatidylcholine at 9 g/day for 3 months, mixed results were seen (Hirsch and Dougherty 1992). A 40% improvement on the open label study was followed by a negative result on the double-blind study. The double-blind study design is noteworthy due to the conclusions after 2 months. Experimental subjects on the active agent dropped out of the double-blind trial with phosphatidylcholine as a result of their severe dislike of the taste of the phosphatidylcholine. Since none of the patients voiced this complaint initially, it seems possible that their sense of smell, and therefore of flavor, improved during treatment, making them more aware of the taste of the active agent. None of the control subjects who dropped out mentioned the licorice taste as a reason (Hirsch et al. 1996). Accordingly, in those with idiopathic hyposmia or anosmia, a 3-month trial of phosphatidylcholine (PhosChol) at 9 g/day in three divided doses may be beneficial.

2.5.2 THIAMINE

While a pilot trial of thiamine 100 mg/day showed no effect, anecdotally, some anosmic and hyposmic patients showed remarkable improvement with this treatment (Hirsch and Baker 2001).

2.5.3 VITAMIN A

Since vitamin A exists in the olfactory epithelium and could be involved in olfactory neuron regeneration, it theoretically could improve hyposmia or anosmia (Duncan and Briggs 1962).

Of 56 studied, in a study of anosmic patients, 89% who underwent intramuscular vitamin A injections regained full or partial olfactory ability. Oral retinoid treatment (Etretinate) has also been reported to be effective (Roydhouse 1988). Patients with cirrhosis and hypovitaminosis A display improvement in both taste and smell thresholds in response to vitamin A treatment (Garrett-Laster et al. 1984).

2.5.4 CAFFEINE

Caffeine inhibits adenosine receptors and thus may facilitate taste sensitivity. Although study results are mixed, there is a suggestion that topical caffeine enhances taste to sweet and bitter (Schiffman et al. 1986; DeMet et al. 1989).

2.5.5 ZINC

Zinc has undergone the peripatetic course as the standard bearer for treatment of smell and taste disorders. The zeitgeist of zinc was in the 1960s and 1970s when a series of articles suggested its efficacy in a wide range of chemosensory disorders (Henkin et al. 1967; Henkin and Bradley 1969; Schechter et al. 1972). Zinc was originally used during the polio epidemic in an attempt to prevent the spread of the disease to victims' families (Peet et al. 1937). Family members were treated intranasally to destroy the receptor neuroepithelium. The stratagem was effective only for several months, since stem cells proliferated and underwent transformation into fully developed bipolar olfactory receptor cells, thus allowing the treated persons to be exposed again to the polio virus. This effect of zinc was the basis for the idea of using zinc on the stem cells of patients with anosmia to stimulate the development of bipolar olfactory receptor cells.

The frequent association between olfactory impairment and exposure to trace metals suggests another rationale for using zinc. Mercury, lead, cadmium, and gold exposure has been associated with olfactory dysfunction (Cometto-Muniz and Cain

1991; Schiffman 1991). Iron deficiency alters taste and food selection. Zinc metabolism is abnormal in altered physiologic states with hyposmia such as liver disease and first-trimester pregnancy (Breskin et al. 1983; Tamura et al. 2000; DeVere and Calvert 2011a). Hypothyroid patients with hyposmia and hypogeusia have been found to have low parotid zinc levels (Henkin et al. 1976). Treatment with Synthroid improves olfaction and taste as it returns parotid zinc levels to normal (Henkin et al. 1976). Patients with post-influenza hypogeusia and hyposmia have low parotid zinc and low serum zinc (Henkin et al. 1976).

Clinical trials have not produced the results that one might anticipate from the observations above. A study of 106 patients with hypogeusia following influenza revealed that although zinc treatment corrected their low serum levels, it did not improve hypogeusia and hyposmia (Henkin et al. 1976). A double-blind, crossover trial did not demonstrate the efficacy of zinc and the treatment of hypogeusia (Henkin et al. 1976). Another paper comparing zinc-treated versus nonzinc-treated patients found no difference in taste ability (Deems et al. 1991a). Moreover, zinc is not necessarily benign; toxicity may occur. At 100 mg of zinc a day, a level at or below suggested therapeutic doses, inhibition of immune function, anemia, and neutropenia have been reported (Fosmire 1990).

We have anecdotally found zinc to be remarkably effective in postcardiac transplantation dysosmia and hyposmia despite the presence of normal zinc levels. Zinc at concentrations beyond those in a multivitamin may wisely be limited to use with laboratory evidence of hypozincemia or specific states where zinc has demonstrated efficacy including cirrhosis, dialysis, D-penicillamine treatment, and age-related macular degeneration (Newsome et al. 1988; Schiffman 1991; Deems et al. 1991b).

The potential use of oral zinc does not imply the utility of intranasal zinc—it is actually the opposite: intranasal zinc (as in the form of Zicam) may actually be an olfactotoxin, significantly impairing olfactory ability (DeCook and Hirsch 2000).

2.5.6 Pentoxifylline

Clinically, pentoxifylline has had efficacy in the treatment of vascular insufficiency in the lower extremities. However, as a phosphodiesterase inhibitor, it may also aid in the treatment of olfactory loss. This is because cAMP is a second messenger in the olfactory epithelium, and phosphodiesterase breaks down cAMP. Thus, with less phosphodiesterase, an increase in cAMP will be present, and there is a greater chance of olfactory neuronal depolarization in response to olfactory stimuli, leading to improved olfactory ability. Of 19 patients treated with pentoxifylline, after 1 h, greater olfactory ability was found, as manifested with reduced odor threshold, while odor identification and odor discrimination were unchanged (Gudziol et al. 2007; Gudziol and Hummel 2009).

2.5.7 Intranasal Calcium Inhibitors

Since calcium reduces olfactory nerve excitability and the duration of discharge, reduction of calcium may act to disinhibit olfactory discharge and improve olfactory ability. This was demonstrated with instillation of intranasal sodium citrate–buffered solution. Transient subjective improvement in olfactory ability was noted in approximately 75% of those treated, lasting up to 3 h (Panagiotopoulos et al. 2005).

2.5.8 THEOPHYLLINE

Traditionally used in the management of asthma, theophylline, a phosphodiesterase inhibitor, may increase olfaction by raising the second messenger cAMP levels. An open-label study of theophylline in 312 hyposmic and hypogeusic patients reported improvement in more than one-half of the patients (Henkin et al. 2009). As nasal mucus cAMP and cGMP increased, so did olfactory ability (Henkin et al. 2011). In order to avoid systemic toxicity, intranasal theophylline treatment at 40 mcg was attempted in 10 patients with hyposmia and hypogeusia. This resulted in improvement in eight patients and was more efficacious than systemic theophylline (Henkin et al. 2012).

2.5.9 PREDNISONE

A mainstay of treatment of olfactory loss has been prednisone—intranasal, systemic, or both. While its mechanism of action has been postulated to be due to its anti-inflammatory effects on nasal polyps, or swollen mucosa at the olfactory epithelium, prednisone efficacy in non-inflammatory conditions has brought such mechanisms into question. Oral dosing varies from a short course of a Medrol Dose Pack to higher doses of 60 mg/day, tapering slowly over 21 days (Davidson et al. 1995). A combination of systemic and intranasal corticosteroids has even been suggested for nonsurgical management of nasal polyposis-induced olfactory loss (Mullol and Alobid 2011).

2.5.10 SNIFF THERAPY

After serendipitously finding that recurrent daily exposure to androstenone induced an ability to detect this odor in a previously androstenone odor-blind lab worker, more formalized attempts to validate and expand this to those with olfactory dysfunction have been entertained (Wysocki et al. 1989). Over 4 months, recurrent exposure two times per day per nostril to four high-intensity common odors (lemon, rose, eucalyptus, and clove) has been demonstrated to improve olfaction to not only these specific smells but also odors in general (Hummel et al. 2009). The exact mechanism of such an effect remains unclear, but it does not appear to be through action at the site of olfactory receptors; rather, it may be through a top-down process—sniff treatment in normosmics unilaterally led to an increase in ipsilateral olfactory bulb volume by 11.3% and by even more, 13.1%, in the untreated nostril (Hummel and Pietsch 2014; Pietsch and Hummel 2014). While such a treatment approach is appealing, attempts by one author (ARH) to demonstrate clinically significant effects of such treatment have, so far, not been successful.

2.5.11   Chiropractic Manipulation

While many anosmic patients have sought nonpharmacologic treatment modalities such as acupuncture and chiropractic manipulation, improvement with such approaches has not been generally reported. However, remission of a one-and-a-half-year course of anosmia and ageusia in a 62-year-old male was reported after atlanto-occipital sub-luxation adjustment (Filosa 1988). The mechanism engendering such improvement remains unclear.

2.5.12   Increasing Patients' Awareness of Altered Eating Habits

Chemosensory disorders in general are linked to changes in food selection. Most notably, there is an aversion of foods that are bitter in taste and sweet in smell, as in dark chocolate, coffee, green peppers, and other green leafy vegetables. Also, a pre-dilection develops toward more textured and trigeminally mediated foods as sensory compensation for loss and in an attempt to recreate a sapid experience with such foods as sushi or hot chili peppers (Costanzo and Zasler 1991; DeVere and Calvert 2011b).

Table 2.2 presents the different types of chemosensory impairment and the result-ing impact on food selection and body weight:

- For congenital chemosensory dysfunction, no significant difference in weight, eating patterns, or food preferences compared to normosmics exists (Croy et al. 2014).
- People with acquired, noncongenital chemosensory dysfunction experience changes in food preferences and a compensatory increase in salt and sugar intake (Croy et al. 2014).
- In elderly women with olfactory dysfunction, there is a reduction in pref-erence for sour, bitter, and spicy foods and low-fat milk and an increased consumption of sweets (Duffy et al. 1995).
- People with dysgeusia tend to ingest intense trigeminal stimuli, like mint, in an attempt to overcome the unpleasant dysgeusia's sensation (DeVere and Calvert 2011b).
- In those with chemosensory loss, approximately 10% gain a substantial amount of weight, possibly increasing food consumption due to either a narcissistic drive for a sensory experience or the lack of sensory-specific satiety, which is highest in those with anosmia (Mattes and Cowart 1994). Alternatively, those with olfactory dysfunction may gain weight due to loss of interoceptive awareness of fullness, leading to unrestrained eating (Krajnik et al. 2014). An approximately equal number lose weight, possibly secondary to lack of interest in food or associated depression or due to the hedonically unpleasant distortion in the taste of foods (Aschenbrenner et al. 2008).
- Dysgeusia triggers, which are most noted and avoided, include meats, fresh fruits, coffee, eggs, carbonated beverages, and vegetables (Markley et al. 1983).

Increasing awareness to the predispositions of food selection may help some patients moderate their food selection.

TABLE 2.2
Change in Nutrition with Chemosensory Disorders

Chemosensory Disorders	Food Complaints	Increased Appetite	Decreased Appetite	Decreased Enjoyment	Increased Use of Sugar, Salt, and Spices	Mean Energy Intake Compared to Normosmics	Mean Micronutrient Intake Compared to Normosmics	Mean Body Weight Compared to Normosmics	% Who Gained 10% or More of Body Weight Prior to Chemosensory Dysfunction	% Who Lost 10% or More of Body Weight Prior to Chemosensory Dysfunction
Anosmia (noncongenital)	50% to 60%	20%	31%	88%	20% to 40% 4% decreased	No change	No change	No change	14%	6.50%
Anosmia (congenital)	20%									
Hyposmia	31% to 80%	30%	10% to 20%	50%	20% to 50% 20% decreased				1.50%	10.60%
Dysosmia and phantosmia	75% to 85%		24%	83%	50%			113%		
Ageusia	100%		100%							
Hypogeusia	75%		67%	33%					Reported	Reported
Dysgeusia and phantageusia	72% to 85%	24%	30% to 67%	42% to 70%	40% to 60% 18% decreased	No change	No change		15% to 20%	15% to 20%

Source: Mattes, R.D., and B.J. Cowart, *Journal of the American Dietetic Association* 94:50–56, 1994; Ferris, A.M. et al., *Nutrition and taste and smell deficits: A risk factor or an adjustment?* In *Clinical Measurement of Taste and Smell.* New York: MacMillan, pp. 264–278, 1986; Mattes-Kulig, D.A., and R.I. Henkin, *Journal of the American Dietetic Association* 85:822–826, 1985; Mattes R.D. et al., *American Journal of Clinical Nutrition* 51:233–240, 1990.

2.6 SUMMARY

An anfractuous invisible universe at the tip of the nose is ripe for exploration. Compromised senses of smell and taste influence food selection, food preparation, dietary patterns, and digestion. Chemosensory impairments tend to have insidious onset, and many patients are therefore unaware that these sensations are diminished or altered. Physicians can diagnose chemosensory disorders using a simple screening test: the AST. Familiarity with the medical conditions and iatrogenic risk factors can increase the clinical suspicion of smell and taste impairment. Diagnosis can bring awareness to patients for altered food habits and issues pertaining to home safety and food preparation. These can assist clinicians in identifying and managing both underlying nutrient disturbances and gustatory dysfunction to foster optimized eating education for improved overall human health.

REFERENCES

Acharya, V., J. Acharya, and H. Luders. 1996. Olfactory epileptic auras. *Neurology* 51:56–61.

Ackerman, B.H., and N. Kasbekar. 1997. Disturbances of taste and smell induced by drugs. *Pharmacotherapy* 17:482–496.

Adams, R.D., and M. Victor. 1989. *Principles of Neurology*. New York: McGraw-Hill.

Adams, R.G., and N. Crabtree. 1961. Anosmia in alkaline battery workers. *British Journal of Industrial Medicine* 18:216–221.

Amoore, J.E. 1986. Effects of chemical exposure on olfaction in humans. In *Toxicology of the Nasal Passages*, 155–190, ed. C.S. Barrow. Washington, DC: Hemisphere Publishing.

Amoore, J.E., and B.G. Ollman. 1983. Practical test kits for quantitatively evaluating sense of smell. *Rhinology* 21:49–54.

Apter, A.J., A.E. Mott, W.S. Cain, J.D. Spiro, and M.C. Barwick. 1992. Olfactory loss and allergic rhinitis. *Journal of Allergy and Clinical Immunology* 90:670–680.

Aschenbrenner, K., C. Hummel, K. Teszmer, F. Krone, T. Ishimaru, H.S. Seo, and T. Hummel. 2008. The influence of olfactory loss on dietary behaviors. *Laryngoscope* 118:135–144.

Bakay, L., and H.L. Cares. 1973. Olfactory meningiomas. *Acta Neurochirurgica Fasc* 26:1–12.

Bartoshuk, L.M., F. Catalanotto, V. Duffy, H. Hoffman, H. Logan, V. Mayo, and D. Snyder. 2007. Damage to taste (otitis media) is associated with dysgeusia, intensified pain experience and increased body mass index. *Chemical Senses* 32:A81.

Bates, B. 1974. *Guide to Physical Examination*. Philadelphia: JB Lippincott.

Bingham, A.F., G.G. Birch, C. deGraaf, J.M. Behan, and K.D. Perring. 1990. Sensory studies with sucrose–maltol mixtures. *Chemical Senses* 15:447–456.

Breskin, M.W., B.S. Worthington-Roberts, R.H. Knopp, Z. Brown, B. Plovie, N.K. Mottet, and J.L. Mills. 1983. First trimester serum zinc concentrations in human pregnancy. *American Journal of Clinical Nutrition* 38:943–953.

Brodal, A. 1969. *Neurological Anatomy in Relation to Clinical Medicine*, 3rd Ed., Vol. 10. New York: Oxford University Press.

Bruyn, G.W. 1986. Glossopharyngeal neuralgia. In *Handbook of Clinical Neurology: Headache*, 4:48:459–473, ed. P.J. Vinken, G.W. Bruyn, H.L. Klawans, and F.C. Rose. New York: Elsevier.

Busenbark, K.L., S.T. Huber, G. Greer, R. Pahwa, and W.C. Koller. 1992. Olfactory function in essential tremor. *Neurology* 42:1631–1632.

Cain, W., and J.E. Cometto-Muniz. 1982. Perception of nasal pungency in smokers and non-smokers. *Psychology & Behavior* 29:727–732.

Casper, R.C., B. Kirschner, H.H. Sandstead, R.A. Jacob, and J.M. Davis. 1980. An evaluation of trace metals, vitamins, and taste function in anorexia nervosa. *American Journal of Clinical Nutrition* 33:1801–1808.

Centers for Disease Control and Prevention (CDC). 2014. Cigarette smoking among adults—United States, 2005–2012. *MMWR Morbidity and Mortality Weekly Report* 63(02):29–34.

Chalke, H.D., and J.R. Dewhurst. 1957. Accidental coal-gas poisoning. *British Medical Journal* 2:915–917.

Cometto-Muniz, J.E., and W.S. Cain. 1991. Influence of airborne contaminants on olfaction and the common chemical sense. In *Smell and Taste in Health and Disease*, Ch. 49, 765–785, ed. T.V. Getchell, R.L. Doty, L.M. Bartoshuk, and J.B. Snow, Jr. New York: Raven Press.

Costanzo, R., and D. Becker. 1986. Smell and taste disorders in head injury and neurosurgery patients. In *Clinical Measurement of Taste and Smell*, 565–568, ed. H.L. Meiselman, and R.S. Rivlin. New York: Macmillan.

Costanzo, R.M., and N.D. Zasler. 1991. Head trauma. In *Smell and Taste in Health and Disease*, Ch. 45, 711–730, ed. T.V. Getchell, L.M. Bartoshuk, R.L. Doty, and J.B. Snow. New York: Raven Press.

Costanzo, R.M., J.D. Ward, and H.F. Young. 1992. Olfaction and head injury. In *Science of Olfaction*, Ch. 20, 546–558, ed. M.J. Serby, and K.L. Chobor. New York: Springer-Verlag.

Croy, I., S. Nordin, and T. Hummel. 2014. Olfactory disorders and quality of life—An updated review. *Chemical Senses* 39:185–194.

Custer, K., B. Raudenbush, E. Robinson, K. Schlegel, and S. Moore. 2014. The effects of soccer ball *heading* frequency and intensity on nasal inspiratory and expiratory function as measured by rhinological patency. In *AChemS XXXVI, The Association for Chemoreception Sciences 36th Annual Meeting Abstract Book*, Bonita Springs, FL 266:130.

Davidson, T.M., and C. Murphy. 1997. Rapid clinical evaluation of anosmia: The alcohol sniff test. *Archives of Otolaryngology—Head & Neck Surgery* 123:591–594.

Davidson, T.M., A. Jalowayski, C. Murphy, and R.J. Jacobs. 1987. Evaluation and treatment of smell dysfunction. *Western Journal of Medicine* 146:434–438.

Davidson, T.M., C. Murphy, and A.A. Jalowayski. 1995. Smell impairment. Can it be reversed? *Postgraduate Medicine* 98:1:107–109.

Davidson, T.M., C. Freed, M.P. Healy, and C. Murphy. 1998. Rapid clinical evaluation of anosmia in children: The Alcohol Sniff Test. *Annals of the New York Academy of Sciences* 855:787–792.

DeCook, C.A., and A.R. Hirsch. 2000. Anosmia due to inhalational zinc: A case report. *Chemical Senses* 25:5:659.

Deems, D.A., R.L. Doty, R.G. Settle, V. Moore-Gillon, P. Shaman, A.F. Mester, C.P. Kimmelman, V.J. Brightman, and J.B. Snow, Jr. 1991a. Smell and taste disorders: A study of 750 patients from the University of Pennsylvania Smell and Taste Center. *Archives of Otolaryngology—Head & Neck Surgery* 117:519–528.

Deems, R.O., M.I. Friedman, L.S. Friedman, and W.C. Maddrey. 1991b. Clinical manifestations of olfactory and gustatory disorders associated with hepatic and renal disease. In *Smell and Taste in Health and Disease*, Ch. 51, 805–816, ed. T.V. Getchell, R.L. Doty, L.M. Bartoshuk, and J.B. Snow, Jr. New York: Raven Press.

DeMet, E., M.K. Stein, C. Tran, A. Chicz-DeMet, C. Sangdahl, and J. Nelson. 1989. Caffeine taste test for panic disorder: Adenosine receptor supersensitivity. *Psychiatry Research* 30:231–242.

DeVere, R., and M. Calvert. 2011a. *Navigating Smell and Taste Disorders*. New York: Demos Medical Publishing Company.

DeVere, R., and M. Calvert. 2011b. Food preparation. In *Navigating Smell and Taste Disorders*, Ch. 6, 81–89. New York: Demos Medical Publishing Company.

Doty, R.L. 1991. Influences of aging on human olfactory function. In *The Human Sense of Smell*, 181–195, ed. D.G. Laing, R.L. Doty, and W. Breipohl. Berlin: Springer-Verlag.

Doty, R.L. 1997. Studies of human olfaction from the University of Pennsylvania Smell and Taste Center. *Chemical Senses* 22:565–586.

Doty, R.L., and M. Ferguson-Segal. 1987. Odor detection performance of rats following d-amphetamine treatment: A signal detection analysis. *Psychopharmacology (Berl)* 93:87–93.

Doty, R.L., P. Shaman, S.L. Applebaum, R. Gilberson, L. Sikorsky, and L. Rosenberg. 1984a. Smell identification ability: Changes with age. *Science* 226:1441–1443.

Doty, R.L., P. Shaman, and M. Dann. 1984b. Development of the University of Pennsylvania Smell identification test: A standardized microencapsulated test of olfactory function. *Physiology & Behavior* 32:489–502.

Doty, R.L., M.G. Newhouse, and J.D. Azzalina. 1985. Internal consistency and short-term test–retest reliability of the University of Pennsylvania Smell Identification Test. *Chemical Senses* 10:297–300.

Doty, R.L., T. Gregor, and C. Monroe. 1986. Quantitative assessment of olfactory function in an industrial setting. *Journal of Occupational Medicine* 28:6:457–460.

Doty, R., P. Reys, and T. Gregor. 1987. Presence of both odor identification and detection deficits in Alzheimer's disease. *Brain Research Bulletin* 18:597–600.

Doty, R.L., D.A. Deems, and S. Stellar. 1988a. Olfactory dysfunction in Parkinsonism: A general deficit unrelated to neurologic signs, disease stage, or disease duration. *Neurology* 38:1237–1244.

Doty, R.L., M. Ferguson-Segall, I. Lucki, and M. Kreider. 1988b. Effects of intrabulbar injections of 6-hydroxydopamine on ethyl acetate odor detection in castrate and non-castrate male rats. *Brain Research* 44:95–103.

Doty, R.L., M. Riklan, D. Deems, C. Reynolds, and S. Stellar. 1989. The olfactory and cognitive deficits of Parkinson's disease: Evidence for independence. *Annals of Neurology* 25:166–171.

Doty, R.L., D.P. Perl, J.C. Steele, K.M. Chen, J.D. Pierce, Jr., P. Reyes, and L.T. Kirkland. 1991. Odor identification deficit of the Parkinsonism–dementia complete of Guam: Equivalence to that of Alzheimer's and idiopathic Parkinson's disease. *Neurology* 41:1:77–80.

Doty, R.L., A. Singh, J. Tetrude, and L.W. Langston. 1992a. Lack of olfactory dysfunction in MPTP-induced Parkinsonism. *Annals of Neurology* 32:97–100.

Doty, R.L., M.B. Stern, C. Pfeiffer, S.M. Gollomp, and H.I. Hurtig. 1992b. Bilateral olfactory dysfunction in early stage treated and untreated idiopathic Parkinson's disease. *Journal of Neurology, Neurosurgery, and Psychiatry* 55:138–142.

Doty, R.L., S.M. Bromley, P.J. Moberg, and T. Hummel. 1997. Laterality in human nasal chemoreception. In *Cerebral in Sensory and Perceptual Processing*, 492–542, ed. S. Christman. Amsterdam: Elsevier.

Drewnowski, A. 1987. Sweetness and obesity. In *Sweetness*, 177–201, ed. J. Dobbing. New York: Springer-Verlag.

Drewnowski, A. 1991. Fat and sugar: Sensory and hedonic aspects of sweet, high-fat foods. In *Chemical Senses: Appetite and Nutrition*, 69–83, ed. M.I. Friedman, M.G. Tordoff, and M.R. Kare. New York: Marcel Dekker.

Duffy, V.B., and A.M. Ferris. 1989. Nutritional management of patients with chemosensory disturbances. *Ear, Nose and Throat Journal* 68:395–397.

Duffy, V.B., J.R. Backstrand, and A.M. Ferris. 1995. Olfactory dysfunction and related nutritional risk in free-living, elderly women. *Journal of the American Dietetic Association* 95:879–884 as quoted in Aschenbrenner, K., C. Hummel, K. Teszmer, F Krone, T.

Ishimaru, H.S. Seo, and T. Hummel. 2008. The influence of olfactory loss on dietary behaviors. *The Laryngoscope* 118:135–144.

Duffy, V.B., M.L. Fernandez, S. Lanier, D. Aggarwal, and L. Bartoshuk. 2006. PROP bitterness and cardiovascular disease (CVD) risk factors in adult women. *Chemical Senses* 31:A37.

Duncan, R.B., and M. Briggs. 1962. Treatment of uncomplicated anosmia by vitamin A. *Archives of Otolaryngology* 75:116–124.

Eccles, R. 1978. The central rhythm of the nasal cycle. *Acta Oto-Laryngologica* 86:464–468.

Eichenbaum, H., T. Morton, H. Potter, and S. Corkin. 1983. Selective olfactory deficits in case H.M. *Brain* 106:2:459–472.

Eskenazi, B., W. Cain, R. Novelly, and R. Mattson. 1986. Odor perception in temporal lobe epilepsy patients with and without temporal lobectomy. *Neuropsychologia* 24: 553–562.

Estrem, S.A., and G. Renner. 1987. Disorders of smell and taste. *Otolaryngologic Clinics of North America* 20:1:133–147.

Filosa, D.A. 1988. A remission of anosmia and ageusia following chiropractic adjustments. *Research Forum* 4:43–45.

Fosmire, G.J. 1990. Zinc toxicity. *American Journal of Clinical Nutrition* 51:225–227.

Fox, J. 1966. The olfactory system: Implications for the occupational therapist. *The American Journal of Occupational Therapy* 4:173–177.

Freed, C.L., A.M. Dalve-Endres, T.M. Davidson, and C. Murphy. 1998. Rapid screening of olfactory function in Down's syndrome. *Chemical Senses* 23:610.

Friedman, M.I., and R.D. Mattes. 1991. Chemical senses and nutrition. Ch. 21, 392. In *Smell and Taste in Health and Disease*, ed. T.V. Getchell, R.L. Doty, L.M. Bartoshuk, and J.B. Snow, Jr. New York: Raven Press.

Fritjers, J.E.R., and E.L. Rasmussen-Conrad. 1982. Sensory discrimination, intensity perception, affective judgment of sucrose-sweetness in the overweight. *Journal of General Psychology* 107:233–247.

Frye, R.E. 2003. Nasal patency and the aerodynamics of nasal airflow: Measurement by rhinomanometry and acoustic rhinometry, and the influence of pharmacological agents. In *Handbook of Olfaction and Gustation, 2nd Ed., Revised and Expanded*, 439–459, ed. R.L. Doty. New York: Marcel Dekker.

Frye, R., B. Schwartz, and R. Doty. 1990. Dose-related effects of cigarette smoking on olfactory function. *Journal of the American Medical Association* 263:1233–1236.

Fuller, G. 1993. *Neurological Examination Made Easy*. Edinburgh: Churchill Livingstone.

Furuta, S., K. Nishimoto, M. Egawa, M. Ohyama, and H. Moriyama. 1994. Olfactory dysfunction in patients with Minamata disease. *American Journal of Rhinology* 8:259–263.

Garrett-Laster, M., R.M. Russell, and P.F. Jacques. 1984. Impairment of taste and olfaction in patients with cirrhosis: The role of vitamin A. *Human Nutrition* 38C:203–214.

Gent, J.P., W.S. Cain, and L.M. Bartoshuk. 1986. Taste and smell management in a clinical setting. In *Clinical Measurement of Taste and Smell*, 107–111, ed. H.L. Meiselman, and R.S. Rivlin. New York: Macmillan.

Goodspeed, R.B., J.F. Gent, and F.A. Catalanotto. 1987. Chemosensory dysfunction. Clinical evaluation results of a taste and smell clinic. *Postgraduate Medicine* 81:251–257, 260.

Green, R.F. 1971. Subclinical pellagra and idiopathic hypogeusia. (Letter). *Journal of the American Medical Association* 218:8:1303.

Griep, M.I., T.F. Mets, K. Collys, D. Verté, G. Verleye, I. Ponjaert-Kristoffersen, and D.L. Massar. 1999. MNA and odor perception. *Nestle Nutr Workshop Ser Clin Perform Programme*, 1:41–59; discussion 59–60.

Grinker, J. 1978. Obesity and sweet taste. *American Journal of Clinical Nutrition* 31:1078–1087.

Gudziol, V., and T. Hummel. 2009. Effects of pentoxifylline on olfactory sensitivity: A post-marketing surveillance study. *Archives of Otolaryngology—Head & Neck Surgery*

135:3:291–295 as quoted in Henkin, R.I., M. Schultz, and L. Minnick-Poppe. 2012. Intranasal theophylline treatment of hyposmia and hypogeusia: A pilot study. *Archives of Otolaryngology—Head & Neck Surgery* 138:11:1064–1070.

Gudziol, V., A.M. Maier, and T. Zahnert. 2007. The influence of pentoxifylline on olfactory function [Poster]. *Chemical Senses* 32:A27–A28.

Guild, A.A. 1956. Olfactory acuity in normal and obese human subjects: Diurnal variations and the effect of D-amphetamine sulphate. *The Journal of Laryngology & Otology* 70:408–414.

Haerer, A.F. 1992. *DeJong's The Neurological Examination, 5th Ed.* Philadelphia: Lippincott.

Hawkes, C. 2006. Olfaction in neurodegenerative disorder. In *Taste and Smell. An Update*, 133–151, ed. T. Hummel, and A. Welge-Lussen. Basel: S. Karger AG.

Hawkes, C.H., and R.L. Doty. 2009. *The Neurology of Olfaction*, Ch. 3, p. 135. Cambridge: Cambridge University Press.

Hawkes, C.H., A. Fogo, and M. Shah. 2005. Smell identification declines from age 36 years and mainly affects pleasant odors. *Chemical Senses* 30:A152–A153.

Henkin, R. 1967. Abnormalities of taste and olfaction in patients with chromatin-negative gonadal dysgenesis. Taste and olfaction in Turner's syndrome. *Journal of Clinical Endocrinology* 27:1437–1440.

Henkin, R.I., and D.F. Bradley. 1969. Regulation of taste acuity by thiols and metal ions. *Proceedings of the National Academy of Science, USA* 62:30–37.

Henkin, R.I., H.R Keiser, I.A. Jaffee, I. Sternlieb, and I.H. Scheinberg. 1967. Decreased taste sensitivity after D-penicillamine reversed by copper administration. *Lancet* 2:1268–1271.

Henkin, R.I., P.J. Schechter, W.T. Friedewald, D.L. Demets, and M. Raff. 1976. A double blind study of the effects of zinc sulfate on taste and smell dysfunction. *American Journal of Medical Science* 272:3:285–299.

Henkin, R.I., R.L. AAmodt, A.K. Babcock, R.P. Agarwal, and A.R. Shatzman. 1981. Treatment of abnormal chemoreception in human taste and smell. In *Perceptions of Behavioral Chemicals*, 229–253, ed. D.M. Norris. New York: Elsevier.

Henkin, R.I., I. Velicu, and L. Schmidt. 2009. An open-label controlled trial of theophylline for treatment of patients with hyposmia. *American Journal of the Medical Sciences* 337:6:396–406 as quoted in Henkin, R.I., M. Schultz, and L. Minnick-Poppe. 2012. Intranasal theophylline treatment of hyposmia and hypogeusia: A pilot study. *Archives of Otolaryngology—Head & Neck Surgery* 138:11:1064–1070.

Henkin, R.I., I. Velicu, and L. Schmidt. 2011. Relative resistance to oral theophylline treatment in patients with hyposmia manifested by decreased secretion of nasal mucus cyclic nucleotides. *American Journal of the Medical Sciences* 34:1:17–22, as quoted in Henkin, R.I., M. Schultz, and L. Minnick-Poppe. 2012. Intranasal theophylline treatment of hyposmia and hypogeusia: A pilot study. *Archives of Otolaryngology—Head & Neck Surgery* 138:11:1064–1070.

Henkin, R.I., M. Schultz, and L. Minnick-Poppe. 2012. Intranasal theophylline treatment of hyposmia and hypogeusia: A pilot study. *Archives of Otolaryngology—Head & Neck Surgery* 1:138:1064–1070.

Hirsch, A.R., and T.J. Trannell. 1988. Concurrence of chemosensory and sexual dysfunction. *Biological Psychiatry* 43:52S.

Hirsch, A.R. 1990a. The nose knows. *Chicago Medicine* 93:14:27–31.

Hirsch, A.R. 1990b. Smell and taste: How the culinary experts compare to the rest of us. *Food Technology* 44:9:96–102.

Hirsch, A.R. 1990c. Open label trial of phosphatidylcholine for olfactory and gustatory problems. *Chemical Senses* 15:5:591–592.

Hirsch, A.R. 1992a. Scentsation, olfactory demographic and abnormalities. *International Journal of Aromatherapy* 4:1:16–17.

Hirsch, A.R. 1992b. Olfaction in migraineurs. *Headache* 32:233–236.

Hirsch, A.R. 1995a. Chronic neurotoxicity of acute chlorine gas exposure. *The 13th International Neurotoxicology Conference, Developmental and Neurotoxicity of Endocrine Disruptors Proceedings Abstract Book* 13.

Hirsch, A.R. 1995b. Neurotoxicity as a result of ambient chemicals: Denham Springs, LA. *International Congress on Hazardous Waste: Impact on Human and Ecological Health.* U.S. Department of Health and Human Services. Atlanta: Public Health Agency for Toxic Substances and Disease Registry, 229.

Hirsch, A.R. 1995c. Neurotoxicity as a result of acute nitrogen tetroxide exposure. [Abstract] *International Congress of Hazardous Waste: Impact on Human and Ecology and Health,* U.S. Department of Health and Human Services, Pub Health Agency for Toxic Substances and Disease Registry, Atlanta, GA, 177.

Hirsch, A.R. 1995d. Subjective hyposmia. *Journal of Neurologic and Orthopaedic Medicine and Surgery* 16:157–161.

Hirsch, AR. 1997. Neurotoxicity in dialysis tubing assembly line workers. *Fifteenth International Neurotoxicology Conference, Little Rock, AR.* Abstract Book, 73:74.

Hirsch, A.R. 1998a. *Scentsational Sex.* Boston: Element Books.

Hirsch, A.R. 1998b. Neurotoxic effects of chlordane/heptachlor termiticide sprayed in an apartment complex. *Sixteenth International Neurotoxicology Abstract Book,* 64.

Hirsch, A.R. 2002a. Hydrogen sulfide exposure without loss of consciousness: Chronic effects in four cases. *Toxicology and Industrial Health* 18:2:51–61.

Hirsch, A.R. 2002b. Neuropsychiatric effects of exposure to pyrethroid insecticides: A review. *Journal of Neurological and Orthopaedic Medicine and Surgery* 22:2:22–26.

Hirsch, A.R. 2003. Neurological effects of TCE in groundwater and soil in Lisle, Illinois. *Soils, Sediments and Water,* 86.

Hirsch, A.R. 2008. Use of gustatory stimuli to facilitate weight loss. *First International Conference on Advance Technologies & Treatments for Diabetes (ATTD) Abstract Book,* Prague, Czech Republic, 39.

Hirsch, A.R. 2009. Parkinsonism: The hyposmia and phantosmia connection. *Archives of Neurology* 66:4:538–539.

Hirsch, A.R., and J.G. Aranda. 1992. Treatment of olfactory loss with amatadine—An open label trial. *Chemical Senses* 17:5:642.

Hirsch, A.R., and J. Baker. 2001. Lack of efficacy of thiamine treatment for chemosensory disorder. *Journal of Psychiatry and Clinical Neuroscience* 13:1:151.

Hirsch, A.R., and G. Bissell. 1998. Effects of acute alcohol inebriation and human olfaction: A preliminary report. *Journal of Neurological and Orthopaedic Medicine and Surgery* 18:114–121.

Hirsch, A.R., and M.L. Colavincenzo. 1999. Failure of physicians to assess olfactory ability in neurologic inpatients. *Chemical Senses* 24:5:607–608.

Hirsch, A.R., and M.L. Colavincenzo. 2000a. Olfactory deficits among Chicago firefighters. *Chicago Medicine* 103:11:18–19.

Hirsch, A.R., and M.L. Colavincenzo. 2000b. The Alcohol Sniff Test compared with the University of Pennsylvania Smell Identification Test. *Chemical Senses* 25:5:655.

Hirsch, A.R., and D.D. Dougherty. 1992. Phosphatidylcholine for olfactory problems. *Chemical Senses* 17:5:643.

Hirsch, A.R., and M.B. Gotway. 1993. Validation of the Chicago Smell Test (CST) in subjective normosmic neurologic patients. *Chemical Senses* 18:570–571.

Hirsch, A.R., and J.J. Gruss. 1998. How successful are malingerers? Dissimulating olfactory dysfunction. *Journal of Neurological and Orthopaedic Medicine and Surgery* 18:154–160.

Hirsch, A.R., and N. Thakkar. 1995. Olfaction in a patient with unclassifiable cluster headache-like disorder. *Headache Quarterly* 6:113–122.

Hirsch, A.R., and T.J. Trannel. 1996. Chemosensory disorders and psychiatric diagnoses. *Journal of Neurological and Orthopaedic Medicine and Surgery* 17:25–30.

Hirsch, A.R., and J.G. Vanderbilt. 1992. Treatment of olfactory loss with amitriptyline. *Chemical Senses* 17:5:643–644.

Hirsch, A.R., and J.P. Wyse. 1993. Posttraumatic dysosmia: Central vs. peripheral. *Journal of Neurological and Orthopaedic Medicine and Surgery* 14:152–155.

Hirsch, A.R., S. Lieberman, and S. Gay. 1991. The syndrome of atmospheric pressure-sensitive paroxysmal unilateral phantosmia. *Chemical Senses* 16:5:535–536.

Hirsch, A.R., J.M. Scott, and S.H. Koch. 1992. Efficacy of group therapy in the treatment approach to chemosensory disorders. *Chemical Senses* 17:5:643.

Hirsch, A.R., M.B. Gotway, and A.T. Harris. 1993. Validation of the Chicago Smell Test (CST) in patients with subjective olfactory loss. *Chemical Senses* 18:571.

Hirsch, A.R., D.D. Dougherty, J.G. Aranda, J.G Vanderbilt, and G.C. Weclaw. 1996. Medications for olfactory loss: Pilot studies. *Journal of Neurological and Orthopaedic Medicine and Surgery* 17:108–114.

Hirsch, M., S. Sherman, A. Roussos, and A.R. Hirsch. 2014. Anosmia with absent alliaceous lacrimation. *AChemS XXXVIth Annual Meeting Abstract Book* 257:127.

Hirsch, N.H., R. Bone, and A.R. Hirsch. 2013. Tests of retronasal smell in children: Which flavored jelly bean works best? *Chemical Senses* 38:7:A625.

Hummel, T., and K. Pietsch. 2014. Changes in olfactory bulb volume following lateralized olfactory training in healthy subjects. In *AChemS XXXVI, The Association for Chemoreception Sciences 36th Annual Meeting Abstract Book*, Bonita Springs, FL, 46:51.

Hummel, T., K. Rissom, J. Reden, A. Hahner, M. Weidenbecher, and K. Bernd-Huttenbrink. 2009. Effects of olfactory training in patients with olfactory loss. *Laryngoscope* 119:3:496–499.

Hutchins, H.L., L.S. Pescatello, G.J. Allen, and V.B. Duffy. 2002. Are 6-*n*-propylthiouracil (PROP) nontasters at risk for high blood pressure? *Chemical Senses* 27:A23–A24.

Jackson, I.V., E.A. Nuttal, I.O. Ibe, and J. Perez-Cruet. 1979. Treatment of tardive dyskinesia with lecithin. *American Journal of Psychiatry* 136:1458–1460.

Jafek, B.W., and D.P. Hill. 1989. Surgical management of chemosensory disorders. *Ear, Nose, and Throat Journal* 66:398–404.

Jafek, B.W., D.T. Moran, and P.M. Eller. 1987. Steroid-dependent anosmia. *Archives of Otolaryngology* 113:547–549.

Javoy-Agid, F., and Y. Agid. 1980. Is the mesocortical dopaminergic system involved in Parkinson disease? *Neurology* 30:12:1326.

Jeppson, P. 1969. Studies on the structure and innervation of taste buds. *Acta Otolaryngologica* 259:1–95.

Kalogiera, L., and D. Dzepina. 2012. Management of smell dysfunction. *Current Allergy and Asthma Reports* 12:2:154–162.

Keller, A., C. Dushdid, M.O. Magnasco, and L.B. Vosshall. 2014. Humans can discriminate more than one trillion olfactory stimuli. *AChemS XXXVI, The Association for Chemoreception Sciences 36th Annual Meeting Abstract Book*, Bonita Springs, FL, 120:77–78.

Knight, A. 1988. Anosmia. *The Lancet* 332:8609:512.

Koss, E., J. Weiffenbach, J. Haxby, and R. Friedland. 1988. Olfactory detection and identification performance are dissociated in early Alzheimer's disease. *Neurology* 38:1228–1232.

Krajnik, J., K. Kollndorfer, L. Notter, C.A. Mueller, and V. Schopf. 2014. The impact of olfactory dysfunction in interoceptive awareness. In *AChemS XXXVI, The Association for Chemoreception Sciences 36th Annual Meeting Abstract Book*, Bonita Springs, FL, 262:128.

Kratskin, I.L., and O. Belluzzi. 2003. Anatomy and neurochemistry of the olfactory bulb. In *Handbook of Olfaction and Gustation. 2nd Ed. Revised and Expanded*, Ch. 7, 139–164, ed. R.L. Doty. New York: Marcel Dekker.

Lacey, J.H., and P.A. Stanley. 1977. Sucrose sensitivity in anorexia nervosa. *Journal of Psychosomatic Research* 21:17–21.

Lehrer, S., E. Levine, and W. Bloomer. 1985. Abnormally diminished sense of smell in women with estrogen receptor positive breast cancer. *Lancet* 2:333.

Levin, H., W. High, and H. Eisenberg. 1985. Impairment of olfactory recognition after closed head injury. *Brain* 108:579–591.

Lewis, C.E., D.R. Jacobs, Jr., H. McCreath, C.I. Kiefe, P.J. Schreiner, D.E. Smith, and D. Williams. 2000. Weight gain continues in the 1990s: 10-year trends in weight and overweight from the CARDIA Study. *American Journal of Epidemiology* 151:1172–1181.

Little, A., R. Levy, P. Chuaqui-Kidd, and D. Hand. 1985. Double blind placebo control trial of high dose lecithin in Alzheimer's disease. *Journal of Neurology, Neurosurgery and Psychiatry* 48:736–742.

Loury, M.C., and D.N. Kennedy. 1991. Chronic sinusitis and nasal polyposis. In *Smell and Taste in Health and Disease*, 517–528, ed. T.V. Getchell, R.L. Doty, L.M. Bartoshuk, and J.B. Snow, Jr. New York: Raven Press.

Mackay-Sim, A. 1991. Changes in smell and taste function in thyroid, parathyroid, and adrenal disease. In *Smell and Taste in Health and Disease*, Ch. 52, 817–827, ed. T.V. Getchell, R.L. Doty, L.M. Bartoshuk, and J.B. Snow, Jr. New York: Raven Press.

Mair, R.G., R.L. Doty, K.M. Kelly, C.S. Wilson, P.J. Langlais, W.J. McEntree, and T.A. Vollmecke. 1986. Multimodal sensory deficits in Korsakoff's psychosis. *Neuropsychologia* 24:831–839.

Markley, E.J., Mattes-Kulig, D.A., and R.I. Henkin. 1983. A classification of dysgeusia. *Journal of the American Dietetic Association* 83:578–580.

Markopoulou, K., K.W. Larsen, E.K. Wszolek, M.A. Denson, A.E. Lang, R.F. Pfeiffer, and Z.K. Wszoelk. 1977. Olfactory dysfunction in familial Parkinsonism. *Neurology* 49:1262–1267.

Mattes, R.D., and B.J. Cowart. 1994. Dietary assessment of patients with chemosensory disorders. *Journal of the American Dietetic Association* 94:50–56.

Meats, P. 1988. Olfactory hallucinations. *British Medical Journal* 290:645.

Meisami, E., L. Mikhail, D. Baim, and K.P. Bhatnagar. 1998. Human olfactory bulb: Aging of glomeruli and mitral cells and a search for the accessory olfactory bulb. *Annals of the New York Academy of Sciences* 855:708–715.

Mela, D.J. 1988. Sensory assessment of fat content in fluid dairy products. *Appetite* 10:37–44.

Middleton, C.B., M.W. Geisler, T.M. Davidson, and C. Murphy. 1998. Relationship between the alcohol sniff test and sensory olfactory event-related potentials: Validation of a psychophysical test. *Chemical Senses* 23:610.

Minski, K.R., L.M. Bartoshuk, J.E. Hayes, H.J. Hoffman, S. Rawal, and V.B. Duffy. 2010. NIH Toolbox: Proposed Food Liking Survey. *Chemical Senses* 35:7:A21.

Moberg, P.J., and R.L. Doty. 1997. Olfactory function in Huntington's disease patients and at-risk offspring. *International Journal of Neuroscience* 89:133–139.

Moberg, P.J., R.L. Doty, B.I. Turetsky, S.T.E. Arnold, R.N. Mahr, R.C. Gur, W. Bilker, and R.E. Gur. 1997. Olfactory identification deficits in schizophrenia: Correlation with duration of illness. *American Journal of Psychiatry* 154:1016–1018.

Mohr, P.D. 1986. Early neurological complications of coronary artery bypass surgery. *British Medical Journal* 292:60–61.

Monath, T., B. Cropp, and A. Harrison. 1983. Mode of entry of a neurotropic arbovirus into the central nervous system. *Laboratory Investigation* 48:399.

Mott, A.E., and D.A. Leopold. 1991. Disorders in taste and smell. *Medical Clinics of North America* 75:1321–1353.

Mullol, J., and I. Alobid. 2011. Combined oral and intranasal corticosteroid therapy: An advance in the management of nasal polyposis? *Annals of Internal Medicine* 154:5:365–367.

Murphy, C., and W.S. Cain. 1980. Taste and olfaction: Independence vs. interaction. *Physiology & Behavior* 24:601–605.

Murphy, C., C.R. Schubert, K.J. Cruickshanks, B.E.K. Klein, R. Klein, and D.M. Nondahl. 2002. Prevalence of olfactory impairment in older adults. *Journal of the American Medical Association* 288:2307–2312.

Murphy, C., R.L. Doty, and H.J. Duncan. 2003. Clinical disorders of olfaction. In *Handbook of Olfaction and Gustation, Second Edition, revised and expanded*, Ch. 22, 461–478, ed. R.L. Doty. New York: Marcel Dekker.

Murphy, C., E. Green, A. Jacobson, L. Haase, E. McIntosh, and A. Buncic. 2014. fMRI of the brain response to chemosensory stimuli in metabolic syndrome. *AChemS XXXVI, The Association for Chemoreception Sciences 36th Annual Meeting Abstract Book*, Bonita Springs, FL, 225:115.

Newsome, D.A., M. Swartz, N.C. Leone, R.C. Elston, and E. Miller. 1988. Oral zinc in macular degeneration. *Archives of Ophthalmology* 106:2:192–198.

Nordin, S., A.U. Monsoh, and C. Murphy. 1995. Unawareness of smell loss in normal aging and Alzheimer's disease: Discrepancy between self-reporting and diagnosed smell sensitivity. *Journal of Gerontology* 50:187–192.

Obrebowski, A., Z. Obrebowska-Karsznia, and M. Gawlinski. 2000. Smell and taste in children with simple obesity. *International Journal of Pediatric Otorhinolaryngology* 55:191–196.

Panagiotopoulos, G., S. Naxakis, and A. Papavasiliou. 2005. A decreasing nasal mucous Ca++ improves hyposmia. *Rhinology* 43:2:130–134, as quoted in *Navigating Smell and Taste Disorders*, Ch. 5, 61–80, ed. R. DeVere, and M. Calvert. New York: Hamilton Printing Company.

Pangborn, R.M., K.E.O. Bos, and J. Stern. 1985. Dietary fat intake and taste responses to fat in milk by under-, normal, and overweight women. *Appetite* 6:25–40.

Parsons, M. 1983. *Color Atlas of Clinical Neurology*, 18. Chicago: Year Book Medical.

Pearson, R., M. Esiri, R. Hiorns, G. Wilcock, and T. Powell. 1985. Anatomical correlates of the distribution of the pathological changes in the neocortex in Alzheimer's disease. *Proceedings of the National Academy of Science, USA* 82:4531–4534.

Peet, M.M., D.H. Echols, and H.J. Richter. 1937. Chemical prophylaxis for poliomyelitis: Technic of applying zinc sulfate intranasally. *Journal of the American Medical Association* 108:2184.

Pietsch, K., and T. Hummel. 2014. Changes in olfactory bulb volume following lateralized olfactory training. *Chemical Senses* 39:1:107.

Post, F. 1975. Dementia, depression, and pseudodementia. In *Psychiatric Aspects of Neurologic Disease*, 99–120, ed. D.V. Benson, and D. Blumer. New York: Grune and Stratton.

Potter, H., and N. Butters. 1980. An assessment of olfactory deficits in patients with damage to prefrontal cortex. *Neuropsychologia* 18:621–628.

Public Health Service. 1979. *Report of the Panel on Communicative Disorders to the National Advisory Neurological and Communicative Disorders and Stroke Council* (NIH Publication No. 79-1914), 319. Washington, DC: National Institute of Health.

Rawal, S., H.J. Hoffman, K.E. Bainbridge, and V.B. Duffy. 2014. Prevalence and risk factors of self-reported chemosensory disorders and preliminary associations with adiposity in United States adults: Results from 2011–2012 National Health and Nutrition Examination Survey (NHANES). In *AChemS XXXVI, The Association for Chemoreception Sciences 36th Annual Meeting Abstract Book*, Bonita Springs, FL, 253:125.

Richardson, B.D., E.A. VanderWoude, R. Sudan, J.S. Thompson, and D.A. Leopold. 2004. Altered olfactory acuity in the morbidly obese. *Obesity Surgery* 14:7:967–969 as quoted in L.D. Stafford, and K. Welbeck. 2011. High hunger state increases olfactory sensitivity to neutral but not food odors. *Chemical Senses* 36:189–198.

Roberts, R. 1986. Alzheimer's disease may begin in the nose and may be caused by aluminosilicates. *Neurobiology of Aging* 7:561–567.

Rodin, J., H.R. Moskowitz, and G.A. Bray. 1976. Relationship between obesity, weight loss, and taste responsiveness. *Physiology & Behavior* 17:591–597.

Rolls, E.T. 2010. Taste, olfactory and food texture reward processing in the brain and obesity. *International Journal of Obesity* 35:550–561.

Roydhouse, N. 1988. Retinoid therapy and anosmia. *New Zealand Medical Journal* 101:465.

Rubert, S.L., M. H. Hollender, and E.G. Mehrof. 1961. Olfactory hallucinations. *Archives of General Psychiatry* 5:121–126.

Sajjadian, A., R.L. Doty, D.N. Gutnick, R.J. Chirurgi, M. Sivak, and D. Perl. 1994. Olfactory dysfunction in amyotrophic lateral sclerosis. *Neurodegeneration* 3:153–157.

Sauberlich, H.E. 1975. Vitamin metabolism and requirements. *South African Medical Journal* 49:2235–2244.

Schechter, P.J., W.T. Friedewald, D.A. Bronzert, M.S. Raff, and R.I. Henkin. 1972. Idiopathic hypogeusia: A description of the syndrome and a single blind study with zinc sulfate. *International Review of Neurobiology Supplement* 1:125–140.

Schiffman, S.S. 1991. Drugs influencing taste and smell perception. In *Smell and Taste in Health and Disease*, Ch. 54, 845–850, ed. T.V. Getchell, R.L. Doty, L.M. Bartoshuk, and J.B. Snow, Jr. New York: Raven Press.

Schiffman, S.S., and Z.S. Warwick. 1988. Flavor enhancement of foods for the elderly can reverse anorexia. *Neurophysiology of Aging* 9:24–26.

Schiffman, S.S., C. Diaz, and T.G. Beeker. 1986. Caffeine intensifies taste of certain sweeteners: Role of adenosine receptor. *Pharmacology Biochemistry and Behavior* 24:429–432.

Schlotfeld, C.R., M.W. Geisler, T.M. Davidson, and C. Murphy. 1998. Clinical application of the alcohol sniff test on HIV positive and HIV negative patients with nasal sinus disease. *Chemical Senses* 23:610.

Schwartz, A., J. Frey, and R. Lukas. 1988. Risk factors in Alzheimer's disease: Is aluminum hazardous to your health? *Barrow Neurologic Institute Quarterly* 4:2.

Schwartz, B.S. 1991. Epidemiology and its application to olfactory dysfunction. In *The Human Sense of Smell*, Ch. 15, 308–339, ed. D.G. Laing, R.L. Doty, and W. Breipohl. Berlin: Springer-Verlag.

Schwartz, B.S., P. Ford, K.I. Bolla, J. Agnew, N. Rothman, and M.L. Bleecker. 1990. Solvent-associated decrements in olfactory function in paint manufacturing workers. *American Journal of Industrial Medicine* 18:697–706.

Scott, A.E. 1989a. Caution urged in treating "steroid-dependent anosmia." *Archives of Otolaryngology Head and Neck Surgery* 115:109–110.

Scott, A.E. 1989b. Clinical characteristics of taste and smell disorders. *Ear, Nose and Throat Journal* 68:297–298.

Scott, A.E., W.S. Cain, and G. Clavet. 1988. Topical corticosteroids can alleviate olfactory dysfunction. *Chemical Senses* 13:735.

Scott, A.E., W.S. Cain, and G. Leonard. 1989. Nasal/sinus disease and olfactory loss at the Connecticut Chemosensory Clinical Research Center. *Chemical Senses* 14:745.

Serby, M. 1987. Olfaction and neuropsychiatry [Abstr.]. Distributed at Dr. Serby's lecture at the Institute for Research and Behavioral Neurosciences, New York, December 12, 1987.

Serby, M., J. Corwin, A. Novatt, P. Conrad, and J. Rotrosen. 1985. Olfaction in dementia. *Journal of Neurosurgery & Psychiatry* 14:848–849.

Serby, M., C. Flicker, B. Rypma, S. Weber, J.P. Rotrosen, and S.H. Ferris. 1989. Scopolamine and olfactory function. *Biological Psychiatry* 28:79–82.

Serby, M., P. Larson, and D. Kalkstein. 1990. Olfactory sense in psychoses. *Biologic Psychiatry* 28:829–830.

Serby, M.J., P.M. Larson, and D. Kalkstein. 1992. Olfaction and neuropsychiatry. In *Science of Olfaction*, Ch. 21, 559–589, ed. M.J. Serby, and K.L. Chobor. New York: Springer-Verlag.

Small, D.M. 2009. Individual difference in the neurophysiology of reward and the obesity epidemic. *International Journal of Obesity* 33:544–548.

Smith, A.D. 1983. Legaloblastic anemias. In *Hematology, 3rd Ed.*, 4343–465, ed. W.J. Williams, E. Beutler, A.J. Erslev, and M.A. Lichtman. New York: McGraw-Hill.

Smith, D.V. 1986. Taste, smell and psychophysical measurement. In *Clinical Measurement of Taste and Smell*, 1–18, ed. H.L. Meiselman, and R.S. Rivlin. New York: Macmillan.

Smith, D.V., and A.M. Seiden. 1995. Olfactory dysfunction. In *The Human Sense of Smell*, Ch. 14, 298, ed. D.G. Laing, R.L. Doty, and W. Briepohl. New York: Springer-Verlag.

Smith, D.V., R.A. Frank, M.L. Pensak, and A.M. Seiden. 1987. Characteristics of chemosensory patients and a comparison of olfactory assessment procedures. *Chemical Senses* 12:698.

Snow, Jr. J., and J. Martin. 1994. Disturbances of smell, taste and hearing. In *Harrison's Principles of Internal Medicine, 13th Ed.*, 109–115, ed. K.J. Isselbacher, E. Braunwald, J.D. Wilson, J.B. Martin, and A.S. Fauci. New York: McGraw Hill.

Snyder, D.J., S.S. O'Malley, S.A. McKee, and L.M. Bartoshuk. 2005. Sex differences in adult obesity risk associated with childhood tobacco exposure. *AChemS XXVIIth Annual Meeting Abstract Book*, 153:39.

Sollai, G., P. Muroni, M. Melis, R. Crnjar, and I. Tomassini-Barbarossa. 2014. A paper screening test to assess oral sensitivity to oleic acid in normo-weight PROP super-tasters, medium tasters and non-tasters. *Chemical Senses* 39:1:103.

Solomon, G.S., W.M. Petrie, J.R. Hart, and H.B. Brackin, Jr. 1998. Olfactory dysfunction discriminates Alzheimer's dementia from major depression. *Journal of Neuropsychiatry and Clinical Neurosciences* 10:1:64–67.

Spitzer, L., and J. Rodin. 1981. Human eating behavior: A critical review of studies in normal weight and overweight individuals. *Appetite* 2:293–329.

Stafford, L.D., and K. Welbeck. 2010. Olfactory sensitivity related to hunger state, BMI and negative mood. *AchemS XXXII Abstract Book*, Poster P353:144.

Stafford, L.D., and K. Welbeck. 2011. High hunger state increases olfactory sensitivity to neutral but not foods. *Chemical Senses* 36:189–198.

Stevens, J.C., and W.S. Cain. 1986. Smelling via the mouth: Effect of aging. *Perception & Psychophysics* 43:3:142–146.

Stevens, J.C., W.C. Cain, and D.E. Weinstein. 1987. Aging impairs the ability to detect gas odor. *Fire Technology* 23:3:198–204.

Sullivan, B., J.E. Hayes, P.D. Faghri, and V.B. Duffy. 2007. Connecting diet and disease risk via food preference. *AChemS XXVIIII Abstract Book*, Poster 158:19.

Sunday, S.R., and K.A. Halmi. 1990. Taste perceptions and hedonics in eating disorders. *Psychology & Behavior* 48:587–594.

Takagi, S.F. 1984. A standardized olfactometer in Japan. A review over 10 years. Preliminary studies for manufacture of a standardized olfactometer. *Annals of New York Academy of Sciences* 510:113–118.

Tamura, T., R.L. Goldenberg, K.E. Johnston, and M. DuBard. 2000. Maternal plasma zinc concentrations and pregnancy outcome. *American Journal of Clinical Nutrition* 71:109–113.

Tepper, B.J., L. Zhao, N. Ullrich, G. Persico, M. Ciullo, V. Colonna, T. Nutile, and P. Gasparini. 2005. Taste blindness to 6-*n*-propylthiouracil (PROP) and body weight in a genetically isolated population in Southern Italy. *AChemS XXVIIth Annual Meeting Abstract Book* 126:32.

Thierry, A.M., Tassin, J.P., Blanc, G., and J. Glowinski. 1976. Selective activation of mesocortical DA system by stress. *Nature* 263:242–244.

Venstrom, D., and J.E. Amoore. 1968. Olfactory threshold in relation to age, sex or smoking. *Journal of Food Science* 33:264–265.

Ward, C.D., W.A. Hess, and D.B. Calne. 1983. Olfactory impairment in Parkinson's disease. *Neurology* 33:943–946.

Warwick, Z.S., S.S. Schiffman, and J.J.B. Anderson. 1990. Relationship of dietary fat content to preferences in young rats. *Physiology & Behavior* 48:581–586.

Weismann, K., E. Christensen, and V. Dreyer. 1979. Zinc supplementation in alcoholic cirrhosis. *Acta Medica Scandinavica* 205:361–366.

Witherly, S.A., R.M. Pangborn, and J.S. Stern. 1980. Gustatory responses and eating duration of obese and lean adults. *Appetite* 1:53–63.

Witt, M., K. Reutter, and I.J. Miller, Jr. 2003. Morphology of the peripheral taste system. In *Handbook of Olfaction and Gustation. 2nd Ed. Revised and Expanded*, Ch. 32, 651–677, ed. R.L. Doty. New York: Marcel Dekker.

Wolfe, J.M. 2006. *Sensation & Perception*. Ch. 13, 32. Sunderland, MA: Sinauer Associates.

Wurtman, R.J. 1979. Sources of choline and lecithin in the diet. In *Nutrition and the Brain*, Vol. 5, 73–81, ed. J.H. Barbeau, J.H. Growden, and R.J. Wurtman. New York: Raven Press.

Wurtman, R.J., F. Hefti, and E. Melamed. 1981. Precursor control of neurotransmitter synthesis. *Pharmacologic Review* 32:315–335.

Wysocki, C.J., K.M. Dorries, and G.K. Beauchamp. 1989. Ability to perceive androstenone can be acquired by ostensibly anosmic people. *Proceedings of the National Academy of Science* 86:7976–7978.

Zegeer, L.J. 1986. The effects of sensory changes in older persons. *Journal of Neuroscience Nursing* 18:6:325–332.

3 Retronasal Olfaction

Jason J. Gruss and Alan R. Hirsch

CONTENTS

3.1   Introduction 65
3.2   Olfactory Anatomy 66
3.3   Chemical Signal 67
3.4   Odorants and Flavors 68
3.5   Role of Sensory Adaptation 69
3.6   Difference between Orthonasal and Retronasal Olfaction 69
3.7   Clinical Testing Retronasal Smell 70
3.8   Response to Chemosensation 73
3.9   Food and Chemosensation 74
3.10 Other Behavioral Realms 75
References 75

3.1   INTRODUCTION

Olfaction is the process by which chemical stimulants are processed into the sensation of smell. In this process, aerosolized chemical stimulants traverse the nose, move into the olfactory cleft, and eventually contact the olfactory sensory neurons. With a sufficient stimulus, the sensory signal of smell is triggered. This is considered a chemosensory process, as the stimulus is a chemical that binds to a receptor. Most of the other human senses use different stimuli. Vision uses light; hearing uses sound waves; and touch uses pressure. All of those sources are not from a chemical stimulus. Using chemicals to stimulate a response is known as chemosensation. Olfaction shares chemosensation with the sense of taste. Smell and taste are strongly linked in this regard. In fact, 90% of taste, or flavor, is actually smell (Hirsch 1992a). Despite the close association, there are significant differences between smell and taste.

The olfactory neurons are located in the nose, just as the taste buds are located on the tongue. Therefore, it may be thought that the sense of smell is mediated via the nostrils, whereas the sense of taste is experienced through the mouth. While this is true, it is only a part of the story. Odorants entering the nose through the nostrils are considered orthonasal, but there is a separate route as well. Odorants can also enter the mouth and stimulate the olfactory sensory neurons retronasally. In this route, odorants from the mouth travel to the nasopharynx then to the sensory neurons. Therefore, an oral source of stimuli, such as food, has the ability to trigger both taste and smell regardless of the strength of the orthonasal stimulus.

Historically, the phenomenon of retronasal olfaction has been confusing to study. Because the nature of smell and taste are so intertwined, research has long struggled at times to isolate each sensory system (Ogle 1870). Researchers have described the olfactory system as being frequently confused with the sensation of taste (Rozin 1982). Indeed, taste–smell confusion has been discovered among research subjects (Murphy et al. 1977; Murphy and Cain 1980). Because of the natural link between these two senses, determining a food's flavor involves complicated, multisensory system processing (Small and Prescott 2005). Along with the determination of chemical flavor, the effects of a food on the sense of touch, temperature, and other sensory input are also simultaneously being processed. Despite the presence of multiple sensory systems, more recently, some have isolated retronasal olfaction for research (Pierce and Halpern 1996). By isolating this system, researchers are beginning to learn how smell and taste overlap, how they differ, and how orthonasal and retronasal olfactions each contribute to the sensory experience.

It has long been established that olfaction plays a significant role in behavior (Dalton 2000). The effects of olfaction on weight have been well demonstrated (Duffy et al. 1995; Hirsch and Gomez 1995). Additionally, olfactory sensations can have powerful effects on emotional state (Joseph 2000) and even sexual arousal (Hirsch 1998; Hirsch and Gruss 1999; Huh et al. 2008). Also, abnormalities in the olfactory process can have significant consequences (Miwa et al. 2001; Hummel and Nordin 2005). The differences between orthonasal olfaction and retronasal olfaction in these important aspects of behavior are still being elucidated.

3.2 OLFACTORY ANATOMY

To understand the function of retronasal olfaction, we must first understand the anatomy of olfaction. Putting aside the issue of retronasal, versus orthonasal, once the stimuli reaches the olfactory epithelium, what happens then?

There is a mucus layer at the top of the nose within which the olfactory cilia reside. Chemical signals are dissolved in the mucus and then reach the receptor organ on the cilia. Not all chemical signals move through the mucus layer equally. Each cilium is connected to its olfactory receptor cell. These cells have terminal filaments that combine the filaments from other olfactory receptor cells. As they combine, these clusters of filaments travel through the cribriform plate of the ethmoid bone, which separates the nasal cavity from the cranium. Once through the cribriform plate, the filaments synapse with the olfactory bulb.

The cortical processing of smell is simultaneously instant and primal, as well as subtle and evocative. When we think of odors, humans have a reaction that is unlike the thoughts of other stimuli. When humans remember auditory stimuli, we are often precise, remembering details. When humans remember odors, these memories evoke stronger emotional responses (Herz and Cupchik 1995). This response is due to the anatomy of olfaction.

The olfactory bulb has two main connections. First, it is linked directly to the primary olfactory cortex. This is unique. All other sensory modalities route through the thalamus. The primary olfactory cortex is found at the junction of the anterior–medial temporal lobe and the ventral–posterior frontal lobe. The primary olfactory cortex connects to several other cortical areas: thalamus, hypothalamus, amygdala, and entorhinal cortex.

In addition to the direct link to the primary olfactory cortex, the olfactory bulb is also linked to the amygdala. This direct connection is significant as the amygdala controls the formation and storage of memories associated with emotional events. The amygdala is also involved in memory consolidation, which plays critical roles in long-term memory formation. It has been well established that damage to the amygdala has been shown to produce significant social and emotional deficits (Brown and Shafer 1888; Kluver and Bucy 1939).

3.3 CHEMICAL SIGNAL

Processing of an odor generally follows the following system: Is it detectable? Is it familiar? Is it good or bad? What odor is this? (Lawless and Engen 1977).

The first step is always detection. In order for olfaction to occur, the chemical signal must be delivered to its receptor. Each receptor is able to interact with a specific group of odorants. Each odor will trigger a combination of receptor neurons. This combination of receptor firing will be one part of the cascade that allows us to first define whether we detect an odorant and, second, to determine whether we can identify the odorant. In order to be detected, the odorant must be soluble to the mucus layer. The nature of the odorant, the viscosity of the mucus layer, and other factors all contribute to the ability of a stimulant to penetrate the mucus layer. When someone has a stuffy nose from a cold, the increased quality of mucus, the increased thickness of the mucus, and the decreased air flow can all reduce the sense of smell.

The ability to detect an odorant is referred to as its threshold. Varying odorants have different concentrations required to reach this threshold (Punter 1983). Additionally, individuals have a different ability to detect odorants. The threshold for orthonasal and retronasal olfaction is also different (Heilmann and Hummel 2004). Orthonasal stimuli are detected at lower thresholds than those same stimuli presented via the retronasal route. This means that detecting an aroma presented to the mouth requires a higher concentration of stimuli. When this concept of retronasal versus orthonasal threshold is related to olfaction during eating, a remarkable effect is seen. Let us assume that minimal orthonasal stimulus is present in the ambient air. Then, a fixed stimulus is presented with each bite of food. Because additional stimulus is needed to reach threshold, as there is minimal orthonasal stimulus, more food is needed. This can occur in many different ways, such as eating in the car, eating prepared foods, etc. There are alternatives to presenting additional food to increase the stimulus. The food may be prepared to have a stronger or longer-lasting stimulus that could be triggered when eaten to stimulate retronasal olfaction. This could be done through mastication or modification with salivation, for example.

Retronasal olfaction occurs during exhalation when air is pushed up to the nose from the pharynx. This is what carries the odorant to the sensory neurons. Turbulence and airflow can alter the delivery of the odorant. A classic example that demonstrates this is to plug the nose when eating a food with strong odor, such as strawberry or banana. After taking a few chews, unplug the nose and then chew more. With the unplugged nose, airflow carries the stimulant to the sensory neurons, and a strong stimulus triggers a response. Since the stimulus is delivered from the mouth to the nose, this is retronasal olfaction. The concentration of stimulus is low initially, and the threshold may not have been reached. Once the airflow starts, the concentration increases. Then, the threshold is reached, and the perception of flavor dramatically increases.

A substance must be volatile enough to allow the transportation of a stimulus to the olfactory sensory organs. Many things can alter a substance's volatility. An example of this would be bread. Hot baking bread coming right out of the oven has a very strong and familiar odor. Two days later, the same bread is much less volatile and presents a much lower stimulus. Using this concept, modern chefs are preparing foods that have specific sensory effects. A chef might prepare a food with minimal aroma until it meets with saliva or until it is chewed. An example of this would be crystallized or dehydrated concentration of specific flavors, such as powders that turn into fruit punch or lemonade with water. Another chef might add a complimentary aroma to a course that is not eaten but only smelled. An example of this would be a bouquet of pine needles. When hot water is added to the needles, the aroma is unmistakable, but the needles need not be eaten for the aroma to add to the flavor. In these ways, orthonasal aroma can be added to alter the flavor of food. Alternatively, retronasal flavors can be added. When a retronasal stimulus is added, there is a sudden change from minimal odor detection to strong odor detection. This contrast results in strong sensory perception, perhaps similar to stepping out of a darkened theater into sunlight.

The following is another question we ask ourselves in this identification process: is this a good odor or a bad odor? This is olfactory hedonics. Familiarity and intensity play a role in the perception of odor quality. Generally, the more familiar the odor is, the more pleasant it is perceived. However, there are differences among individuals due to experience. One example would be an otherwise pleasant odor that is associated with an unpleasant experience. For example, if a specific food (fried fish) caused an episode of illness, there could be a learned aversion to the odor. Also, odor preferences are different between childhood and adulthood. There is also evidence of cultural preferences for certain odors.

3.4 ODORANTS AND FLAVORS

Odorants are also known as fragrances or aromas. These chemical stimuli are found in many different substances. They have many different structures and are organized into several different groups. These groups include

- Esters such as geranyl acetate or rose; also benzyl acetate or strawberry
- Linear terpenes such as citronella or lemongrass
- Cyclic terpenes such as camphor
- Aromatics such as vanilla
- Amines such as cadaverine, the smell of rotting flesh
- Alcohols such as menthol

There is a plethora of other groups and combinations of odorants.

In comparison to the large list of odors, the sense of taste is limited to salt, sweet, sour, bitter, umami, and possibly some fats. Through the study of anosmics, researchers have learned that the perception of taste can be altered by the sense of smell.

In addition to taste buds and olfactory sensory neurons, the trigeminal nerve has receptors in the olfactory epithelium that are responsible for tactile, pressure, pain, and temperature sensation in the areas of the mouth, eyes, and nasal cavity. Some chemical sensory stimuli also affect the trigeminal nerve. In this way, menthol is sensed both by the olfactory neurons as *mint* and by the trigeminal nerve as *cool* in moderate concentrations and *hot* at high concentrations. Mustard, chili powder, and onion are other common examples of chemicals that can stimulate the trigeminal nerve.

3.5   ROLE OF SENSORY ADAPTATION

Sensory stimuli are powerful. However, over time, our senses become dulled to repeated stimuli. Conversely, there is a stronger response to new stimuli. This has been described as sensory adaptation and novelty, respectively. This adaptation is a useful one. As we are exposed to a stimulus, we become familiar with it; we achieve a behavioral equilibrium. We know the stimulus is there should we choose to focus on it. However, the familiar stimulus is not a distraction. A *new* stimulus is then able to more easily attract our attention.

This phenomenon is certainly true regarding olfactory stimuli. Adaptation can be achieved by exposure to a strong stimulus or exposure to a stimulus for a long period of time. For example, people are often unaware of the normal smell of their house until they return from a vacation. Also, people instantly notice the smell of a new house but stop noticing it after a few minutes. Similarly, when someone applies perfume, the initial smell can be powerful, but this decreases after a few minutes. However, when they interact with someone, this new person is quite likely to notice the fragrance.

3.6   DIFFERENCE BETWEEN ORTHONASAL
AND RETRONASAL OLFACTION

Historically, the phenomenon of retronasal olfaction has been confusing to study, as the sensation of taste is so closely linked (Ogle 1870). The olfactory system is frequently confused with the sensation of taste (Rozin 1982). Indeed, taste–smell confusion routinely occurs among research subjects (Murphy et al. 1977; Murphy and Cain 1980). Because of this natural correlation, determining a food's flavor involves a complicated multisensory system processing (Small and Prescott 2005). Despite the presence of multiple sensory systems, isolated retronasal olfaction has been studied (Pierce and Halpern 1996; Heilmann et al. 2002). Moreover, retronasal olfaction plays a critical role in food hedonics (Lim and Padmanabhan 2013).

3.7 CLINICAL TESTING RETRONASAL SMELL

As described above, flavor is a combination of different senses, including olfactory, gustatory, and irritation or pungency (Bresslin 2006; Small 2008; Spense 2012). The smell component of flavor comes from retronasal smell—odors that flow from the mouth, through the oropharynx, to the olfactory nerves at the roof of the nose (Adams and Taylor 2012) (see Figure 3.1).

As such, retronasal smell is a chemosensory example of ventriloquist illusion (Veldhuizen et al. 2010). In this, speech is falsely localized to the moving mouth of the dummy rather than the puppeteer. With this model, while eating, retronasal odors are falsely localized to the oral cavity rather than to the nose.

How much of the flavor of food is due to this retronasal smell varies depending on the food (Ruijschop et al. 2008). This was demonstrated by Mozell over half a century ago (Mozell et al. 1969). He set off to determine how much of perceived flavor or *taste* was actually due to retronasal smell. In order to do this, he both blocked the nose (with nose plugs) and pumped air backward, from the nostrils through the nose, down the nasal pharynx, and out the mouth, thus definitively preventing any odorants during ingestion from reaching the olfactory nerves. He tested 21 sophomore medical students who had fasted for half an hour. They were all subjectively normosmic (believed they had a normal sense of smell) and had a normal terpineol olfactory test. The flavors tested were coffee, port wine, red wine, vinegar, maraschino cherry, whiskey, lemon juice, dark molasses, onions, garlic powder, apricot nectar, pineapple juice, dill pickle gherkins, salt, sucrose, and distilled water. To reduce influence of texture, if not already in a liquid form, the foods were liquefied. In a random order, all the flavors were presented two times to the same subject, with the nasal pathway occluded, then with the pathway open, or vice versa. Under these conditions, subjects were queried as to the identification of each flavor. For all flavors, identification was better with, than without, retronasal olfaction. Furthermore, without retronasal smell, 11 flavors were never identified including coffee, cherry, molasses, garlic, apricot, pineapple, root beer, chocolate, cranberry juice, dill pickle, and sugar water. Of these, with retronasal smell, correct identification was seen in over 77% of subjects to coffee, chocolate, and cherry. Ninety-five percent could identify coffee with retronasal smell, whereas 0% could without retronasal smell.

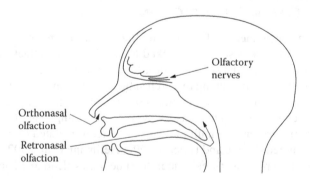

FIGURE 3.1 Pathway of retronasal olfaction.

In a study of retronasal smell in 15 subjects, of 8 different odors, correct identification, given odor name choice, was 100% for bananas and wintergreen; 99.2% for peanuts and chocolate; 98.8% for coffee; 97.9% for orange and cinnamon; and 97.5% for lemon (Wininger and Halpern 1999).

When similar foods diluted by 50% to avoid the ceiling effect were tested, with retronasal smell, in 9 women and 11 men (ages 18–31), identification was seen for the following: wintergreen, 77.5%; strawberry and bananas, 35%; cinnamon, 70%; orange, 62.5%; canola oil, 57.5%; coffee, 47.5%; and lemon, 42.5% (Puttanniah and Halpern 2001).

Furthermore, it had been observed, but not quantitated, that retronasal olfactory input enhances not just identification but also actually the intensity of perceived flavor or taste (Djordjevic et al. 2004). Such intensification can even occur at subthreshold levels of odor wherein odors presented to the nose were of such low intensity that they could not be consciously detected but still increased the perceived intensity of the food being concurrently tasted (Breslin et al. 2001; Labbe et al. 2007).

However, judgment of intensity, as opposed to identification, may not be correlated. Engen observed, "If the set is to judge intensity rather than quality, and one asks the person to judge the intensity of something tasted, then olfactory input seems to play a different role" (Engen 1982, p. 149).

Chewing enhances such retronasal smell-induced flavor sensation by up to 100% (deWijk and Prinz 2005), thus implying that a greater intensity would be seen if a viscous substance, such as jelly beans, were used as opposed to liquefied flavors that Mozell et al. (1969) used. The process of eating also influences the degree of retronasal smell. Depending on the study, swallowing reduces or increases the amount of retronasal smell and thus the importance of testing with chewing but without swallowing (Halpern 2003; Leclerq and Blancher 2012). Mozell's approach of both blocking with nose plugs and injecting air up the nostrils to prevent retronasal smell goes beyond the current standard approach to inhibit retronasal smell—just the use of nose plugs (Halpern 2004; Ruijschop et al. 2008). These function like the occlusion of one end of a manometer, thus preventing odor flow down a closed tube, to the olfactory epithelium. Such a process has equal efficacy but is technically much simpler to perform.

The use of jelly beans as a standard testing agent in retronasal smell is not new. Over a decade ago, ratings of jelly bean retronasal flavor intensity were found to correlate with other aspects of chemosensation including the following: taste intensity rating, taste status (supertaster or normal taster), number of fungiform papillae, rings of intensity of bitter when quinine hydrochloride is placed on the tip of the tongue, and orthonasal smell (Duffy et al. 2003).

It is important to be able to easily test retronasal smell since smell loss can occur in retronasal smell, whereas orthonasal smell remains normal (Cowart et al. 1999, 2003). No frequently utilized clinical tests of retronasal smell currently exist (Bartoshuk et al. 1983). Bartoshuk (oral communication, 2011) observed that cappuccino Jelly Belly jelly beans are the best testing agent to clinically assess retronasal smell.

Hirsch et al. (2013) set out to demonstrate this in a study of 42 normosmic (Brief Smell Identification Test 3/3) children. In a randomized fashion, they rated 10 jelly bean flavors on a 10-point visual analog scale form intensity of flavor with and without the presence of nose clips.

Significant differences ($p < 0.05$) were found between the means of the following: cappuccino, 5.3; popcorn, 5.2; mint chocolate chip ice cream, 5.1; cinnamon, 4.4; grape, 4.2; mango chili, 4.1; bubblegum, 4.1; Tabasco, 4.0; 7UP, 3.6; and cotton candy, 2.9.

These results confirmed Mozell et al.'s (1969) findings of coffee flavor having the most retronasal component. While it is known that different food flavors have specific retronasal smell components, why cappuccino had the greatest is unclear. Part of the reason may be due to the lack of trigeminal impact (Prescott 1999). This is independent of the olfactory pathway, and trigeminal sensation is so intense that it would overwhelm olfactory influence (Labbe et al. 2008). Such is seen with the irritant jelly bean flavor, jalapeño, or tabasco, with little effect on retronasal smell. The relative absence of trigeminal nerve stimulation in cappuccino helps to explain its efficacy in testing of retronasal smell. On the other hand, the importance of sensory integration between bitter taste and sweet retronasal smell has been noted for espresso coffee (Chiralertpong et al. 2008). Such is even recognized by the public in TV commercials promoting the delicious aroma of coffee.

Thus, the flavor intensity difference with Jelly Belly cappuccino jelly beans, with and without nose clips, is a clinically useful test for retronasal smell: the Jelly Bean Difference Test.

Traditionally, retronasal smell has been considered equivalent to orthonasal smell, just coming from a different direction (Wolfe et al. 2006). However, the validity of such an assumption has come under question. Retronasal olfaction has been demonstrated to evoke different sensations when odors were presented orthonasally (Frasnelli et al. 2008). Olfactory thresholds are different: orthonasal detection threshold is lower than retronasal detection threshold (Melzner et al. 2011). Projections of retronasal smell have been found to proceed to different areas of the brain than orthonasal smell (Small et al. 2005). The reason for such differences has been postulated to be due to different olfactory epithelium stimulation with orthonasal as opposed to retronasal smell, or due to different time sequences of activation (Engen 1982). Retronasal smell enhances the identification of intraoral flavor as well as the intensity (Puttanniah and Halpern 2001). Such intensification has been demonstrated to have an additive or superadditive influence (White and Prescott 2007). While retronasal smell has acted to increase the perceived taste of a flavor, taste has similarly been shown to enhance the perceived retronasal olfactory component (Welge-Lüssen et al. 2009). In the above examples, congruency between taste and smell has been a major factor in the impact of retronasal smell (Labbe and Martin 2009). Retronasal smell has been shown to decrease intraoral trigeminal stimulation (Frasnelli et al. 2004). Alternatively, trigeminal stimuli can act to increase retronasal smell (Dragich and Halpern 2005). The extent of retronasal smell can even impact upon true taste perception (Fujimaru and Lim 2013). Alternatively, chorda tympani anesthetization blocking taste reduces retronasal smell by 50% (Stamps and Bartoshuk 2010).

Formalized chemosensory tests of orthonasal smell are utilized clinically. These include tests of identification (University of Pennsylvania Smell Identification Test, Quick Smell Identification Test [QSIT], Pocket Smell Identification Test, Brief Smell Identification Test, and Sniffin' Sticks) and tests of detection (Phenyl Ethyl Alcohol Threshold Test, Sniffin' Sticks, Alcohol Sniff Test) (Doty 1975, 2003, 2007; Doty et al. 1984, 1986, 1996; Kobal et al. 1996; Davidson and Murphy 1997; Jackman and Doty 2005; Hummel et al. 2007).

Despite the plethora of orthonasal olfactory and gustatory testing, clinical retronasal olfactory testing remains minimal (Bartoshuk et al. 1983). Such testing is important since in pathological states, it is unclear how closely retronasal and orthonasal smell correlates. While anatomy implies a close linkage, it has been suggested that retronasal smell may be impacted with preservation of orthonasal smell or vice versa (Cowart et al. 2003).

Thus, in those with chemosensory dysfunction, the linkage between orthonasal smell and retronasal smell was investigated.

Twenty-four consecutive patients at a smell and taste clinic who were aware of what cappuccino flavor should taste like, presenting with chemosensory complaints, underwent orthonasal testing with the QSIT and retronasal olfactory testing of Jelly Belly cappuccino-flavored jelly beans with and without Snuffer nose clips (Roussos et al. 2014). In this testing, subjects were instructed to chew normally without swallowing and to rate on a visual analog scale the intensity of the cappuccino.

Independent of the chemosensory diagnosis, there was no statistically significant correlation between the QSIT score and retronasal smell difference.

Unlike Duffy, Roussos et al. found that in those with chemosensory dysfunction, orthonasal and retronasal smell were not found to be correlated (Duffy et al. 1999). This suggests that these processes involve distinct pathways or mechanisms whereby one can be affected while the other is not (Pierce and Halpern 1996). Such results suggest that along with orthonasal olfactory testing, retronasal olfactory testing should be used as a way of detecting olfactory dysfunction (Cowart et al. 1999).

Jelly Belly-flavored cappuccino jelly beans with and without nose clips are an easy, quick, and inexpensive clinical test for assessment of retronasal olfactory function. Serial testing of retronasal, like orthonasal function, may be useful in determining the response to therapy or the progression of disease.

3.8 RESPONSE TO CHEMOSENSATION

There is a wide individual variation in response to a given odor. Olfaction plays a role in many aspects of life. One of the most familiar responses is the response to food odors. There are a multitude of other odors that elicit a response. Odors that are familiar and nostalgic can return an individual to the emotional state associated with that odor (Hirsch 1992b). Examples of this could be holiday odors such as Thanksgiving turkey or the smell of a Christmas tree. Other examples might be the fragrance worn by a loved one. There are some fragrances that have a stimulating response or a calming effect. These fragrances certainly do not produce the same effect in every person just as not everyone will agree on what art is beautiful or what music is soothing. Familiarity and hedonics play a role in how stimuli will trigger a response in most sensory modalities.

3.9 FOOD AND CHEMOSENSATION

The olfactory component of the dining experience is significant. The ambient aroma alone can drastically alter the experience. Dining alfresco on a busy street clogged with traffic and car exhaust contributes to the perceived flavor of the food. While many restaurants use flowers to decorate their tables, few of them use strongly scented bouquets. Similarly, the familiar smells of the family kitchen can induce a strong emotional response (Hirsch 1999). However, eating is a multisensory experience. While the focus of this chapter is olfaction, it should be noted that ambient sound, visual stimuli, and many other sensations will contribute to the experience of any meal.

The trappings and the environment that surround a meal all serve to prepare a person for the experience of consuming food. Pleasant food odors typically produce salivation. Salivation is a preparatory step in eating. This also begins to prepare the gastrointestinal system for the food about to arrive. The milieu of sensory input has an emotional response as well. This can all occur before the food is even in sight.

Once the food is served and eating begins, the tactile components of sensation are elicited. With chewing comes salivation. Retronasal olfaction is strongest here. Orthonasal olfaction occurs throughout the pre-eating phase. As discussed earlier, there may be an extinguishing of the orthonasal component due to the timing of exposure. Retronasal olfaction will increase as oral stimulus is presented. The retronasal olfactory stimulus will extinguish after the food is swallowed.

The drive to eat is biologically considered hunger. In modern experience, the drive to eat is more complicated. Food is often more readily available. A wide variety of available food creates an environment where food with strong hedonics is nearly always an option. In such an environment, there should be little surprise that obesity is endemic. The biological trigger to eat, the need to meet the caloric needs of the body, can easily be dwarfed by the brain processing of the pleasant stimuli of food.

However, there is another feature to hunger that has also been studied. In some people, appetite can be decreased to a level where dangerous weight loss occurs. Patients with diseases such as cancer and elderly patients with diminished sense of smell and taste are two examples. In these populations, decreased appetite can lead to significant medical problems.

Along with hunger, there should be discussion of satiety. Satiety can be described as the signal to stop eating. It is controlled in several ways. There is chemosensory satiety, which is the signal to stop eating due to sufficient chemosensory input. There is also gastric fullness, which is the stretch response of a filled stomach. There are other forms of satiety that can focus on negative feedback, such as revulsion, nausea, etc. These are often triggered through chemosensory mechanisms but can be triggered by other stimuli. For example, the taste of spoiled milk may trigger nausea and stop a person from eating. Alternatively, watching someone else become physically ill from ingesting spoiled milk may also trigger satiety without any chemosensory input.

Chemosensory satiety relies on the chemosensory stimulus. Threshold, hedonics, and fatigue—all of them play a role.

Eating speed plays a role in calorie intake and flavor perception (Hollowood et al. 2000). If a stimulus is rapidly extinguished, or if food is rapidly ingested due to behavior, the slower chemosensory input will have a diminished response. Essentially, eating faster will mean decreased sensory input and greater calorie consumption.

The ability to safely modify appetite and satiety has important clinical consequences in weight management. Increasing appetite or decreasing satiety would lead to weight gain, just as decreasing appetite or increasing satiety would lead to weight loss.

Appetite has been shown to be altered by several medications. Megestrol has been approved to treat unintended weight loss; some antidepressants have been used to stimulate weight gain especially in elderly populations (Fox et al. 2012).

3.10   OTHER BEHAVIORAL REALMS

The role of olfaction has been shown to affect relaxation and alertness (Martin 1998). Additionally, research has shown that olfactory stimuli can affect performance with some tasks (Becker et al. 1995; Hirsch and Johnston 1996). The role of general olfactory function and mood has also been examined (Negoias et al. 2010). However, there has been limited research examining how retronasal olfaction specifically affects human behaviors. As research in retronasal smell expands, there should be additional developments in the ability to determine how retronasal olfaction contributes to mood, alertness, social interaction, cognition, and other aspects of the human experience.

REFERENCES

Adams, S., and A.J. Taylor. 2012. Oral processing and flavor sensing mechanisms. In *Food Oral Processing. Fundamentals of Eating and Sensory Perception*, eds. J. Chen, and L. Engelen, 177–202. Chichester: John Wiley & Sons.

Bartoshuk, L.M., J. Gent, F.A. Catalanotto, and R.B. Goodspeed. 1983. Clinical evaluation of taste. *American Journal of Otolaryngology* 4:257–260.

Becker, N., C. Chambliss, C. Marsh, and R. Montemayor. 1995. Effects of mellow and frenetic music and stimulating and relaxing scents on walking by seniors. *Perceptual and Motor Skills* 80:411–415.

Breslin, P.A., N. Doolittle, and P. Dalton. 2001. Subthreshold integration of taste and smell: The role of experience in flavor integration. *Chemical Senses* 26:282:1035.

Bresslin, P.A. 2006. The integration of multiple sensory modalities and the creation of flavor. [Abstract]. *AChemS XXVIIIth Annual Meeting* 305:77.

Brown, S., and E. Shafer. 1888. An investigation into the functions of the occipital and temporal lobes of the monkey's brain. *Philosophical Transactions of the Royal Society of London: Biological Sciences* 179:303–327.

Chiralertpong, A., T.E. Acree, J. Barnard, and K.J. Siebert. 2008. Taste–odor integration in espresso coffee. *Chemical Perception* 1:147–152.

Cowart, B.J., B.P. Halpern, and E.K. Varga. 1999. A clinical test of retronasal olfactory function. *Chemical Senses* 24:608.

Cowart, B.J., B.P. Halpern, D. Rosen, C.T. Klock, and E.D. Pribitkin. 2003. Differential loss of retronasal relative to orthonasal olfaction in a clinical population. *Chemical Senses* 24:A65.

Dalton, P. 2000. Psychophysical and behavioral characteristics of olfactory adaptation. *Chemical Senses* 25:487–492.

Davidson, T.M., and C. Murphy. 1997. Rapid clinical evaluation of anosmia. The alcohol sniff test. *Archives of Otolaryngology—Head and Neck Surgery* 123:6:591–594.

deWijk, R.A., and J. Prinz. 2005. Effects of oral movements on perceived food flavors. *Chemical Senses* 30:A169.

Djordjevic, J., R.J. Zatorre, and M. Jones-Gotman. 2004. Effects of perceived and imagined odors on taste detection. *Chemical Senses* 29:199–208.

Doty, R.L. 1975. An examination of relationships between pleasantness, intensity, and concentration of 10 odorous stimuli. *Perception & Psychophysics* 17:492–496.

Doty, R.L. 2003. *The Odor Memory Test™ Administration Manual*. Haddon Heights, NJ: Sensonics, Inc.

Doty, R.L. 2007. Office procedures for quantitative assessment of olfactory assessment of olfactory function. *American Journal of Rhinology* 21:460–473.

Doty, R.L., P. Shaman, and M. Dann. 1984. Development of the University of Pennsylvania Smell Identification Test: A standardized microencapsulated test of olfactory dysfunction. *Physiology & Behavior* 32:489–502.

Doty, R.L., T.P. Gregor, and R.G. Settle. 1986. Influence of intertribal interval and sniff bottle volume on phenyl ethyl alcohol detection thresholds. *Chemical Senses* 11:259–264.

Doty, R.L., A. Marcus, and W.W. Lee. 1996. Development of the 12-item cross cultural smell identification test (CC-SIT). *Laryngoscope* 106:353–356.

Dragich, A.M., and B.P. Halpern. 2005. Retronasal smelling: An oral cavity component. *Chemical Senses* 30:A202.

Duffy, V., J. Backstrand, and A. Ferris. 1995. Olfactory dysfunction and related nutritional risk in free-living, elderly women. *Journal of the American Dietetic Association* 95:879–884.

Duffy, V.B., W.S. Cain, and A.M. Ferris. 1999. Measurement of sensitivity to olfactory flavor: Application in a study of aging and dentures. *Chemical Senses* 24:671–678.

Duffy, V.B., A.K. Chapo, H.L. Hutchins, D. Snyder, and L.M. Bartoshuk. 2003. Retronasal olfactory intensity: Association with taste. *Chemical Senses* 28:A29.

Engen, T. 1982. *The Perception of Odors*. New York: Academic Press.

Fox, C.B., A.K. Treadway, A.T. Blaszczyk, and R.B. Sleeper. 2012. Megestrol acetate and mirtazapine for the treatment of unplanned weight loss in the elderly. *Pharmacotherapy* 29:4:383–397.

Frasnelli, J., S. Heilmann, and T. Hummel. 2004. Responsiveness of human nasal mucosa to trigeminal stimuli depends on the site of stimulation. *Neuroscience Letter* 62:1:65–69.

Frasnelli, J., M. Ungermann, and T. Hummel. 2008. Ortho- and retronasal presentation of olfactory stimuli modulates odor percepts. *Chemosensory Perception* 1:9–18.

Fujimaru, T., and J. Lim. 2013. Enhancement of odor intensity and hedonics by taste: Roles of nutritive taste and congruency. *AChemS XXXV Annual Meeting, abstract book* P29:40.

Halpern, B.P. 2003. When are oral cavity odorants available for retronasal olfaction? In *Handbook of Flavor Characterization: Sensory, Chemical, and Physiological Techniques*, eds. K.D. Deibler, and J.F. Delwiche, 51–63. New York: Marcel Dekker.

Halpern, B.P. 2004. Retronasal and orthonasal smelling. *ChemoSense* 6:1–7.

Heilmann, S., and T. Hummel. 2004. A new method for comparing orthonasal and retronasal olfaction. *Behavioral Neuroscience* 118:2:412–419.

Heilmann, S., G. Strehle, K. Rosenheim, M. Damm, and T. Hummel. 2002. Clinical assessment of retronasal olfactory function. *Archives of Otolaryngology—Head and Neck Surgery* 128:414–418.

Herz, R., and G. Cupchik. 1995. The emotional distinctiveness of odor-evoked memories. *Chemical Senses* 20:517–528.

Hirsch, A.R. 1992a. Scentsation, olfactory demographic and abnormalities. *International Journal of Aromatherapy* 4:1:16–17.

Hirsch, A.R. 1992b. Nostalgia: A neuropsychiatric understanding. *Advances in Consumer Research* 19:390–395.

Hirsch, A.R. 1998. Scent and sexual arousal. *Medical Aspects of Human Sexuality* 1:3:9–12.

Hirsch, A.R. 1999. Garlic therapy. *Harper's Magazine* 298:1788:32.

Hirsch, A.R., and R. Gomez. 1995. Weight reduction through inhalation of odorants. *Journal of Neurological and Orthopaedic Medicine and Surgery* 16:28–31.

Hirsch, A.R., and J.J. Gruss. 1999. Human male sexual response to olfactory stimuli. *Journal of Neurological and Orthopaedic Medicine and Surgery* 19:14–19.

Hirsch, A.R., and L.H. Johnston. 1996. Odors and learning. *Journal of Neurological and Orthopaedic Medicine and Surgery* 17:2:119–126.

Hirsch, N.H., R. Bone, and A.R. Hirsch. 2013. Tests of retronasal smell in children: Which flavored jelly bean works best? *Chemical Senses* 38:7:A625.

Hollowood, T.A., R.S. Linforth, and A.J. Taylor. 2000. The relationship between carvone release and the perception of mintyness in gelatine gels. In *Flavor Release*, eds. D.D. Roberts, and A. Taylor, Ch. 30, 370–380. Washington, D.C.: American Chemical Society.

Huh, J., K. Park, I.S. Hwang et al. 2008. Brain activation areas of sexual arousal with olfactory stimulation in men: A preliminary study using functional MRI. *Journal of Sexual Medicine* 5:3:619–625.

Hummel, T., and S. Nordin. 2005. Olfactory disorders and their consequences for quality of life. *Acta Otolaryngologica* 125:116–121.

Hummel, T., G. Kobal, H. Gudziol, and A. Mackay-Sim. 2007. Normative data for the "Sniffin' Sticks" including tests of odor identification, odor discrimination, and olfactory thresholds: An upgrade based on a group of more than 3000 subjects. *European Archives of Oto-Rhino-Laryngology* 264:3:237–243.

Jackman, A.H., and R.L. Doty. 2005. Utility of a 3-item smell identification test in detecting olfactory dysfunction. *Laryngoscope* 115:2209–2212.

Joseph, R. 2000. Olfactory limbic system. In *Neuropsychiatry, Neuropsychology, Clinical Neuroscience, 3rd Ed.*, New York: Academic Press.

Kluver, H., and P. Bucy. 1939. Preliminary analysis of function of the temporal lobe in monkeys. *Archives of Neurology* 42:979–1000.

Kobal, G., B. Sekinger, S. Barz, S. Roscher, and S. Wolf. 1996. "Sniffin' Sticks": Screening of olfactory performance. *Rhinology* 34:222–226.

Labbe, D., and N. Martin. 2009. Impact of novel olfactory stimuli at supra- and subthreshold concentrations on the perceived sweetness of sucrose after associative learning. *Chemical Senses* 34:645–651.

Labbe, D., A. Rytz, C. Morgennegg, S. Ali, and N. Martin. 2007. Subthreshold olfactory stimulation can enhance sweetness. *Chemical Senses* 32:205–214.

Labbe, D., F. Gilbert, and N. Martin. 2008. Impact of olfaction on taste, trigeminal, and texture perceptions. *Chemical Perception* 1:217–226.

Lawless, H., and T. Engen. 1977. Associations to odors: Interference, mnemonics, and verbal labeling. *Journal of Experimental Psychology: Human Learning & Memory* 3:52–59.

Leclerq, S., and G. Blancher. 2012. Multimodal sensory integration during sequential eating—Linking chewing activity, aroma release, and aroma perception over time. *Chemical Senses* 37:689–700.

Lim, J., and A. Padmanabhan. 2013. Retronasal olfaction in vegetable liking and disliking. *Chemical Senses* 38:1:45–55.

Martin, G.N. 1998. Human electroencephalographic (EEG) response to olfactory stimulation: Two experiments using the aroma of food. *International Journal of Psychophysiology* 30:3:287–302.

Melzner, J., T. Bitter, O. Guntinas-Lichius, R. Gottschall, M. Walther, and H. Gudziol. 2011. Comparison of the orthonasal and retronasal detection thresholds for carbon dioxide in humans. *Chemical Senses* 36:435–441.

Miwa, T., M. Furukawa, T. Tsukatani, R.M. Costanzo, L.J. DiNardo, and E.R. Reiter. 2001. Impact of olfactory impairment on quality of life and disability. *Archives of Otolaryngology—Head and Neck Surgery* 127:5:497–503.

Mozell, M.M., B.P. Smith, P.E. Smith, R.L. Sullivan, Jr., and P. Swender. 1969. Nasal chemoreception in flavor identification. *Archives of Otolaryngology* 90:131–373.

Murphy, C., and W.S. Cain. 1980. Taste and olfaction: Independence vs interaction. *Physiology & Behavior* 24:601–605.

Murphy, C., W.S. Cain, and L.M. Bartoshuk. 1977. Mutual action of taste and olfaction. *Sensory Processes* 1:3:204–211.

Negoias, S., I. Croy, and J. Gerber. 2010. Reduced olfactory bulb volume and olfactory sensitivity in patients with acute major depression. *Neuroscience* 169:1:415–421.

Ogle, W. 1870. Anosmia, or cases illustrating the physiology and pathology of the sense of smell. *Medico-Chirurgical Transactions* 53:263–290.

Pierce, J., and B.P. Halpern. 1996. Orthonasal and retronasal odorant identification based upon vapor phase input from common substances. *Chemical Senses* 21:5:529–543.

Prescott, J. 1999. Introduction to the trigeminal sense: The role of pungency in food flavours. In *Tastes and Aromas: The Chemical Senses in Science and Industry*, eds. G.A. Bell, and A.J. Watson, 38–49. Sydney: University of New South Wales Press.

Punter, P.H. 1983. Measurement of human olfactory thresholds for several groups of structurally related compounds. *Chemical Senses* 7:215–235.

Puttanniah, V.G., and B.P. Halpern. 2001. Retronasal and orthonasal identification of odorants: Similarities and differences. *Chemical Senses* 26:802.

Roussos, A., M.O. Soto, S. Freels, and A.R. Hirsch. 2014. Comparison of orthonasal to retronasal smell in those with chemosensory dysfunction. In *AChemS XXXVIth Annual Meeting Abstract Book* 292:139–140.

Rozin, P. 1982. "Taste–smell confusions" and the duality of the olfactory sense. *Perception & Psychophysics* 31:4:397–401.

Ruijschop, R.M., A.E.M. Boelrijk, J.A. de Ru, C. de Graaf, and M.S. Westerterp-Plantenga. 2008. Effects of retro-nasal aroma release on satiation. *British Journal of Nutrition* 99:1140–1148.

Small, D.M. 2008. Flavor and the formation of category-specific processing in olfaction. *Chemical Perception* 1:136–146.

Small, D.M., and J. Prescott. 2005. Odor/taste integration and the perception of flavor. *Experimental Brain Research* 166:345–357.

Small, D.M., J.C. Gerber, Y.E. Mak, and T. Hummel. 2005. Differential neural responses evoked by orthonasal versus retronasal odorant perception in humans. *Neuron* 47:593–605.

Spense, C. 2012. Multi-sensory integration and the psychophysics of flavor perception. In *Food Oral Processing. Fundamentals of Eating and Sensory Perception*, eds. J. Chen, and L. Engelen, 203–223. Chichester: John Wiley & Sons.

Stamps, J.J., and L.M. Bartoshuk. 2010. Trigeminal input may compensate for taste loss during flavor perception. *Chemical Senses* 35:A80.

Veldhuizen, M.G., T.G. Shepard, M.F. Wang, and L.E. Marks. 2010. Coactivation of gustatory and olfactory signals in flavor perception. *Chemical Senses* 35:121–133.

Welge-Lüssen, A., A. Husner, M. Wolfensberger, and T. Hummel T. 2009. Influence of simultaneous gustatory stimuli on orthonasal and retronasal olfaction. *Neuroscience Letter* 454:124–128.

White, T.L., and J. Prescott. 2007. Chemosensory cross-modal stroop effects: Congruent odors facilitate taste identification. *Chemical Senses* 32:337–341.

Wininger, D.A., and B.P. Halpern. 1999. Retronasal and orthonasal odorant identification without sniffing. *Chemical Senses* 24:600.

Wolfe, J.M., K.R. Kluender, D.M. Levi et al. 2006. *Sensation & Perception*. 341–343. Sunderland, MA: Sinauer Associates.

4 Taste and Food Choice

Thomas R. Scott

CONTENTS

4.1 Introduction 81
4.2 Gustatory Functional Anatomy 83
    4.2.1 Receptors 83
        4.2.1.1 Papillae 83
        4.2.1.2 Taste Buds 83
        4.2.1.3 Receptor Cells 84
    4.2.2 Peripheral Nerves 84
    4.2.3 Central Taste System 84
        4.2.3.1 Nucleus of the Solitary Tract 84
        4.2.3.2 Thalamic Taste Area 84
        4.2.3.3 Primary Taste Cortex 84
        4.2.3.4 Beyond Primary Taste Cortex 86
4.3 Gustatory Control of Eating 87
    4.3.1 Organization of the Taste System 87
    4.3.2 Enduring Changes in Taste Based on Experience 88
    4.3.3 Transient Changes in Taste Based on Physiological Needs 90
    4.3.4 Momentary Changes in Taste Based on Level of Hunger 90
4.4 Conclusion 95
References 96

4.1 INTRODUCTION

The acquisition of nutrients is the most basic of biological requirements. Each creature must regularly assimilate an array of nutrients to serve the biochemical processes that define its existence. The single purpose of human appetite is to begin the alchemy of turning other organisms into humans.

The sexual motive is nearly as ancient as feeding but more simply satisfied and less urgent. Indeed, successful reproduction is predicated on satisfactory nutrition, for insemination requires energy, and pregnancy only strains nutritional resources, which therefore must prove themselves adequate for conception to occur. Sex is an activity of the fed. Thirst is a newcomer among biological drives. It evolved only in the past few hundred million years, as our ancestors emerged from the seas with the demand that they continue to bathe each cell in the very fluids that they had forsaken.

The search for and acquisition of nutrients is a complex and relentless task that has constituted a central pressure on the evolution of sensory, motor, and cognitive capacities of animals. In the lethal contest between predator and prey, three major types of sensory systems have evolved on each side: vision, sensitivity to vibration (touch, hearing, and lateral line systems), and chemical sensitivity.

The chemical senses are the most primitive of these three, having evolved specialized sensory organs as long as 500 million years ago in coelenterates (Garcia and Hankins 1975). They remain the dominant sensory systems across the animal kingdom as well as within the class Mammalia. We humans are unusual mammals in placing such reliance on vision and hearing. We come to this from our primate heritage, aloft in trees or raised up by our bipedal gait. The collection of sensory systems on our heads is lifted away from the odiferous earth and provided the long views that give value to vision. Yet, chemical senses are central to mammalian evolution and so should have pervasive, if sometimes subtle, influences on human behavior. In accord with their age and status, smell and taste largely manage the two most fundamental biological functions: eating to preserve the individual and reproduction to preserve the species. The sense of taste has become more specialized to serve eating, whereas the sense of smell, reproduction.

Animals sense chemicals that originate both within and beyond the body. Internal communication is accomplished largely through the release of chemicals from one site and their recognition at another, whether it is 200 Å away as in synaptic transmission, or perhaps a meter away as with leptin, insulin, cytokines, or glucose. In contrast, the capacity to detect chemicals from *outside* the body is only poorly developed. Significant deviations from a pH of 7 can lead to sensations of acidity or causticity anywhere on the skin, and certain toxins (e.g., poison ivy, poison oak) may elicit a histamine response. The skin, however, is only a crude chemical detector. The exceptions to this are the points where most chemicals enter the body through the nose and mouth. Here, chemoreception is refined, complex, and subtle, for decisions must be made about which chemicals to admit. Thus, smell and taste are the beginnings of a long chemosensory tube that extends from the face through the intestines, with receptors along its length that are sensitive to the products released by digestion. Consequently, the chemical senses should be responsive to feedback from the gut that is a continuation of their own function—an implication to be confirmed later in this chapter. This system represents a core of chemosensitivity that mediates between the vast array of chemicals around us and the subset of them that serve our tightly regulated biochemical needs.

Chemoreceptors in the mouth are not fundamentally different from those in the rest of the body. The recognition of glucose by a taste receptor and by a β-cell in the pancreas both proceed by similar mechanisms, leading to a perception of sweetness in one case to a release of insulin in the other. The passage of sodium ions through amiloride-sensitive channels produces a salty taste on the tongue but sodium resorption in the kidney. The umami taste of monosodium glutamate and the recognition of glutamate throughout the central nervous system are probably managed by the same receptor, albeit tuned to different concentrations.

What distinguishes the chemical senses is not that they recognize these molecules but that they do so before the irrevocable decision to swallow has been made. Taste is located at the interface between the uncontrolled external chemical world and our highly regulated biochemical environment, and its primary role is to reduce the former to the latter. While preliminary assessments are provided by other senses—notably touch, vision, and olfaction—and by central processes of familiarity and cultural norms, nonetheless, each chemical that enters the mouth goes before a gustatory judge whose only verdicts are swallow or not swallow.

As a chemical gatekeeper, taste provides an assessment of the nutritional value or toxic consequences of a potential food. This input is sent to at least four locations: to the gut to help mediate gastrointestinal reflexes; to the hindbrain to control the somatic reflexes for ingestion or rejection; to the thalamus and insular cortex for a cognitive appreciation of the taste; and to the orbitofrontal cortex (OFC) and ventral forebrain to be integrated with sight, smell, and texture to generate a hedonic response that provides among our most intense pleasure or disgust (Lat: bad taste). It is the hedonic value that determines whether a bite will be extended to a meal, and a meal to a diet.

4.2 GUSTATORY FUNCTIONAL ANATOMY

4.2.1 Receptors

Humans vary by a factor of 100 in the number of taste receptor cells they possess, but the mean is about 300,000 (Miller 1986). They are gathered in groups of approximately 50 in goblet-shaped taste buds, of which the mean number in humans is about 6000. Approximately two-thirds are located on the dorsal surface of the tongue where they are housed in small swellings called papillae (Lat: nipple).

4.2.1.1 Papillae

On the front of the tongue are approximately 200 *fungiform* (Lat: mushroom-shaped) papillae, each of which contains from 0 to 36 buds, with a mean of 3. Thus, a typical person has approximately 600 taste buds in fungiform papillae. On each lateral margin of the tongue are five to seven folds referred to as *foliate* (Lat: leaf-shaped) papillae. The groove between each pair of swellings may contain 100 buds for a total of 1200. On the posterior tongue are 7–11 *circumvallate* (Lat: surrounded by a trench) papillae arranged in the form of a chevron. The moat that surrounds each papilla is lined with taste buds, a mean of 250 per papilla, or approximately 2200 altogether. Beyond these 4000 buds, on the tongue surface are another 2000 embedded in the soft palate, pharynx, larynx, and epiglottis. Without papillae to fix their locations, they are broadly distributed.

4.2.1.2 Taste Buds

Taste buds are of similar shape and composition wherever they occur in the mouth. Each is a collection of perhaps 50 taste cells, arranged like sections of an orange. The resulting globular structure is approximately 30 μm in diameter and 50 μm in length. At the base of the bud is a sturdy membrane surrounded by flattened cells that join to create a shell in which the bud nestles. Thus, each bud is practically isolated with no apparent electrical or diffusional interaction with its neighbors. At the top is a 6-μm-diameter pore through which the microvilli of its 50 receptor cells project to sample the environment.

4.2.1.3 Receptor Cells

Taste receptor cells are created continuously from basal cells at the periphery of the bud to migrate toward the center, where they are dispatched after an average life span of 10 days.

4.2.2 PERIPHERAL NERVES

The peripheral anatomy of the taste system offers such complexity that it was not clarified until the 1930s. Four cranial nerves drain the diverse gustatory receptive fields, and the information they carry is mixed with that from touch and motor fibers that travel in parallel with taste axons.

Taste fibers innervating the front of the tongue exit as part of cranial nerve V (trigeminal) but soon depart to join nerve VII (facial). They are joined by axons from the soft palate to form the sensory component of the predominantly motor nerve VII. At their central terminus, they enter the rostral division of the nucleus of the solitary tract (NST).

Fibers serving the midregion and posterior region of the tongue join nerve IX (glossopharyngeal) and proceed to the NST. Those that serve the esophagus and epiglottis become part of nerve X (vagus) and pass to the NST.

4.2.3 CENTRAL TASTE SYSTEM

4.2.3.1 Nucleus of the Solitary Tract

While the course of peripheral taste nerves remained controversial into the twentieth century, their destination did not (Figure 4.1). All three terminate in orderly fashion in the rostral division of the NST in caudal medulla (Pfaffmann et al. 1961; Makous et al. 1963; Travers and Smith 1979; Scott et al. 1986a). This crucial structure receives taste input in its rostral half, touch, and temperature immediately lateral to taste, and visceral afferents more medially and caudally. Thus, information concerning taste, which largely determines which chemicals enter the body, appropriately terminates in close contiguity with touch and temperature from the mouth (permitting an early integration of some components of flavor) and with fibers from the viscera through which the consequences of having swallowed a chemical may be reported.

4.2.3.2 Thalamic Taste Area

Fibers from the NST in primates project to a small region in the medial thalamus (Figure 4.1). Approximately one-third of the cells here respond to taste stimulation (Pritchard et al. 1989), while others are activated by touch and temperature in the mouth and by visceral stimulation of the vagus nerve. Thus, the intimate relationship whereby taste is located between oral touch on the one side and visceral sensations on the other is apparently maintained.

4.2.3.3 Primary Taste Cortex

Taste realizes its cortical representation along the sharp bend that extends from the anterior insula to the frontal operculum, most commonly known as insular

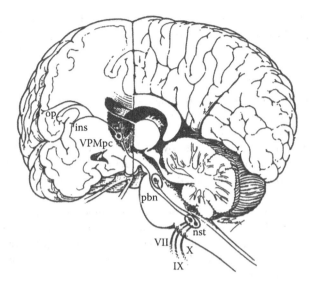

FIGURE 4.1 The human brain, showing the sensory pathways for taste through primary taste cortex (insula). ins: insula; nst: nucleus of the solitary tract; op: operculum; pbn: parabrachial nucleus; VPMpc: parvicellular division of the ventroposteromedial nucleus of the thalamus. (From Pritchard, T.C. The primate gustatory system. In *Taste and Smell in Health and Disease*, eds. T.V. Getchell, R.L. Doty, L.M. Bartoshuk, and J.B. Snow, Jr., 109–125. New York: Raven Press, 1991.)

cortex (Figure 4.1). The area has been explored extensively, revealing that only approximately 6% of its cells respond to taste stimuli (Scott et al. 1986b). This begs the question of what the vast majority of cells in *taste cortex* are engaged in if not taste.

For one, they respond to a variety of somatosensory components of a stimulus, including viscosity, temperature, fat content, grittiness, astringency, and capsaicin (Critchley and Rolls 1996; Rolls 2005). Verhagen et al. (2004) reported that 53% of the insular neurons that responded to oral stimulation were sensitive to viscosity and that another 35% were tuned to stimulus temperature, with individual cells assigned specific temperature ranges. Variations in grittiness and fat content each elicited activity from 8% of the insular cells. Half the neurons responded to only one of these components; half were either bimodal or multimodal.

Others are activated by jaw movements or touch in the mouth. Functional magnetic resonance imaging (MRI) studies have revealed that humans shown expressions of disgust experienced activation of the insula. Thus, the same area that houses taste neurons also has cells that permit a visual appreciation of the social expression of a taste experience (Phillips et al. 1997). The insular cortex also receives visceral sensations and sends axons to regions that guide both oral and visceral reflexes associated with foods. It houses the components of the *ingestive cortex*.

Functional MRI studies using humans have confirmed that the insula is activated by water (deAraujo et al. 2003), stimulus viscosity (deAraujo and Rolls 2004), temperature (Guest et al. 2007), and texture (deAraujo and Simon 2009). More unexpectedly, photographs of food activated the insula, whereas those of nonfood objects did not (Simmons et al. 2005).

It is likely that visceral sensory information also reaches the primary taste cortex. Insular neurons are activated by stimulation of the visceral regions of the esophagus (Weusten et al. 1994; Aziz et al. 1995) and of the throat (Roper et al. 1993), as well as by general visceral arousal induced by phobic anxiety (Rauch et al. 1995). Thus, insular neurons appear to be involved in stimulation by food, beginning with its appearance (vision) and perhaps smell, to contact with the tongue and through the digestive process.

Just as both somatic and visceral sensory systems appear to project into the insula, both oral skeletal and visceral muscles are influenced by its activity. Positron emission tomography (PET) scans revealed insular activation as subjects were instructed to move their mouths and tongues during speech (Raichle 1991), implying involvement in oromotor functions. Seizures that began in the anterior insula (AI) induced vomiting (Fiol et al. 1988) as did electrical stimulation of the insula in experimental animals (Oppenheimer et al. 1992).

Beyond this range of sensory and motor activity, central processes were also implicated. The insula was activated not only by taste stimuli but also by the subject's imagining sweetness or saltiness (Levy et al. 1999). Subjects who were misled and told that the subsequent taste would not be bitter showed less activity to quinine in insula than when they expected bitterness (Nitschke et al. 2006). When subjects were instructed to try to detect a taste that was in fact absent, their taste-related attention elicited an insular response (Veldhuisen et al. 2007). Similar insular responses were seen in those shown images of expressions of disgust (Phillips et al. 1997; Wicker et al. 2003; Jabbi et al. 2008). Finally, when both anticipating and consuming food, obese subjects showed larger activation in the insula than those who were lean (Stice et al. 2008). Thus, imagination, expectation, attention, anticipation, and emotion are brought into the set of features that can affect activity in the insula.

4.2.3.4 Beyond Primary Taste Cortex

In the macaque, neurons in the insular cortex project forward to end in various subdivisions of the OFC. These fibers are joined by those from vision, olfaction, and touch to form a sensory network from which an integrated appreciation of flavor can be extracted. The insula also projects to the central nucleus of the amygdala (CNA), which has robust reciprocal connections with OFC. The amygdala is an important site for processing taste information as well as for the motivational aspects of eating (Scott et al. 1993). Both OFC and CNA—receiving parallel input and themselves interconnected—project to the lateral hypothalamic area (LHA), which is also involved in the motivation to eat.

Finally, all forebrain taste areas send projections back to the NST, establishing a circuit through which higher-order functions such as conditioning can affect the reflexive acceptance or rejection of foods.

4.3 GUSTATORY CONTROL OF EATING

4.3.1 ORGANIZATION OF THE TASTE SYSTEM

All sensory systems must build receptors that are sensitive to the physical environment that they are charged to monitor. So with taste, where there are at least six receptor mechanisms. Four are committed to detecting the major components of our diet: carbohydrates (sweet, starch), fats, proteins (umami), and sodium (salty); the two others are vigilant to the primary threats to our biochemical welfare: acidity (sour) and toxins (bitter). Two of the mechanisms—for salty and sour—rely on the passage of small sodium and hydrogen ions through molecular membranes. The other four require specialized protein receptors.

This federation of receptor mechanisms stands in contrast to the strategies of vision, hearing, and olfaction, each of which employs a single receptor process, though with receptors that are tuned to different parts of the physical dimension that they are assigned to detect (e.g., red versus blue). Taste is more akin to the skin senses where touch, pressure, temperature, pain, and others are separate sensations. Failed attempts to integrate the basic taste sensations at the receptor level have even led to the suggestion that taste is not a single sense but a series of half a dozen senses housed in a common location.

Yet, there *is* a common organizing principle of taste. It eluded researchers because gustatory physiologists adopted the vision model to investigate their discipline, seeking to establish the relationship between the physical stimulus (wavelength) and the perceptual result (color). Taste is faced with a different requirement. Alone among the senses, it must evaluate whether a stimulus will become part of the body. Taste is charged not only with detecting a stimulus as other sensory systems are but also with predicting the impact of that chemical on the animal's physiological welfare. The organizing principle of taste is not physical but physiological (Scott and Mark 1987).

The high degree of effectiveness with which taste manages this obligation is demonstrated in a behavioral study in which naïve rats under 18-h fluid deprivation were offered 15-s exposures to a wide sample of chemicals that appear in the natural environment (Scott and Giza 2000). In these brief tests, with neither experience nor post-ingestive feedback to guide them, rats rejected chemicals in direct proportion to toxicity. Rats inherit a taste system that permits accurate judgments about toxicity across a broad range of chemicals with diverse physical characteristics. While strychnine and cadmium possess entirely different molecular structures and poison the consumer by wholly different mechanisms, the taste system, as the chemical guardian of the body, has the receptors to be vigilant to both. Moreover, the more assiduously a chemical was rejected by rats, the more likely it was to be described by humans as *bitter* or *nauseous*; chemicals avidly accepted by rats were labeled *food-like* or *pleasant*. Thus, the neural dimension of nutrition versus toxicity is directly related to acceptance versus rejection behavior in rats and is perceptually coded in the hedonics of pleasant or unpleasant experiences by humans. With only a few exceptions, the better a chemical tastes, the more nutritious it is.

This basic assessment of whether a substance is nutritious or toxic is developed at birth, as demonstrated by the reactions of newborns to the delivery of sweet, salty, sour, or bitter tastes to tongues that had only moments before been cleared of amniotic fluid (Steiner 1973). Sugars elicited licking and swallowing; quinine evoked gaping, rejection, and crying. Indeed, saccharin injected into the amniotic fluid 6 weeks before birth results in greater sucking and swallowing behavior in the fetus.

Anencephalic neonates, born with no forebrain, reacted identically to healthy babies, demonstrating that these acceptance–rejection reflexes are orchestrated in the hindbrain. The critical location would appear to be the NST. This is the major hindbrain recipient of sensory information that originates within the body, including taste, respiration, blood pressure, blood pH, gastrointestinal activity, and pain (Smith and Scott 2003). Efferents from NST regulate somatic reflexes both for acceptance and rejection and autonomic reflexes associated with digestion.

To control somatic reflexes, clusters of cells in the ventral regions of gustatory NST send projections to the retrofacial area, trigeminal motor nucleus, nucleus ambiguus, and hypoglossal nucleus. The contrary behavioral reactions of acceptance and rejection may be driven by anatomically distinct taste inputs (Grill and Norgren 1978). The greater superficial petrosal and chorda tympani nerves are most sensitive to sweet and salty stimuli and could activate circuits that evoke acceptance responses. The glossopharyngeal nerve is responsive to sour and bitter qualities and could stimulate a separate population of NST taste cells from which rejection reflexes were organized.

Autonomic reflexes are controlled by a second set of axons from the ventral gustatory NST, which travels caudally to the viscerosensory NST, to the salivatory nuclei, and to the dorsal motor nucleus of the vagus, to invoke parasympathetic processes associated with digestion (Travers 1993). These include salivation, gastric reflexes, and cephalic phase releases of digestive enzymes and insulin. The dorsal motor nucleus of the vagus, whose output controls these processes, lies directly beneath the NST and sends apical dendrites toward the taste area, though their contact with taste cells of the NST has not yet been demonstrated. These cephalic phase reflexes prepare the digestive system for the nutrients that they are destined to receive when a sweet or other foodlike taste is registered in the NST.

Thus the sense of taste is organized to perform a general differentiation of toxins from nutrients and that this is accomplished at a brainstem level and is intact at or before birth in humans. Moreover, this analysis drives somatic reflexes of swallowing or rejection, parasympathetic reflexes that anticipate the digestive process, and inform the hedonic reaction to the tasted chemical. While providing a broad and effective system for maintaining the biochemical welfare of the species, this organization would not allow for the idiosyncratic allergies or biochemical needs of the individual, or be sensitive to changes in those needs over time. The effects of experience—conditioned aversions or preferences—and of age, reproductive status, disease state, mineral needs, and level of satiety all affect behavioral reactions to foods. To serve these requirements, the taste code must be plastic.

4.3.2 ENDURING CHANGES IN TASTE BASED ON EXPERIENCE

An animal's experience has a pronounced and enduring effect on behavioral reactions to taste stimuli. The taste experiences of suckling rats establish preferences that persist into adulthood (Galef and Henderson 1972; Capretta and Rawls 1974). Preferences also develop through association of taste with positive visceral reinforcement such as the delivery of a nutrient of which the animal has been deprived (Rozin and Rogers 1967; Revusky et al. 1971; Booth et al. 1974). An efficient experimental paradigm has been developed to create conditioned preferences in rats (Sclafani and Nissenbaum 1988). Animals fitted with gastric cannulae are offered two taste solutions equally preferred. Upon licking one, water is delivered into the stomach, whereas with the other, a rich nutrient mix is delivered. After several days of trials, the rats overwhelmingly select whichever taste solution was associated with the receipt of nutrients. Such learned preferences among humans probably serve to bind members of a culture together through culinary identity. Each of the major cuisines of the world is characterized by unique flavors delivered with a nutritive carbohydrate load. Conditioned preferences for those tastes serve as the basis for the culinary rituals and social interactions identified with that culture.

The activity of single taste neurons in the NST of rats reflects the neural changes that may underlie these conditioned preferences. Upon undergoing the experimental procedure described above, rats developed preferences for the taste solution associated with the gastric infusion of nutrients, as expected. Responses to these, as well as innately appetitive (e.g., glucose) and aversive (e.g., quinine) tastes, were then monitored in the NST. It was revealed that whichever taste had become preferred, its neural profile was less like those of aversive and more like those of appetitive stimuli (Giza et al. 1997). Thus, in rats, the taste system itself is altered at the brainstem level to reflect gustatory experiences, and this alteration may provide the basis for food preferences that develop throughout life.

Contrasted with the subtlety of conditioned preferences is the potent and instantaneous aversion resulting from a single pairing of a novel taste with nausea: the conditioned taste aversion (CTA). As opposed to gently guiding the animal toward tastes that have been associated with nutrients, the CTA is an intense alarm to protect the animal that survives its first encounter with a toxin from ever consuming that substance again (Garcia et al. 1955). It is so readily established, potent, and enduring that the CTA protocol has become a standard tool for studying taste behavior and physiology.

The mechanisms underlying the development of CTAs have been studied mainly in rats. Taste-evoked activity in the NST (Chang and Scott 1984; McCaughey et al. 1997) and in the parabrachial nucleus (PBN) (Shimura et al. 1997) rises to a taste that is paired with nausea. In the NST, that increase is associated with a reorganization of inputs such that the incriminated taste no longer elicits swallowing reflexes and parasympathetic activity designed to ingest and assimilate the chemical but rather induces the opposite: rejection reflexes. In the PBN, the evoked activity shifts from a subnucleus associated with positive hedonics to one normally activated by aversive tastes (Yamamoto 1993). Discrete subnuclei of the PBN are hypothesized to send separate projections to forebrain areas that analyze taste quality and hedonics. Thus, the shift in representation of the offending taste could serve as the basis for its reversed hedonics—from appealing to disgusting—established in the brainstem but manifested in the forebrain.

4.3.3 TRANSIENT CHANGES IN TASTE BASED ON PHYSIOLOGICAL NEEDS

An animal's choice of foods is related to its physiological condition. The *body wisdom* demonstrated in cafeteria studies by Richter appear to be related to taste-directed changes in food preferences. Animals deprived of thiamine (Seward and Greathouse 1973), threonine (Halstead and Gallagher 1962), or histidine (Sanahuja and Harper 1962) will experiment with different tasting foods until chancing upon one that supplies the missing nutrient.

Another need, reflected in a more constant and perhaps innate preference, is for sodium, whose concentration must be maintained at approximately 0.14 M to serve its functions of electrical conductance and the provision of osmotic force. Mammals seek out and consume salt and, when plentiful, do so in excess of need, as the American diet demonstrates (Richter 1936; Denton 1976). This preference becomes exaggerated under conditions of sodium deficiency. Humans depleted by pathological states (Wilkins and Richter 1940) or experimental manipulation (McCance 1936) show a pronounced craving for salt. Similarly, rats subjected to uncontrolled urinary sodium loss following adrenalectomy (Clark and Clausen 1943; Epstein and Stellar 1955) to acute loss of plasma volume (Stricker and Jalowiec 1970) or to sodium dietary restriction (Fregley et al. 1965) show sharp increases in sodium consumption. This compensatory response to the physiological need for salt results from a change in the hedonic value of tasted sodium. Concentrations that are rejected when the animal is sodium-replete are avidly accepted when deprived. This change in taste-based behavior can also be traced to changes in the neural response to salt.

The activity generated by sodium in the peripheral taste nerves declines when a rat is in particular need of salt (Contreras 1977; Contreras and Frank 1979), a result that should lead to the observed shift of the acceptance curve for sodium to higher concentrations. Beyond this, however, recordings in the NST reveal that the central nervous system has added a more complex adaptation to the need for sodium. NST responses to sodium in salt-deprived rats declined moderately, as expected from the peripheral nerve reports. But an analysis of the contributions of individual neurons revealed that salt-responsive neurons showed a precipitous reduction in evoked activity and that this was partially offset by an increased response in neurons normally tuned to sweet tastes. Thus, the net effect was to transfer the burden of signaling sodium from salty- toward sweet-oriented cells (Jacobs et al. 1988). Thus, sodium might taste *sweet* or, if sweetness is only a human construct, perhaps *good* to such a rat. This interpretation transcends a mere change in intensity perception and explains the eagerness with which deprived rats consume sodium, an avidity not created simply by decreasing the concentration of sodium, as the peripheral nerve work would imply. Whether based on changes in intensity or on a shift in perceived quality, however, it is clear that adaptive alterations in taste preferences are governed by modifications in the sensory code.

4.3.4 MOMENTARY CHANGES IN TASTE BASED ON LEVEL OF HUNGER

While the appreciation of amino acid or sodium deficiency occurs and may be restored over a period of days, the availability of glucose and other sources of energy is of an almost hourly concern. There must be an accommodation of the decision to swallow or reject, and in the hedonic evaluation that drives that decision, as the dangers of malnutrition weigh against those of ingesting a toxin. Common experience reinforces the results of psychophysical studies: as hunger increases, foods become more palatable; with satiety, they are less so (Campbell 1958; Cabanac 1971; Rolls et al. 1981). There is now a body of data from rats and primates that demonstrate the neural mechanisms underlying these changes.

The first effect of consuming a meal is gastric distension. Experimentally distending a rat's stomach with air causes the taste response to sucrose, recorded in the NST, to decline, implying a less rewarding experience to the rat (Glenn and Erickson 1976). The next effect of a meal is to raise blood sugar levels. When these were increased experimentally through an intravenous infusion of glucose, taste responses to sugar in the NST also declined (Giza and Scott 1984). Similar but smaller effects on taste activity were seen with modest infusions of insulin (Giza and Scott 1987a) or glucagon (Giza et al. 1993), both of which result in the greater availability of glucose to the muscles, though by different mechanisms. Thus, each procedure that delivered glucose to the body caused a transient reduction in sensitivity to sugars in the NST. This implies a partial loss of the pleasure that sustains eating, making termination of a meal more likely.

If sensory activity in NST, deep in the hindbrain, declines with satiety, the perceived intensity of a taste should also be reduced. This has indeed been shown to occur in rats (Giza and Scott 1987b). Humans, however, respond differently. They report that the hedonic value of foods decreases with satiety, but intensity judgments are affected to a lesser extent or not at all (Thompson et al. 1976; Sharma et al. 1977). This prompted a series of studies in macaques, who had proven to be worthy surrogates for human gustation (Smith-Swintosky et al. 1991), on the impact of satiety at various synaptic levels, from the hindbrain to the cortex.

The initial recordings were from the NST to mimic those from the rat. A neuron was isolated, and its responses to sugar, salt, acid, and quinine were recorded. The monkey was then fed 50-mL aliquots of glucose, after each of which the responses to the same four taste stimuli in the NST were reassessed (Yaxley et al. 1985). As the monkey proceeded through this sequence toward satiety, and as avid acceptance of the glucose eventually progressed to active rejection, the responsiveness of NST neurons remained constant. In contradiction to the findings in the rats, the hindbrain taste neurons in primates were not influenced by the induction of satiety (Figure 4.2).

The recordings proceeded to the primary taste cortex in the anterior insula with the same result (Yaxley et al. 1988). Even as the macaque progressed from eager acceptance of glucose to total rejection, the responsiveness of taste cells in the insular cortex to each of the four basic tastes remained constant. The insula has proven to house taste cells that give the most precise cognitive evaluation of stimulus quality (Scott and Plata-Salamán 1999). These results would imply that this evaluation is unfettered with implications for liking or disliking these tastes.

From the insula, projections proceed forward to the OFC, where taste has at least two representations (Carmichael and Price 1996). The first, with the higher concentration of taste cells, and purer representation of taste, is toward the midline, in the

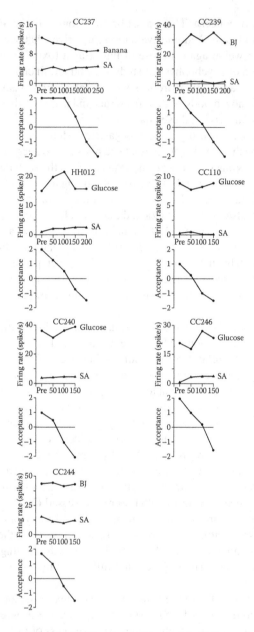

FIGURE 4.2 Seven independent trials of the effects of feeding monkeys to satiety on the neural response to the satiating solution in the NTS. SA: spontaneous activity. Under the neural response data for each trial, the willingness of the monkey to accept (+2) or reject (−2) the solution is shown as a function of the amount of solution delivered. The satiating solution was 20% glucose in each case except for the two trials of blackcurrant juice (BJ) and one of banana. Monkeys were fed 50 mL of the solution and tested neurally and behaviorally after each aliquot. Pre: the discharge rate of each neuron before the satiety trials began. (From Yaxley, S. et al., *Brain Res*, 347:83–95, 1985.)

medial OFC (Pritchard et al. 2005). Here, taking a macaque from hunger to satiety caused variable effects on the responsiveness of taste cells. Most showed a decline in sensitivity, but others were unmodified, just like those at earlier synaptic levels. Moreover, when a decline occurred, it was generic to all stimuli (Pritchard et al. 2007). In addition, a subpopulation of neurons that had been silent began responding to taste stimuli as the monkey neared satiety, implying the existence of an active component to satiety. These cells may blunt hunger.

The transitional state found in the medial OFC—a partial reflection of hedonic decline, though not specific to the satiating stimulus—was refined in the caudolateral OFC to which the medial OFC may project. Here, taste cells were tuned more narrowly than at earlier synapses and responded more specifically to changing hedonics (Rolls et al. 1989). Feeding a macaque to satiety on glucose was associated with a total loss of response to glucose in the caudolateral OFC, whereas the activity evoked by other stimuli was nearly unchanged (Figure 4.3). Just as humans report the loss of appeal of foods that they have consumed to satiety, they still derive pleasure from others, which is a phenomenon dubbed as sensory-specific satiety (Rolls et al. 1983; Rolls 1986). Thus, a filling entrée may still be complemented by an appealing dessert.

Cells in the caudolateral OFC demonstrated other properties that relate to human food choices. A portion of the taste cells also responded to the sight, smells, and textures of foods, though not to those of nonfood objects (Rolls et al. 1998, 1999; Verhagen et al. 2003). They would be ideally informed to integrate sensory activity into an amalgam that we know as flavor. Thus, in the caudolateral OFC of macaques are neurons equipped to evaluate the full sensory experience of eating and to reflect—perhaps direct—changes in the desirability of foods as a meal progresses.

Imaging studies using PET and functional MRI have been conducted on human subjects to identify areas associated with taste, flavor, and reward. Neurons in the OFC were generally activated by affectively charged stimuli (deAraujo et al. 2003; Small et al. 2003) or by the subject's level of hunger (Gautier et al. 2000; Del Parigi et al. 2002). Whether a function of the technical approach (single-neuron electrophysiology versus imaging) or a true species difference, the region associated with hunger and satiety in humans appears considerably larger than in macaque. In humans, most of the caudal OFC is activated by hunger and part of the anterior OFC by satiety (Tataranni et al. 1999). It is likely that the broad distribution of activity associated with eating in the human OFC reflects the activation of reward systems rather than flavor perception per se (O'Doherty et al. 2002; Kringelbach and Rolls 2004).

The caudolateral OFC is part of a complex that also includes the ventral forebrain regions, specifically the central nucleus of the amygdala (Scott et al. 1993) and the LHA (Norgren 1970; Burton et al. 1976). Recordings from each of these regions reveal activity much like that in the caudolateral OFC, with reduced responsiveness to a taste on which a macaque is fed to satiety (Karádi et al. 1992; Yan and Scott 1996).

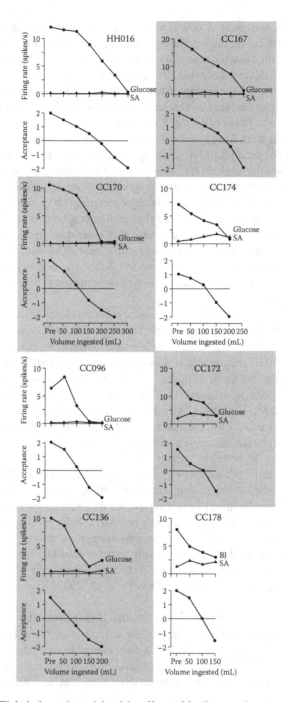

FIGURE 4.3 Eight independent trials of the effects of feeding monkeys to satiety on the neural response to the satiating solution in the caudolateral orbitofrontal cortex. The organization and abbreviations are as in Figure 4.2. (From Rolls, E.T. et al., *Eur J Neurosci*, 1:53–60, 1989.)

4.4 CONCLUSION

A progression from *recognition* to *analysis* to *integration* takes place as we proceed up the nervous system. Recognition occurs at the receptors. Early analysis at the level of the NST permits the control of reflexes for acceptance or rejection, as well as of the parasympathetic reflexes that anticipate digestive processes. Cells in the NST and PBN enable the associative processes involved in appetitive and aversive conditioning and in the mediation of sodium appetite. In the rat, these hindbrain gustatory relays also reflect changes in physiological condition of the animal, from satiety to hunger over a period of hours, or the reverse over just minutes of eating.

In primates, represented in behavioral and neural imaging studies of humans and in electrophysiological experiments in macaques, the reflexive responses to taste stimuli appear to be managed in the hindbrain as in rats. Taste quality is most accurately represented in the primary taste cortex in the insula. Beyond this level, integration is the major theme both with other sensory systems and with central motivational states. In the caudolateral OFC, taste activity converges with that of the sight, smell, and texture of foods and is subject to modification according to the monkey's level of hunger. These properties are extended to subsequent processing stages in the amygdala and hypothalamus. Thus, what begins as an analysis of chemical structure at the receptor becomes a component of the assessment of flavor and serves to drive the motivational systems that guide the selection and consumption of foods.

Throughout the history of scientific research on feeding, human and animal studies have approached the topic from different perspectives, asked different questions, and employed different techniques. Humans were addressed in psychophysical studies, and animals in those that were behavioral and electrophysiological. There are three levels of ambiguity that intervene when investigators attempt to relate human and animal data on feeding.

Species differences between humans and the dominant animal model—the rat—comprise the first level. Differences in how humans and rats process orosensory information have been demonstrated both anatomically and functionally. Norgren and his colleagues (Norgren and Leonard 1971; Norgren 1976) have reported that PBN is a major obligatory synaptic relay for taste in rats, whereas gustatory fibers appear to bypass the PBN in primates. This difference gains significance in that the PBN in rats sends dual projections, both to the thalamocortical axis and to a series of ventral forebrain sites, such that the cognitive and hedonic components of a food may be processed in parallel. Lacking the relay in the PBN, taste in primates proceeds from the NST to the thalamus and the insular cortex before being relayed to the OFC and the ventral forebrain, thus implying serial rather than parallel processing.

This presumed strategic difference has functional consequences. Manipulations of hunger levels affected gustatory responsiveness in the hindbrains of rats (Giza and Scott 1984, 1987a; Giza et al. 1993) but not primates (Yaxley et al. 1985). Rather, these inevitable impacts are reserved for later processing in primates after a cognitive analysis of taste quality has presumably been performed. This implies that primates may identify a taste and then independently determine its hedonic value, whereas in rats, these functions may be one. With the hindbrain accepting the responsibility of modifying its responsiveness to suit the animal's momentary needs, the rat may simply eat what tastes good and reject the rest.

Second is the neural level: the cortex versus the hindbrain. When a psychophysicist requests a verbal reply from a human subject, it is the cortex that is engaged. In contrast, most electrophysiology in rats has been performed in hindbrain relays: NST and PBN. The rat's thalamic taste relay is small and difficult to access, and cortical taste responses have been compromised by the use of anesthetics (see the anesthetic effects below). Thus, the majority of information from humans is cortically mediated and so vastly more processed than responses from the rodent's hindbrain.

Anesthetic effects comprise the third level. Taste, being phylogenetically old, lies deep in the nervous system, near the midline. It requires penetrating surgery to access taste nuclei, and so general anesthesia. The resultant impact of suppressing activity at higher-order levels of the CNS is felt in hindbrain nuclei, whose responses are typically exaggerated by relief from the tonic inhibition normally placed on them by forebrain neurons. Therefore, anesthesia may both impair recordings from the rodent cortex and adulterate the quality of data obtained from hindbrain nuclei.

There have been signal advances from both the animal and human sides of this dichotomy that have served to reduce the ambiguities that we face in interpreting gustatory data. Electrophysiological recordings may now be obtained from unanesthetized or lightly anesthetized rats, which are implanted with chronic recording chambers and actively licking tastants. But the major advance in mediating between human and animal studies is the development of an awake primate recording model. Species differences are minimized, as verified by reports demonstrating that taste processing in the macaque cortex is nearly identical to the taste experiences reported by humans in psychophysical studies (Scott and Plata-Salamán 1999). The macaque cortex is readily accessible and may be investigated through hundreds of recording tracks over a period of months, providing an analog to extended psychophysical tests with humans. Anesthetics are not required for the painless recording procedures, and the monkeys sit comfortably, tasting a variety of stimuli and offering behavioral reactions to them.

Just as studies of animals are becoming more expansive to approach those in humans, neural imaging experiments in humans now permit an investigation of activity elicited in the nervous system by taste stimuli, a domain formerly restricted to animal studies. As mentioned above, PET and functional MRI experiments now provide insights into responses of the human nervous system to orosensory stimulation. The constraints with these techniques lie in the lack of precise localization of activated neurons and in the very newness of a field that is still seeking accepted standards against which further data may be compared. Nonetheless, imaging studies will eventually extend the study of human responses to orosensory stimulation from the psychophysical to the neural to complete the bridge between human and animal studies.

REFERENCES

Aziz, Q., P.L. Furlong, J. Barlow et al. 1995. Topographic mapping of cortical potentials evoked by distension of the human proximal and distal oesophagus. *Electroencephalogr Clin Neurophysiol* 96:219–229.

Booth, D.A., R. Stoloff, and J. Nicholls. 1974. Dietary flavor acceptance in infant rats established by association with effects of nutrient composition. *Physiol Psychol* 2:313–319.

Burton, M.J., E.T. Rolls, and F. Mora. 1976. Effects of hunger on the responses of neurons in the lateral hypothalamus to the sight and taste of food. *Expl Neurol* 51:668–676.

Cabanac, M. 1971. Physiological role of pleasure. *Science* 173:1103–1107.

Campbell, B.A. 1958. Absolute and relative sucrose preference thresholds in hungry and satiated rats. *J Comp Physiol Psychol* 51:795–800.

Capretta, P.J. and L.H. Rawls. 1974. Establishment of a flavor preference in rats: Importance of nursing and weaning experience. *J Comp Physiol Psychol* 86:670–673.

Carmichael, S.T. and J.L. Price. 1996. Sensory and premotor connections of the orbital and medial prefrontal cortex of macaque monkeys. *J Comp Neurol* 363:642–664.

Chang, F.C. and T.R. Scott. 1984. Conditioned taste aversions modify neural responses in the rat nucleus tractus solitarius. *J Neurosci* 4:1850–1862.

Clark, W.G. and D.F. Clausen. 1943. Dietary "self-selection" and appetites of untreated and treated adrenalectomized rats. *Am J Physiol* 139:70–79.

Contreras, R. 1977. Changes in gustatory nerve discharges with sodium deficiency: A single unit analysis. *Brain Res* 121:373–378.

Contreras, R. and M. Frank. 1979. Sodium deprivation alters neural responses to gustatory stimuli. *J Gen Physiol* 73:569–594.

Critchley, H.D. and E.T. Rolls. 1996. Responses of primary taste cortex neurons to the astringent tastant tannic acid. *Chem Senses* 21:125–135.

deAraujo, I.E.T. and E.T. Rolls. 2004. Representation in the human brain of food texture and oral fat. *J Neurosci* 24:3086–3093.

deAraujo, I.E.T and S.A. Simon. 2009. The gustatory cortex and multisensory integration. *Int J Obes* 33:534–543.

deAraujo, I.E.T., M.L. Kringelbach, E.T. Rolls, and F. McGlone. 2003. Human cortical responses to water in the mouth, and the effects of thirst. *J Neurophysiol* 90:1865–1876.

Del Parigi, A., J.F. Gautier, and K. Chen. 2002. Neuroimaging and obesity: Mapping the brain responses to hunger and satiation in humans using positron emission tomography. *Ann NY Acad Sci* 967:389–397.

Denton, D.A. 1976. Hypertension: A malady of civilization? In *Systemic Effects of Hypertensive Agents*, ed. M.P. Sambhi, pp. 577–583. New York: Stratton Intercontinental Medical Books.

Epstein, A.N. and E. Stellar. 1955. The control of salt preference in adrenalectomized rat. *J Comp Physiol Psychol* 46:167–172.

Fiol, M.E., I.E. Leppik, R. Mireles, and R. Maxwell. 1988. Ictus emeticus and the insular cortex. *Epilepsy Res* 2:127–131.

Fregley, M.J., J.M. Harper, and E.P. Radford, Jr. 1965. Regulation of sodium chloride intake by rats. *Am J Physiol* 209:287–292.

Galef, Jr., B.G. and P.W. Henderson. 1972. Mother's milk: A determinant of the feeding preferences of weaning rat pups. *J Comp Physiol Psychol* 78:213–219.

Garcia, J. and W.G. Hankins. 1975. The evolution of bitter and the acquisition of toxiphobia. In *Olfaction and Taste, vol. V*, eds. D.A. Denton and J.P. Coughlan, pp. 39–45. New York: Academic Press.

Garcia, J., D.J. Kimmeldorf, and R.A. Koelling. 1955. Conditional aversion to saccharin resulting from exposure to gamma radiation. *Science* 122:157–158.

Gautier, J.F., K. Chen, and A.D. Salbe. 2000. Differential brain responses to satiation in obese and lean men. *Diabetes* 49:838–846.

Giza, B.K. and T.R. Scott. 1984. Blood glucose selectively affects taste-evoked activity in the rat nucleus tractus solitarius. *Physiol Behav* 31:643–650.

Giza, B.K. and T.R. Scott. 1987a. Intravenous insulin infusions in rats decrease gustatory-evoked responses to sugars. *Am J Physiol* 252:R994–R1002.

Giza, B.K. and T.R. Scott. 1987b. Blood glucose level affects perceived sweetness intensity in rats. *Physiol Behav* 41:459–464.

Giza, B.K., R.O. Deems, D.A. VanderWeele, and T.R. Scott. 1993. Pancreatic glucagon suppresses gustatory responsiveness to glucose. *Am J Physiol* 265:R1231–R1237.

Giza, B.K., K. Ackroff, S.A. McCaughey, A. Sclafani, and T.R. Scott. 1997. Preference conditioning alters taste responses in the nucleus of the solitary tract of the rat. *Am J Physiol* 273:R1230–R1240.

Glenn, J.F. and R.P. Erickson. 1976. Gastric modulation of gustatory afferent activity. *Physiol Behav* 16:561–568.

Grill, H.J. and R. Norgren. 1978. The taste reactivity test. II. Mimetic responses to gustatory stimuli in chronic thalamic and chronic decerebrate rats. *Brain Res* 143:281–297.

Guest, S., F. Grabenhorst, G. Essick et al. 2007. Human cortical representation of oral temperature. *Physiol Behav* 92:975–984.

Halstead, W.C. and B.B. Gallagher. 1962. Autoregulation of amino acids intake in the albino rats. *J Comp Physiol Psychol* 55:107–111.

Jabbi, M., J. Bastiaansen, and C. Keysers. 2008. A common anterior insula representation of disgust observation, experience and imagination shows divergent functional connectivity pathways. *PLoS ONE* 3:8:e2939.

Jacobs, K.M., G.P. Mark, and T.R. Scott. 1988. Taste responses in the nucleus tractus solitarius of sodium-deprived rats. *J Physiol* 406:393–410.

Karádi, Z., Y. Oomura, H. Nishino, T.R. Scott, and L. Lénárd. 1992. Responses of lateral hypothalamic glucose-sensitive and glucose-insensitive neurons to chemical stimuli in behaving rhesus monkeys. *J Neurophysiol* 67:389–400.

Kringelbach, M.L. and E.T. Rolls. 2004. The functional neuroanatomy of the human orbitofrontal cortex: Evidence from neuroimaging and neurophysiology. *Prog Neurobiol* 72:341–372.

Levy, L.M., R.I. Henkin, C.S. Lin, A. Finley, and D. Shellinger. 1999. Taste memory induces brain activation as revealed by functional MRI. *J Comput Assist Tomog* 23:499–505.

Makous, W., S. Nord, B. Oakley, and C. Pfaffmann. 1963. The gustatory relay in the medulla. In *Olfaction and Taste*, ed. Y. Zotterman, pp. 381–393. New York: Pergamon Press.

McCance, R.A. 1936. Experimental sodium chloride deficiency in man. *Proc R Soc Lond* 119:245–268.

McCaughey, S.A., B.K. Giza, L.J. Nolan, and T.R. Scott. 1997. Extinction of a conditioned taste aversion in rats. II. Neural effects in the nucleus of the solitary tract. *Physiol Behav* 61:373–379.

Miller, Jr., I.J. 1986. Variation in human fungiform taste bud densities among regions and subjects. *Anat Rec* 216:474–482.

Nitschke, J.B., G.E. Dixon, I. Sarinopoulos et al. 2006. Altering expectancy dampens neural response to aversive taste in primary taste cortex. *Nat Neurosci* 9:435–442.

Norgren, R. 1970. Gustatory responses in the hypothalamus. *Brain Res* 21:63–70.

Norgren, R. 1976. Taste pathways to hypothalamus and amygdala. *J Comp Neurol* 166:17–30.

Norgren, R. and C.M. Leonard. 1971. Taste pathways in rat brainstem. *Science* 173:1136–1139.

O'Doherty, J.P., R. Deichmann, and H.D. Critchley. 2002. Neural responses during anticipation of a primary taste reward. *Neuron* 33:815–826.

Oppenheimer, S.M., A. Gelb, J.P. Girvin, and V.C. Hachinski. 1992. Cardiovascular effects of human insular cortex stimulation. *Neurol* 42:1927–1932.

Pfaffmann, C., R. Erickson, G. Frommer, and B. Halpern. 1961. Gustatory discharges in the rat medulla and thalamus. In *Sensory Communication*, ed. W.A. Rosenblith, pp. 455–473. Cambridge, MA: MIT Press.

Phillips, M.L., A.W. Young, C. Sr. et al. 1997. A specific neural substrate for perceiving facial expressions of disgust. *Nature* 389:495–498.

Pritchard, T.C. 1991. The primate gustatory system. In *Taste and Smell in Health and Disease*, eds. T.V. Getchell, R.L. Doty, L.M. Bartoshuk, and J.B. Snow, Jr., pp. 109–125. New York: Raven Press.

Pritchard, T.C., R.B. Hamilton, and R. Norgren. 1989. Neural coding of gustatory information in the thalamus of *Macaca mulatta*. *J Neurophysiol* 61:1–14.

Pritchard, T.C., E.M. Edwards, C.A. Smith, E.E. Nedderman, G.J. Schwartz, and T.R. Scott. 2005. Gustatory neural responses in the medial orbitofrontal cortex of the Old World monkey. *J Neurosci* 25:6047–6056.

Pritchard, T.C., G.J. Schwartz, and T.R. Scott. 2007. Taste in the medial orbitofrontal cortex of the macaque. *Ann NY Acad Sci* 1121:121–135.

Raichle, M.E. 1991. Memory mechanisms in the processing of words and word-like symbols. Exploring brain functional anatomy with positron tomography. *Ciba Foundat Symp* 163:198–204.

Rauch, S.L., C.R. Savage, N.M. Alpert et al. 1995. A positron emission tomographic study of simple phobic symptom provocation. *Arch Gen Psychiat* 52:10–28.

Revusky, S.H., M.H. Smith, and D.V. Chalmers. 1971. Flavor preferences: Effects of ingestion-contingent intravenous saline or glucose. *Physiol Behav* 6:341–343.

Richter, C.P. 1936. Increased salt appetite in adrenalectomized rats. *Am J Physiol* 115:55–161.

Rolls, B.J. 1986. Sensory-specific satiety. *Nutr Rev* 44:93–101.

Rolls, B.J., E.T. Rolls, E.A. Rowe, and K. Sweeney. 1981. Sensory-specific satiety in man. *Physiol Behav* 27:137–142.

Rolls, E.T. 2005. Taste and related systems in primates including humans. *Chem Senses* 30:i76–i77.

Rolls, E.T., B.J., Rolls, and E.A. Rowe. 1983. Sensory-specific and motivation-specific satiety for the sight and taste of food and water in man. *Physiol Behav* 30:185–192.

Rolls, E.T., Z.J. Sienkiewicz, and S. Yaxley. 1989. Hunger modulates the responses to gustatory stimuli of single neurons in the caudolateral orbitofrontal cortex of the macaque monkey. *Eur J Neurosci* 1:53–60.

Rolls, E.T., H.D. Critchley, A. Browning, and I. Hernadi. 1998. The neurophysiology of taste and olfaction in primates and umami flavor. *Ann NY Acad Sci* 855:426–437.

Rolls, E.T., H.D. Critchley, A.S. Browning, I. Hernadi, and L. Lénárd. 1999. Responses to the sensory properties of fat of neurons in the primate orbitofrontal cortex. *J Neurosci* 19:1532–1540.

Roper, S.N., M.F. Lévesque, W.W. Sutherling, and J. Engel, Jr. 1993. Surgical treatment of partial epilepsy arising from the insular cortex. *J Neurosurg* 79:226–229.

Rozin, P. and W. Rogers. 1967. Novel-diet preferences in vitamin-deficient rats and rats recovered from vitamin deficiency. *J Comp Physiol Psychol* 63:421–428.

Sanahuja, J.C. and A.E. Harper. 1962. Effect of amino acid imbalance on food intake and preference. *Am J Physiol* 202:165–170.

Sclafani, A. and J.W. Nissenbaum. 1988. Robust conditioned flavor preference produced by intragastric starch infusions in rats. *Am J Physiol* 255:R672–R675.

Scott, T.R. and B.K. Giza. 2000. Issues of gustatory neural coding: Where they stand today. *Physiol Behav* 69:65–76.

Scott, T.R., and G.P. Mark. 1987. The taste system encodes stimulus toxicity. *Brain Res* 414:197–203.

Scott, T.R., and C.R. Plata-Salamán. 1999. Taste in the monkey cortex. *Physiol Behav* 67:489–511.

Scott, T.R., S. Yaxley, Z.J. Sienkiewicz, and E.T. Rolls. 1986a. Gustatory responses in the nucleus tractus solitarius of the alert cynomolgus monkey. *J Neurophysiol* 55:182–200.

Scott, T.R., S. Yaxley, Z.J. Sienkiewicz, and E.T. Rolls. 1986b. Gustatory responses in the frontal opercular cortex of the alert cynomolgus monkey. *J Neurophysiol* 56:876–890.

Scott, T.R., Z. Karadi, Y. Oomura, H. Nishino, and C.R. Plata-Salamán. 1993. Gustatory neural coding in the amygdala of the alert macaque monkey. *J Neurophysiol* 69:1810–1820.

Seward, J.P. and S.R. Greathouse. 1973. Appetitive and aversive conditioning in thiamine-deficient rats. *J Comp Physiol* 83:157–167.

Sharma, K.N., H.L. Jacobs, and V. Gopal. 1977. Nutritional state/taste interactions in food intake: Behavioral and physiological evidence for gastric/taste modulation. In *The Chemical Senses and Nutrition*, eds. M.R. Kare and O. Maller, pp. 167–187. New York: Academic Press.

Shimura, T., H. Tanaka, and T. Yamamoto. 1997. Salient responsiveness of parabrachial neurons to the conditioned stimulus after the acquisition of taste aversion learning in rats. *Neurosci* 81:239–247.

Simmons, W.K., A. Martin, and L.W. Barsalou. 2005. Pictures of appetizing foods activate gustatory cortices for taste and reward. *Cereb Cort* 15:1602–1608.

Small, D.M., M.D. Gregory, and Y.E. Mak. 2003. Dissociation of neural representation of intensity and affective valuation in human gestation. *Neuron* 39:701–711.

Smith, D.V. and T.R. Scott. 2003. Gustatory neural coding. In *Handbook of Olfaction and Gustation, 2nd Edition*, ed. R.L Doty, pp. 731–758. New York: Marcel Dekker.

Smith-Swintosky, V.L., C.R. Plata-Salamán, and T.R. Scott. 1991. Gustatory neural coding in the monkey cortex: Stimulus quality. *J Neurophysiol* 66:1156–1165.

Steiner, J.E. 1973. The gustofacial response: Observation on normal and anencephalic newborn infants. *Symp Oral Sens Percept* 4:254–278.

Stice, E., S. Spoor, C. Bohon, M. Veldhuisen, and D. Small. 2008. Relation of reward from food intake and anticipated food intake to obesity: A function magnetic imaging study. *J Abnorm Psychol* 117:124–135.

Stricker, E.M. and J.E. Jalowiec. 1970. Restoration of intravascular fluid volume following acute hypovolemia in rats. *Am J Physiol* 218:191–196.

Tataranni, P.A., J.F. Gautier, and K. Chen. 1999. Neuroanatomical correlates of hunger and satiation in humans using positron emission tomography. *Proc Nat Acad Sci* 96: 4569–4574.

Thompson, D.A., H.R. Moskowitz, and R.G. Campbell. 1976. Effects of body weight and food intake on pleasantness for a sweet stimulus. *J Appl Physiol* 41:77–83.

Travers, J.B. and D.V. Smith. 1979. Gustatory sensitivities in neurons of the hamster nucleus tractus solitarius. *Sens Proc* 3:1–26.

Travers, S.P. 1993. Orosensory processing in neural systems of the nucleus of the solitary tract. In *Mechanisms of Taste Transduction*, eds. S.A. Simon and S.D. Roper, pp. 339–394. Boca Raton, FL: CRC Press.

Veldhuisen, M.G., G. Bendor, R.T. Constable, and D.M. Small. 2007. Trying to detect taste in a tasteless solution: Modulation of early gustatory cortex by attention to taste. *Chem Senses* 32:569–581.

Verhagen, J.V., E.T. Rolls, and M. Kadohisa. 2003. Neurons in primate orbitofrontal cortex respond to fat texture independently of viscosity. *J Neurophysiol* 90:1514–1525.

Verhagen, J.V., M. Kadohisa, and E.T. Rolls. 2004. The primate insular/opercular taste cortex: Neural representation of the viscosity, fat, texture, grittiness, temperature, and taste of food. *J Neurophysiol* 92:1685–1699.

Weusten, B.L.A.M., H. Fransson, G.H. Wieneke, and A.J.P.M. Smout. 1994. Multichannel recording of cerebral potentials evoked by esophageal balloon distension in humans. *Digest Dis Sci* 39:2074–2083.

Wicker, B., C. Keysers, J. Plailly, J.P. Royet, V. Gallese, and G. Rizzolatti. 2003. Both of us disgusted by my insula: The common neural basis of seeing and feeling disgust. *Neuron* 40:655–664.

Wilkins, L. and C.P. Richter. 1940. A great craving for salt by a child with corticoadrenal insufficiency. *J Am Med Assoc* 114:866–868.

Yamamoto, T. 1993. Neural mechanisms of taste aversion learning. *Neurosci Res* 16:181–185.

Yan, J. and T.R. Scott. 1996. The effect of satiety on responses of gustatory neurons in the amygdala of alert cynomolgus macaques. *Brain Res* 740:193–199.

Yaxley, S., E.T. Rolls, Z.J. Sienkiewicz, and T.R. Scott. 1985. Satiety does not affect gustatory activity in the nucleus of the solitary tract of the alert monkey. *Brain Res* 347:83–95.

Yaxley, S., E.T. Rolls and Z.J. Sienkiewicz. 1988. The responsiveness of neurons in the insular gustatory cortex of the macaque monkey is independent of hunger. *Physiol Behav* 42:223–229.

5 Psychophysical Measurement of Human Oral Experience

Derek J. Snyder and Linda M. Bartoshuk

CONTENTS

5.1   Introduction 103
5.2   Thresholds vs. Intensity: How Should Oral Experience Be Measured?....... 104
    5.2.1   Threshold Procedures 104
        5.2.1.1   Chemical Taste Thresholds.. 106
        5.2.1.2   Electrogustometry.. 107
    5.2.2   Direct Scaling of Suprathreshold Intensity 108
        5.2.2.1   Magnitude Estimation.. 108
        5.2.2.2   Measuring Oral Sensory Differences: Magnitude
                Matching 109
        5.2.2.3   Measuring Oral Sensory Differences: Labeled Scales 113
5.3   Methods of Oral Sensory Evaluation.. 119
    5.3.1   Whole Mouth Oral Sensation 120
    5.3.2   Videomicroscopy of the Tongue.. 121
    5.3.3   Spatial Taste Testing 122
        5.3.3.1   Clinical Correlates of Localized Taste Loss...................... 122
    5.3.4   Retronasal Olfaction 125
5.4   Conclusion 126
References... 126

5.1   INTRODUCTION

Nutritional health relies on food choices reflecting a balanced diet, and oral sensation plays a significant role in the initiation, consolidation, and expression of these choices both acutely and over time. While many other factors contribute to dietary choice, this relationship makes intuitive sense—your perception of food guides your intake of it, which guides its effect on you. However, defining and quantifying this relationship have proven vexing: not only is food intake famously difficult to measure accurately, but oral sensation and affect also show astonishing individual variation even under healthy conditions. Part of the problem, of course, is that individual experience is subjective: we can describe our experiences, but we cannot directly share them, and it is difficult to compare descriptions that may mean different things to different people. Nevertheless, over the past several decades, advances in psychophysical scaling have demonstrated that individual differences in oral sensation (when measured properly) are not simply measurement artifacts but reflect true physiological variation with potent behavioral health impact. This evolutionary process supports the idea that perceptual experiences can be measured and compared, but it has also revealed widespread measurement practices that obscure links among chemosensation, diet, and health. As such, a better understanding of oral sensory measurement promises to clarify both the extent of its variation and its role in human nutrition across the lifespan.

This chapter examines the development of contemporary methods of oral sensory assessment, with particular emphasis on suprathreshold intensity scales that span the full range of oral sensory function. In addition to the gold standard technique of magnitude estimation, useful suprathreshold tools include labeled scales, which are often used incorrectly to compare experiences between individuals and groups. When measured correctly, suprathreshold methods of oral sensation have proven especially useful as part of a multivariate testing process (e.g., multiple standards, genetic testing, oral anatomy) that permits confirmation of results and (where necessary) correction for unexpected scaling problems. Through ongoing calibration and refinement, this approach aims to identify streamlined and predictive measures of oral sensation suitable for expansion from the laboratory and specialty clinic into broader health-related and consumer settings.

5.2 THRESHOLDS VS. INTENSITY: HOW SHOULD ORAL EXPERIENCE BE MEASURED?

When we enjoy a meal, we can tell easily if the soup is too salty or if the coffee is too weak. These judgments demonstrate that intensity is a continuous concept involving graded intervals of strength rather than a binary presence or absence of sensation—yet debate continues regarding the ability of various measurement strategies to capture sensory experience. Some psychophysicists avoid suprathreshold methods because they believe that the degrees of intensity cannot be measured accurately (e.g., Brindley 1960; Laming 1997), whereas others contend that thresholds offer insufficient information about the range of sensory function (e.g., Moskowitz 1977b). In the case of oral sensation, neither of these views is entirely correct: taste threshold differences carry important clinical and research implications when interpreted carefully, and suprathreshold measures hold unique diagnostic and predictive capabilities when used correctly.

5.2.1 THRESHOLD PROCEDURES

Thresholds have been used for sensory evaluation ever since Fechner described them in his *Elemente der Psychophysik* (Fechner 1860/1966), one of the first published works of experimental psychology. Although thresholds present both conceptual and practical challenges (e.g., Engen 1972; Lawless and Heymann 2010), their basic definition is straightforward: the absolute or detection threshold for a stimulus is the lowest concentration at which its presence can be detected as something, whether or not its quality can be determined. The recognition threshold, which is often slightly higher than the absolute threshold, is the lowest concentration at which the primary quality of a stimulus (e.g., sweet, painful) can be identified. Finally, the difference threshold is the smallest increase in suprathreshold stimulus concentration that can be detected (i.e., the *just noticeable difference* [jnd]). Clinical assessments of gustatory function typically focus on the absolute threshold, whereas food and consumer scientists often use difference thresholds to evaluate flavor changes or off-tastes.

In the most basic version of the taste threshold procedure, participants report whether or not they perceive a taste sensation from a given stimulus (i.e., *yes* or *no*). Concentration is raised from an undetectable level until the participants report a sensation, and then it is decreased from a clearly detectable level until the participants report an absence of sensation. (Taste stimuli are generally presented in logarithmic steps, which approximate equal intervals of perceived intensity.) Over a series of ascending and descending runs, the average concentration of transition points serves as an estimate of threshold (McBurney and Collings 1977). One popular variant of this method involves the presentation of ascending series only, which was introduced to address concerns about adaptation to suprathreshold stimuli during descending series (e.g., Pangborn et al. 1964).

While elegant, this procedure raises concerns that warrant serious consideration. Test efficiency is extremely important; too few trials render the procedure unreliable, but too many trials can lead to adaptation and fatigue. In addition, signal detection theory (Green and Swets 1966) shows that individuals use different criteria when deciding how much sensory change warrants a response: one person may respond to the slightest hint of change, while another may want to be extremely confident that change has occurred before responding. As a result, participants show bias toward responses already made (i.e., habituation errors), but they may also change their responses prematurely when they believe that an actual change is imminent (i.e., anticipation errors). Shifts in these criteria can occur over many trials, highlighting the need for concise testing methods.

Efforts to balance task difficulty, bias, and test duration have yielded several refinements to threshold measurement. In the *up–down* or *staircase* method, stimulus concentration depends on the outcome of the previous trial; positive responses proceed to a lower concentration and negative responses to a higher one (Cornsweet 1962), which improves test efficiency by focusing on observations near threshold. Forced-choice discrimination protocols address response bias by requiring the participants to identify a target stimulus on each trial. When up–down and forced-choice elements are combined (e.g., Jesteadt 1980), shifting the number of correct vs. incorrect trials required to change concentration reduces the likelihood of chance (i.e., false-positive) performance at a particular concentration (Wetherill and Levitt 1965), and a reduction in the ratio of target vs. background stimuli in each trial lowers chance performance and may counteract stimulus adaptation (e.g., Lawless et al. 1995; Murphy et al. 1995). These modifications have proven especially useful in the chemical senses, which adapt and fatigue easily compared to other sensory systems (e.g., Linschoten et al. 1996). On the other hand, the fact that thresholds are so susceptible to change reflects a fundamental yet underappreciated concept in signal detection: thresholds are a statistical construct and not a fixed biological constant.

They must be considered in the context of the specific methods used, and they can be compared only with values measured similarly.

Two approaches dominate modern taste threshold measurement: chemical taste thresholds typically involve whole mouth sampling of dilute solutions (although regional testing is also feasible), whereas electrogustometry involves localized taste sensations elicited by weak electrical current applied to specific regions of the tongue.

5.2.1.1 Chemical Taste Thresholds

One of the most widely accepted methods for determining taste detection thresholds is an up–down, two-alternative, forced-choice (2-AFC) staircase (Wetherill and Levitt 1965; McBurney and Collings 1977). This test comprises multiple trials of two stimuli in which participants distinguish the tastant from water. Testing begins at a stimulus concentration that can be perceived, proceeding to a lower concentration (in logarithmic steps) following two correct trials and a higher concentration following one incorrect trial. Such an arrangement produces a series of *reversals* over time, and the geometric mean of the second through seventh reversal concentrations is defined as threshold. To avoid adaptation effects (e.g., McBurney and Pfaffmann 1963; Bartoshuk 1974; Hertz et al. 1975), participants should rinse thoroughly before sampling any test solution.

More streamlined methods for taste detection threshold measurement include the three-drop and eight-cup techniques. In the three-drop technique, one drop of tastant and two drops of water are presented in each trial, and threshold is defined as the lowest concentration at which the participant chooses the target correctly in at least two of three trials (Henkin et al. 1963). The eight-cup technique is a sorting task in which four cups of the tastant and four cups of water are presented; threshold is defined as the lowest concentration at which the participant separates the cups into the tastant and water groups without error (Harris and Kalmus 1949a). Weiffenbach (1983) found that the three-drop technique produces significantly higher detection thresholds for NaCl and sucrose than does the eight-cup technique, but both are far less stringent than the up–down 2-AFC staircase (Frank et al. 2003).

Recognition thresholds for taste are distinct from detection thresholds, as a concentration range exists in which dilute solutions can be discriminated from water but cannot be qualitatively identified. However, the challenge in determining taste detection and recognition thresholds for a given person is that the two test procedures must be equivalent in difficulty to permit valid comparison. Signal detection theory has been used to develop up–down, forced-choice recognition threshold measures that match the task demands of the detection threshold (Collings 1974), but these measures remain biased because individuals do not choose randomly among taste qualities when guessing (Weiffenbach 1983). Another challenge to the interpretation of taste threshold results is that taste solutions can produce tactile sensations (e.g., tingle, burn), suggesting that individuals with severe taste loss retain partial ability to discriminate between the tastant and water. Accordingly, instructions for participants must be explicit in terms of the types of sensation to be reported.

Chemical taste thresholds are used widely in research and clinical settings, where they have revealed regional and whole mouth losses associated with aging, health status, and medication use (e.g., Cowart 1989; Schiffman 1997; Mojet et al. 2001;

Heath et al. 2006; Ileri-Gurel et al. 2013), as well as individual differences associated with genetic taste status (e.g., Reed et al. 1995; Desai et al. 2011). One reason thresholds are so popular is that they are expressed in terms of a physical unit of intensity (i.e., molarity), which promotes a false impression of objectivity over suprathreshold ratings. In fact, thresholds are neither more reliable nor more accurate than other sensory measures, since they are statistical approximations of ever-changing sensitivity (Lawless and Heymann 2010). Accordingly, test–retest reliability for chemical taste thresholds is low (Stevens et al. 1995; McMahon et al. 2001), with many trials required to achieve a stable result. Even with abbreviated methods, one of the biggest drawbacks of taste thresholds is efficiency; measuring them requires a significant amount of time and yields only the lower boundary of the psychophysical function. By comparison, suprathreshold procedures generate the entire taste function in much less time.

More broadly, taste thresholds may lack validity as a measure of overall taste function, particularly at suprathreshold levels consistent with real-world sensation. Conceptually speaking, the use of thresholds in lieu of suprathreshold measures assumes that there is strong concordance between threshold and suprathreshold experiences. While such a relationship exists for olfactory sensation (e.g., Cain and Stevens 1989), taste thresholds and suprathreshold taste intensity can dissociate in substantial and unexpected ways, compromising the prediction of suprathreshold sensation from threshold values alone. Some manipulations (e.g., sodium lauryl sulfate, a detergent found in many toothpastes) suppress taste sensation uniformly across the perceptible range (DeSimone et al. 1980), but others affect specific regions of the dose–response function: radiation therapy impairs taste sensation at high concentrations while leaving it intact near threshold (Bartoshuk 1978), and taste thresholds shift without affecting suprathreshold taste intensity during both aging (Bartoshuk et al. 1986) and adaptation (McBurney 1966; McBurney and Bartoshuk 1973; Bartoshuk 1974, 1978). This disagreement alone does not preclude the use of threshold testing, as it remains useful to identify taste anomalies regardless of their effect on real-world experience: compensatory oral sensory interactions may sustain whole mouth suprathreshold sensation following nerve damage, rendering individuals unaware of the underlying sensory disturbance (e.g., Bartoshuk et al. 1987; Lehman et al. 1995); if present, abnormal taste thresholds would signal a need for further examination. That said, normal taste thresholds should not be interpreted in isolation as evidence of stable function but should be confirmed with more extensive suprathreshold and/or spatial testing.

5.2.1.2 Electrogustometry

Another measure of taste sensitivity, known as electrogustometry, involves the application of weak anodal electric currents to specific regions of the mouth (Mackenzie 1955; Krarup 1958). Electric taste has been attributed to various proposed mechanisms (Bujas 1971; DeSimone et al. 1981, 1984; Kashiwayanagi et al. 1981), the most likely of which involves the transport of positively charged ions in saliva toward taste receptors, concentrating them to levels where they can be detected (Herness 1985). Because saliva is mildly acidic and contains salts, electrogustometry typically evokes sour or salty taste sensations (e.g., Bujas 1971; Grant et al. 1987; Murphy et al. 1995).

Electrogustometry is widely recognized for its convenience. It is portable; avoids the use of chemical solutions; permits regional stimulation of taste bud fields; and provides values that can be compared across individuals, time points, locations within the mouth, or treatment conditions (e.g., Frank and Smith 1991). Compared to chemical taste thresholds, electrogustometry shows high test–retest reliability and bilateral correspondence (Murphy et al. 1995), suggesting that it may be especially useful in clinical and other brief access settings. To this end, normative data have been described for some groups (e.g., Tomita et al. 1986), and electric taste thresholds have identified taste losses associated with aging, denervation, and disease (Groves and Gibson 1974; Grant et al. 1987; Le Floch et al. 1990; Ovesen et al. 1991; Murphy et al. 1995; Nakazato et al. 2002; Pavlidis et al. 2013).

Nevertheless, several factors warrant a cautious approach to electric taste threshold data, especially when they are used to approximate the full range of taste function (e.g., Stillman et al. 2003). First, electrogustometry chiefly stimulates sour and salty taste rather than nonionic modalities like sweetness and bitterness (Frank and Smith 1991). Mounting data indicate that oral sensory alterations are often quality-specific but target bitter taste preferentially (Grushka et al. 1986; Lehman et al. 1995; Yanagisawa et al. 1998; Bartoshuk et al. 2002a). Thus, methods that fail to assess bitter taste may fail to identify relevant damage. Second, electrogustometric thresholds correlate well with regional chemical taste thresholds (Krarup 1958; Tomita et al. 1986) but not whole mouth ones (Murphy et al. 1995), and suprathreshold functions for electrical and chemical taste show poor agreement (Salata et al. 1991). As with chemical taste thresholds, electrogustometry should not be discounted simply because it is discontinuous with real-world taste experience, but its limitations for comprehensive taste evaluation should be considered.

5.2.2 DIRECT SCALING OF SUPRATHRESHOLD INTENSITY

While threshold methods provide only the lower limit of physical energy that can be perceived (e.g., decibels of sound, molar concentration), suprathreshold or *direct* scaling methods measure perceived intensity across the full dynamic range of sensation (e.g., Stevens 1946).

5.2.2.1 Magnitude Estimation

Fechner assumed that the jnd was the basic unit of psychological intensity, so he created a suprathreshold scale in which stimulus intensity was described in terms of the number of jnds above the absolute threshold. This view prevailed for nearly a century until S.S. Stevens observed that the jnd does not multiply like a proper unit: a 10-jnd stimulus is not twice as intense as a 5-jnd stimulus; it is actually more intense (Stevens 1961), demonstrating that suprathreshold scales based on thresholds provide a distorted view of intensity experiences.

Stevens (1956) introduced direct scaling methods with ratio properties, the most popular of which is magnitude estimation. In this procedure, subjects provide a number reflecting the perceived intensity of a stimulus; they then give a number twice as large to a stimulus that is twice as intense, a number half as large to a stimulus half as intense, and so on. The size of the numbers is irrelevant; only the ratios among numbers carry a meaning. Accordingly, when magnitude estimate data are pooled, they are typically *normalized* to bring ratings into a common register while preserving the ratios among them. This practice ensures that one individual's data are not unduly weighted just because they used larger numbers (Marks 1974).

Over several years, Stevens used magnitude estimation to compare the growth rates of psychophysical functions across sensory modalities (Stevens and Galanter 1957; Stevens 1959, 1962), but he was not particularly interested in studying how functions for specific stimuli vary among people. This distinction is important because magnitude estimates describe only how perceived intensity varies with stimulus intensity within an individual; they cannot reflect meaningful differences of absolute perceived intensity between individuals or groups (Marks 1974). Because group comparisons are such a basic element of scientific inquiry, this limitation has often been overlooked, even though its consequences on experimental validity are severe. As Section 5.2.2.2 shows, the identification of robust variation in oral sensation has played a vital role in efforts to scale group differences accurately.

5.2.2.2 Measuring Oral Sensory Differences: Magnitude Matching

5.2.2.2.1 Individual Differences in Oral Sensation

Discovered by the chemist A.L. Fox (1931), individuals differ significantly in their ability to taste thiourea compounds like phenylthiocarbamide (PTC) and 6-*n*-propylthiouracil (PROP) (e.g., Fox 1932; Barnicot et al. 1951); most individuals perceive some degree of bitterness (i.e., tasters), but others are *taste blind* and perceive nothing (i.e., nontasters). Early reports suggested that nontasting is a recessive trait with a single genetic locus (Snyder 1931; Blakeslee 1932), whereas other studies measured the proportion of tasters by race, sex, and disease (e.g., Parr 1934; Kalmus and Farnsworth 1959; Sunderland and Cartwright 1968; Whissell-Buechy and Wills 1989). In response to a proliferation of methods used to measure PTC/PROP sensitivity, Harris and Kalmus (1949b) introduced a threshold technique that became the preferred index of taste blindness for over 25 years, primarily because it generates a bimodal distribution of PTC/PROP detection thresholds that easily distinguishes between nontasters and tasters (Olson et al. 1989; Whissell-Buechy 1990). In the 1960s, Fischer (1967) used this technique to explore the behavioral impact of taste blindness, revealing links between PTC/PROP sensitivity and food preferences, alcohol and tobacco use, and body weight and composition (Fischer et al. 1961, 1963). These studies were among the first to use PROP as a substitute for PTC in studies of taste blindness, as PROP is odorless and has well-defined safety limits as a thyroid medication (Wheatcroft and Thornburn 1972; Lawless 1980).

Encouraged by the potential benefits of direct scaling, Bartoshuk sought to compare the suprathreshold bitterness of PTC between nontasters and tasters. This comparison, however, presents a problem: magnitude estimates have relative meaning when subjects are used as their own controls (e.g., McBurney and Bartoshuk 1973), but how can absolute ratings of bitterness (or, for that matter, any sensation) be compared across groups? The answer to this question involves measuring PTC bitterness (or, more generally, any sensation of interest) relative to an unrelated standard.

Although magnitude estimates are often normalized to obtain group functions, this procedure was something new: bringing data into a common range invokes an arbitrary standard that conveys no information about absolute perceived intensity, but group comparisons refer to a standard that is assumed to be equally intense (on average) to all of the groups. Provided this assumption holds, normalization to an unrelated standard yields valid across-group differences in absolute perceived intensity for stimuli of interest. In other words, if "10" denotes the intensity of a standard to nontasters and tasters, PTC ratings of "40" for tasters and "20" for nontasters indicate a twofold intensity difference.

Crucially, appropriate standards for comparison must be identified in order to quantify oral sensory variation with accuracy. This ongoing search has been influenced by research on *cross-modality matching*, the ability to match qualitatively different sensations (Stevens and Marks 1965). Because thioureas share a common chemical moiety, the N–C=S functional group, Bartoshuk supposed that the taste intensity of a nonthiourea compound should be equal, on average, to nontasters and tasters. Based on this logic, group averages of PTC bitterness could be compared by rating it relative to, say, NaCl saltiness. When tested with this procedure, tasters find PTC and PROP more bitter than do nontasters (Hall et al. 1975; Lawless 1980), and subsequent reports document robust oral sensory variation that extends far beyond thiourea compounds: tasters broadly perceive more intense taste and oral tactile sensations (e.g., Bartoshuk 2000), and a subset of tasters known as *supertasters* consistently gives the highest ratings to taste stimuli, oral irritants (e.g., capsaicin, alcohol), fats, and retronasal odors (e.g., Prescott et al. 2004; Bartoshuk et al. 2004c).

5.2.2.2.2 Magnitude Matching

The discovery of supertasters not only certified the extent of individual differences in oral sensation but also presented a challenge: if supertasters of PROP perceive NaCl more intensely than do others, then NaCl is a poor standard for PROP-related comparisons, which makes differences based on PROP status inaccurate. This problem was resolved by introducing stimuli from nontaste modalities as standards. For example, if taste and hearing are assumed to be unrelated, taste stimuli can be rated relative to auditory intensity. This procedure, known as *magnitude matching* (Marks and Stevens 1980; Stevens and Marks 1980; Marks et al. 1988), confirmed the suspicion that the salty taste of NaCl varies with taster status (Bartoshuk et al. 1998). In effect, magnitude matching approaches the problem of group comparisons by changing the task: because oral sensations cannot be compared directly across PROP taster groups, subjects instead rate oral stimuli relative to a non-oral standard. As long as variability in the standard remains independent of variability in PROP bitterness, oral sensory experiences scaled in this fashion are comparable across taster groups.

The ability to measure accurate differences in oral sensation has revealed rich associations among sensory experience, dietary behavior, and disease risk (e.g., Duffy 2007; Snyder et al. 2008a; Tepper et al. 2009). For example, PROP bitterness is associated with reduced vegetable preference and intake (Drewnowski et al. 2000; Duffy et al. 2001; Dinehart et al. 2006), which are known risk factors for colon cancer; it is also associated with an increased presence of colon polyps (Basson et al.

2005). PROP intensity also predicts avoidance of high-fat foods, and some studies have shown that supertasters have lower body mass and more favorable cardiovascular health (Tepper and Ullrich 2002; Duffy 2004).

5.2.2.2.3   Genetic Factors in Oral Sensory Variation

Early family studies showed that non taster parents produce non taster children, so taste blindness was thought for decades to stem from a single gene (Snyder 1931; Blakeslee 1932; Whissell-Buechy 1990). However, modern genetic analysis suggests a much more complex genetic basis for PTC/PROP bitterness (e.g., Bufe et al. 2005). Candidate genes for taste blindness have been identified on chromosomes 5p15, 7, and 16p (Reed et al. 1999; Drayna et al. 2003), and detailed mapping of chromosome 7q has revealed sequence polymorphisms in a taste receptor gene (T2R38) that account for up to 85% of observed differences in PTC threshold sensitivity (Kim et al. 2003; Wooding et al. 2004). These relationships distinguish between nontasters and tasters, but their ability to detect supertasters is limited: medium tasters and supertasters have similar PTC/PROP thresholds (e.g., Bartoshuk 2000), and T2R38 polymorphisms do not fully predict differences in suprathreshold PROP intensity observed between these groups (Hayes et al. 2008). As such, PROP supertasting cannot be explained completely by threshold sensitivity or T2R38 genetics.

Viewed broadly, rising PROP intensity is associated with greater intensity for virtually all oral sensory stimuli (e.g., Prescott et al. 2004; Bartoshuk et al. 2004c). In addition, supertasters express the highest density of fungiform papillae, structures on the anterior tongue that contain taste buds and oral somatosensory end organs (Bartoshuk and Duffy 1994). Taken together, these differences indicate that PTC/PROP taster status arises from two independent conditions: T2R38 expression and fungiform papilla density (Hayes et al. 2008). According to this view, PROP supertasters carry the taster variant of the T2R38 gene (which confers the ability to taste PTC/PROP) and they express a high density of fungiform papillae (which amplifies all oral sensory input; Bartoshuk et al. 2001). Several gene products govern fungiform papilla development (e.g., sonic hedgehog, bone morphogenic proteins, epidermal growth factor, Wnt/β-catenin signaling molecules), but their combined influence on papilla density has yet to be fully understood (e.g., Liu et al. 2009). Nevertheless, the evidence is strong that oral sensory variation arises from the expression of multiple genes mediating receptor activity and underlying anatomy.

Although PTC/PROP bitterness has figured prominently in descriptions of oral sensory variation, it is important to remember that it is a single, highly robust example of the sensory variation that occurs for virtually all oral stimuli. The common theme is that individual differences in sensation for any oral stimulus probably result from genetic variation in a specific receptor or transduction element, which is then amplified by differences in fungiform papilla density. Recent identification of sequence polymorphisms associated with variation in sweet, umami, and fat perception supports this view (Raliou et al. 2009; Shigemura et al. 2009; Fushan et al. 2010; Keller et al. 2012), as does an emerging interaction among PROP bitterness, T2R38 genetics, and sequence variation in the taste bud trophic factor gustin (Calò et al. 2011). As new oral sensory gene variants and expression patterns are found, it is likely that taster status will be defined more broadly based on genotype–phenotype relationships across multiple aspects of oral sensation and anatomy.

5.2.2.2.4 Taster Status Classification

Valid consensus values for the classification of PROP status are lacking mainly because improvements in genetic and psychophysical testing have superseded previous estimates. Consequently, existing criteria are both idiosyncratic and variable, generating vigorous debate over which classification scheme best reflects true differences in oral sensation (e.g., Prutkin et al. 2000; Drewnowski 2003; Rankin et al. 2004). Central to this issue, the validity of any boundary value depends on the instrument used to measure it, and so when suprathreshold psychophysical tools produce distorted comparisons among subjects, the resulting criteria for sorting are also distorted. (Thresholds have remained a popular measure for precisely this reason, even though they also distort real-world sensory experience, albeit for different reasons.) Measurement scales may be numerous, but not all are created equal: for oral sensory evaluation, magnitude matching remains the *gold standard* technique.

Broadly speaking, the most effective assessment strategies integrate multiple converging correlates of function. As advances in anatomy and genetics permit more detailed analysis, the best methods for oral sensory evaluation will incorporate these data in order to complement and enrich sophisticated psychophysical measurement. Based on laboratory and questionnaire data collected over many years, this multivariate approach has yielded working guidelines for the determination of PROP status (Snyder et al. 2006):

- Nontasters and tasters of PROP are distinguished by genetic analysis of T2R38 (Kim et al. 2003), which reliably predicts PROP threshold differences (i.e., >0.2 mM for nontasters; <0.1 mM for tasters) (Bartoshuk 1979; Bartoshuk et al. 1994a). In a sample of 1400 healthy lecture participants, this difference corresponds roughly to a boundary value on the general labeled magnitude scale (gLMS; see Section 5.2.2.3.3) of *weak* (i.e., 17 out of 100) for filter papers impregnated with saturated PROP (~0.058 M). Consistent with previous estimates (Harris and Kalmus 1949b; Bartoshuk et al. 1994a), this cutoff yields ~25% nontasters in the sample.
- Supertasters of PROP are distinguished from medium tasters by psychophysical criteria. Population estimates of PROP taster status are based on a single-locus model, and thus this boundary value will remain arbitrary until the full genetic basis of PROP bitterness is clarified. If nontasters represent the lowest 25% of PROP paper ratings, a working definition of supertasting might include the top 25% of ratings, suggesting a gLMS boundary value of 80.
- Individuals with taster genotypes and nontaster PROP ratings probably reflect oral sensory pathology (see Section 5.3.3.1). In these cases, oral anatomy can often be used to identify supertasters (e.g., Bartoshuk et al. 2004a) who show high fungiform papilla density (i.e., over 100 papillae/cm^2) (Bartoshuk et al. 1994a) despite their low PROP responses.

As the parameters of oral sensory variation have expanded, the use of thiourea bitterness as a marker of generalized oral sensory ability has been cast into question because correlations with it are imperfect and sometimes quite low. Consequently, alternative measures of PROP intensity have been proposed, including the ability to perceive specific taste cues from thermal or irritant stimuli (Green and George 2004; Green and Hayes 2004). While these methods show promise, their broader predictive ability remains uncertain because, like thiourea bitterness, they favor associations with a particular taste modality. Meanwhile, a broader concept of taster status has emerged that frames supertasting as an elevated response across multiple stimuli rather than a single class of compounds (Lim et al. 2008; Reed 2008; Hayes and Keast 2011). New measures like these may prove more predictive than PROP intensity, but they will require extensive study to determine boundary values, interactions with genetics and anatomy, and clinical and consumer significance. For the time being, PROP bitterness remains a useful (if flawed) screening tool as the best characterized index of individual differences in oral sensation.

Regardless of how taster group classifications are determined, some researchers persistently claim that oral sensation has little effect on sensation, food behavior, or health (e.g., Kranzler et al. 1998; Drewnowski 2003). Upon closer examination, many of these contrary reports fail to replicate because they use methods known to distort or eliminate main effects, including inappropriate group comparisons, poor scale instructions, and the use of threshold rather than suprathreshold taste tests (e.g., Bartoshuk 2000; Bartoshuk et al. 2005). These problems are often reinforced by the inappropriate use of labeled intensity scales.

5.2.2.3 Measuring Oral Sensory Differences: Labeled Scales

Measurement scales labeled with intensity descriptors (e.g., weak, strong, very strong) enjoy widespread medical, scientific, and consumer use. Although many of these category scales have reportedly been validated, the fact that a scale measures what it was intended to measure does not guarantee its ability to produce valid group comparisons. In fact, several reports have determined that category scales distort results when their labels fail to denote equal perceived intensities to everyone.

Category scales date back at least to the astronomer Hipparchus (190–120 BC). Today, category scales in common use include the Likert scale (Likert 1932) and the Natick 9-point scale (Peryam and Girardot 1952; Jones et al. 1955). When adapted for sensory use, these scales are typically anchored by adjectives spaced equally along a line (e.g., 1 = none, 3 = slight, 5 = moderate, 7 = strong, 9 = extreme), as shown in Figure 5.1 (Kamen et al. 1961). The visual analog scale (VAS), a line labeled at its endpoints with the minimum and maximum intensity of a particular experience (e.g., Aitken et al. 1963; Hetherington and Rolls 1987), follows similar logic but lacks interior descriptors; it is essentially a category scale without categories. Multiple versions of these scales have been used in oral sensory research, differing in terms of gradation, labeling, and stimulus specificity (Lawless and Heymann 2010).

5.2.2.3.1 Properties of Intensity Labels

Intensity descriptors are used throughout everyday life to compare one's experiences with those of others (e.g., "This food tastes *strong* to me. Does it taste *strong*

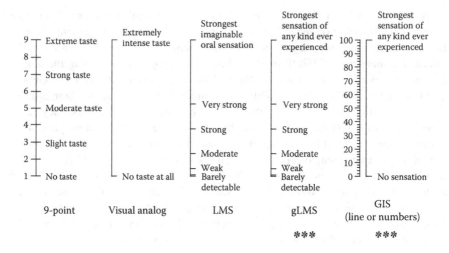

FIGURE 5.1 Labeled scales used for oral sensory evaluation. Asterisks indicate scales enabling valid group comparisons of oral sensation; scales without asterisks require an independent standard for such comparisons. Note the change in context from imaginable to experienced events in recent versions of the gLMS/GIS. LMS = labeled magnitude scale; gLMS = general labeled magnitude scale; GIS = global intensity scale.

to you?"). Because these words are used so frequently, they were incorporated as anchors on intensity scales.

Ratings from category scales generally have ordinal but not ratio properties (Stevens and Galanter 1957) because the equidistant spacing of labels does not reflect their actual perceived intensity (e.g., Lasagna 1960; Berry and Huskisson 1972): A sensation rated "8" on the Natick 9-point scale is more intense than a sensation rated "4," but it is not necessarily twice as intense. For this reason, the 9-point scale is prone to ceiling effects (Lucchina et al. 1998; Bartoshuk 2000). Borg (1970, 1982) addressed this problem by deriving a category scale with ratio properties, and subsequent efforts to define scale labels empirically have generated similar *quasi-logarithmic* spacing across multiple sensory and hedonic domains (Moskowitz 1977a; Gracely et al. 1978; Borg 1990; Green et al. 1993; Schutz and Cardello 2001). This common spacing suggests that virtually all experiences possess similar intensity properties regardless of their source or affective basis.

Another feature of intensity labels is that they convey relative and variable magnitude. Adjectives modify nouns, and so their absolute meaning is flexible, particularly in terms of size. Stevens (1958) illustrated this concept, noting, "Mice may be called large or small, and so may elephants, and it is quite understandable when someone says it was a large mouse that ran up the trunk of the small elephant (p. 633)." As Stevens shows, *large* and *small* carry relative meaning until their nouns are specified, and their absolute meanings become clear only when placed in context: a large mouse will always be smaller than a small elephant.

Intensity descriptors operate in a similar fashion: the word *strong* varies in magnitude depending on whether it refers to a strong odor, a strong gust of wind, or a strong pain. However, many comparisons made with labeled scales implicitly assume that scale descriptors denote the same absolute intensity regardless of the object described. Extending this view, some have proposed that sensory ranges are essentially the same for all modalities and all people (Teghtsoonian 1973; Borg 1982), but in fact, they—and their incorporated intensity descriptor meanings—vary both among groups of people and among different sensory modalities (e.g., Bartoshuk et al. 2002b). In the chemical senses, magnitude matching has been used to demonstrate that intensity descriptors for oral cues retain relative spacing across PROP intensity groups; yet their absolute intensity is greater for supertasters than for nontasters, which is consistent with the idea that supertasters have a broader oral sensory intensity range than do nontasters (Bartoshuk et al. 2004c).

In short, labeled scales maintain their relative spacing, but they are elastic in terms of the domain to be measured and the individual's experience with that domain. Because conventional labeled scales fail to account for this elasticity, they can be used for within-subject comparisons or for across-group comparisons in which groups are assigned randomly; but across-group comparisons are invalid whenever subject classification (e.g., sex, age, weight, clinical status) produces groups for which scale labels denote different absolute intensities.

5.2.2.3.2 Consequences of Invalid Comparisons

Figure 5.2 illustrates errors that arise with the false assumption that intensity descriptors denote the same absolute intensity to everyone. (This figure is idealized,

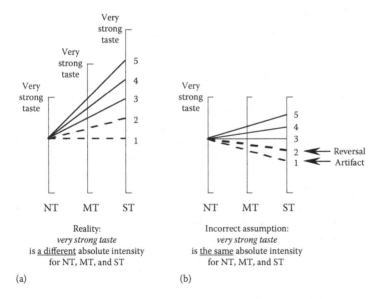

(a)
(b)

FIGURE 5.2 Consequences of invalid comparisons. (a) Taste functions measured with magnitude matching that reflect differences among NT, MT, and ST. (b) Effect of incorrectly assuming that *very strong taste* indicates the same absolute perceived intensity to NT, MT, and ST: valid effects appear truncated and may reverse direction inaccurately. (Modified from Bartoshuk, L.M. et al., *Physiol Behav* 82:109–114, 2004.)

but similar effects occur with experimental measures of taste and food intensity [Bartoshuk et al. 2004a].) Figure 5.2a shows stimuli that produce equal perceived intensities to PROP nontasters. The diverging lines connecting nontaster and supertaster ratings indicate PROP effects of differing sizes (e.g., Bartoshuk et al. 2004c). In Figure 5.2b, the label *very strong taste* is treated as if it denotes the same average intensity to nontasters and supertasters, resulting in a compression of supertaster data relative to nontaster data: some effects are blunted (effects 4 and 5), and some disappear (effect 3); but some appear to go in the opposite direction (effects 1 and 2) in a phenomenon known as a reversal artifact (e.g., Bartoshuk and Snyder 2004).

Even though the limitations of labeled scales for group comparison have been noted by investigators in several fields (e.g., Narens and Luce 1983; Manis et al. 1991; Biernat and Manis 1994; Birnbaum 1999; Bartoshuk et al. 2002b, 2005), some critics argue that group effects with meaningful impact should be sufficiently robust to be observed across any and all methods used to measure them (Drewnowski 2003). Claims like these are distortions themselves, as biobehavioral effects do not cease to exist simply because a chosen measurement tool fails to detect them. Verification is certainly warranted in such cases, but so too is careful evaluation of methodology. In particular, the popularity of a scale does not necessarily make it the right tool for the task at hand, and some widely used scales are simply not designed for valid group comparisons. Although improved labeled scaling shows promise, contrary reports arising from invalid methods remain significant obstacles to research efforts in the chemical senses.

5.2.2.3.3 General Labeled Magnitude Scale

Category scales assume ratio properties when real-world experience defines the spacing among labels. Considering that intensity categories maintain their relative differences across individuals and modalities, perhaps stretching this common intensity scale to its maximum would produce a labeled scale suitable for comparisons of oral sensory intensity. By this point, the labeled magnitude scale (LMS) had been developed specifically to measure oral sensations (Green et al. 1993). As shown in Figure 5.1, the LMS is a ratio scale anchored by empirically spaced intensity descriptors, including the top anchor *strongest imaginable [oral] sensation*. To generalize the LMS for experiences beyond oral sensation, Bartoshuk and colleagues replaced its top anchor with the label *strongest imaginable sensation of any kind*.

This scale, now known as gLMS, shares a similar logic to magnitude matching: the top anchor of the gLMS is meant to function as a standard, so it must remain unrelated to oral sensation to ensure valid comparisons of chemosensory function. This requirement appears to hold for studies of oral sensory experience: participants rarely describe oral sensations as their strongest imaginable sensory experience (Bartoshuk et al. 2002b), and the gLMS and magnitude matching produce similar oral sensory differences among PROP taster groups (Bartoshuk et al. 2004b). Chemosensory data collected with the gLMS also show strong test–retest reliability (Galindo-Cuspinera et al. 2009).

The gLMS was developed for sensory use; however, it also shows promise as a hedonic scale. Based on the empirical finding that intensity labels for sensation and affect are spaced similarly (e.g., Moskowitz 1977a; Schutz and Cardello 2001), a *hedonic gLMS* was created by extending two gLMSs in opposite directions from a common midpoint; *neutral* is in the center, *strongest imaginable disliking* is the low endpoint, and *strongest imaginable liking* is the high endpoint (Bartoshuk et al. 2002b). This scale, shown in Figure 5.3, has been used successfully in recent studies of food affect: overall food acceptance increases with body mass index, suggesting that the obese experience greater palatability from foods than do the non-obese (Bartoshuk et al. 2006). Also, supertasters of PROP experience greater overall food liking and disliking than do nontasters, which may explain their selective food preferences (Bartoshuk et al. 2010). As with the sensory gLMS, the hedonic gLMS is appropriate for group comparisons because oral sensory cues rarely elicit affective ratings at the endpoints of the scale (Bartoshuk et al. 2010). Other hedonic scales may perform similarly to the gLMS in terms of group comparisons, provided that their boundary labels are explicitly framed in terms of all affective experience; promising candidates shown in Figure 5.3 include the labeled affective magnitude scale (Schutz and Cardello 2001) and the labeled hedonic scale (Lim et al. 2009).

Because the gLMS incorporates an internal standard, the data collected with it should not require normalization—but when the top of the gLMS is related to an experience of interest, comparisons using raw gLMS ratings are invalid. With regard to chemosensation, this problem may arise in studies of trigeminal function, as the gLMS fails as a standard for measures of pain intensity because pain is often associated with the top of the scale. Consequently, it is prudent to embed several candidate standards in sensory scaling experiments; if one standard fails, others may succeed. For example, *brightest light ever seen* has emerged as a suitable standard for pain psychophysics (Bartoshuk et al. 2004a).

The standards used in the laboratory often require cumbersome and expensive equipment, yet scale labels rely on memories of perceived intensity. Accordingly, remembered sensations have been proposed as standards in lieu of sampled stimuli. While the precise relationship between real and remembered intensity is unclear (e.g., Algom 1992), it appears that remembered oral sensations reflect effects observed with actual stimuli (e.g., Stevenson and Prescott 1997; Fast et al. 2001). The incorporation of real and remembered stimuli as standards brings flexibility to data management; raw gLMS scores may be used (which invokes an internal standard), or they may be normalized to other variables (which converts the gLMS to a magnitude-matching task), allowing confirmation of effects across a variety of assumptions. Taken together, these multimodal ratings coalesce into a snapshot of one's sensory and affective world, enabling individual differences of interest to resolve on a diffuse yet stable background (Bartoshuk et al. 2004c).

5.2.2.3.4   *Global Intensity Scales: Beyond the gLMS*

The observation that intensity descriptors are used similarly across multiple dimensions of experience (sensory and hedonic, real and remembered) suggests a cognitive model for intensity perception. We learn the relative spacing among intensity descriptors early in life, and these ratios remain constant. However, the absolute range covered by intensity descriptors is variable, so we stretch or compress our descriptive vocabulary to fit the extremes of whatever we wish to describe. As such,

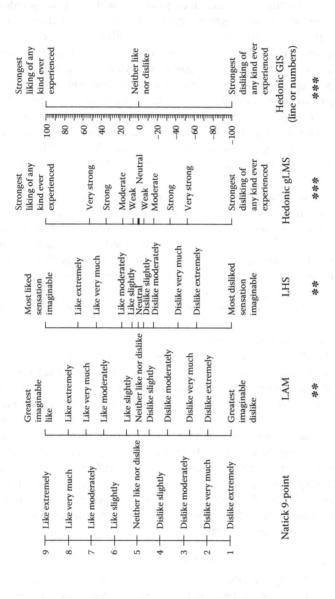

FIGURE 5.3 Labeled scales used for hedonic evaluation. Asterisks indicate scales enabling group comparisons of food-related affect; scales without asterisks require an independent standard for such comparisons. Note the change in context from imaginable events (*) to experienced events (**) in recent versions of the gLMS/GIS. LAM = labeled affective magnitude scale; LHS = labeled hedonic scale; gLMS = general labeled magnitude scale; GIS = global intensity scale.

we may use the same words to describe just about anything, but our experience with the object at hand is critical in guiding our frame of reference.

That said, some descriptors may be more important than others; some may clarify and others may confuse. For example, the word *imaginable* is included in the top anchors of many intensity scales (e.g., *worst imaginable pain*), but it may cloud the common meaning conferred by a standard. Do all people imagine the same maximum intensity regardless of what they actually experience? When subjects rated both the most intense sensation of any kind ever experienced and the strongest sensation imaginable, the two were highly correlated when expressed relative to the brightest light ever seen (Fast et al. 2002). As such, *imaginable* sensations may not be appropriate standards for comparisons of experience, and the term has been removed from recent iterations of the gLMS. As shown in Figure 5.3, boundary labels now refer to the strongest intensity ever experienced.

Another example involves the intermediate descriptors spaced empirically along the length of the scale. In practical terms, the gLMS requires users to express intensity in terms of a specific experience representing the outer limit of their intensity range. While stretching the intensity range to its maximum is precisely the feature that permits cross-modality matching, it may add confusion to the interpretation of intermediate scale labels, which as adjectives require context to establish absolute meaning. This notion suggests that all scale labels could be abandoned except for those at the endpoints. The result (for sensation) would be a line spanning from *no sensation* to the *strongest sensation of any kind ever experienced*. An even more basic approach would be to use numerical ratings (e.g., 0 to 100 for sensation; −100 to +100 for affect) provided that the appropriate endpoint meanings are defined clearly. Recent data indicate that these minimalist *global intensity scales* (GIS), shown in Figure 5.3, perform similarly to the gLMS (Snyder et al. 2008b). Similar to the gLMS, GIS values are suitable for group comparisons unless the strongest sensation ever experienced shows a group difference, in which case an alternative standard would be used.

5.3 METHODS OF ORAL SENSORY EVALUATION

Because it carries such broad behavioral and health implications, chemosensory evaluation shows considerable promise as a diagnostic aid in epidemiology, food and nutritional science, and the health professions. Comprehensive assessments of oral sensory function have been used mainly in basic and clinical research, but there is growing appreciation among food and consumer professionals regarding the role of oral sensory viability in product development and nutritional health.

Several afferent nerves carry sensory information from the mouth, each carrying a particular array of information from a particular area (e.g., Pritchard and Norgren 2004). The chorda tympani (CT), a branch of the facial nerve (cranial nerve VII), carries taste information from the anterior, mobile tongue; the lingual branch of the trigeminal nerve (V) carries pain, tactile, and temperature information primarily from the same region (Lewis and Dandy 1930; Zahm and Munger 1985). Multimodal information (i.e., taste, touch, pain, temperature) is carried from the posterior tongue by the glossopharyngeal nerve (IX), from the palate by the greater superficial petrosal nerve (another branch of VII), and from the throat by the vagus (X) (Fay 1927; Reichert 1934; Kanagasuntheram et al. 1969; Norgren 1984). Taste and oral somatosensory cues combine centrally with retronasal olfaction to produce the composite experience of flavor (e.g., Rozin 1982; McBurney 1986). This spatial distribution of input has led researchers to consider the impact of localized oral sensory damage, so modern protocols for oral sensory evaluation typically include judgments of intensity and quality for both regional and whole mouth stimuli.

5.3.1 WHOLE MOUTH ORAL SENSATION

In whole mouth gustatory testing, chemical stimuli are sipped and swished to stimulate all oral taste bud fields simultaneously, with a water rinse prior to each stimulus. Laboratory tests of oral sensation involve presentation of chemical solutions at concentrations across the functional range of perception (e.g., Bartoshuk et al. 1998; Tepper et al. 2001), but most clinical tests have streamlined this process to a single concentration for each of the common taste qualities (i.e., sucrose, NaCl, citric acid, quinine hydrochloride) (e.g., Frank et al. 2003). In addition, multiple concentrations may be used to derive suprathreshold taste functions, and other oral stimuli may be administered to evaluate oral tactile sensation (e.g., capsaicin, alcohol) or specific individual differences (e.g., PROP). Intensity ratings are typically measured with magnitude matching or the gLMS/GIS with appropriate standards, so stimuli unrelated to oral sensation (e.g., sound, remembered sensations) should be included.

Liquids are inconvenient for clinical, field, or large-scale use, so alternative methods of stimulus delivery have been developed, including paper strips, tablets, and edible films (Adler 1972; Hummel et al. 1997; Mueller et al. 2003; Smutzer et al. 2008). In early studies, PTC crystals were placed directly on the tongue (Fox 1932) or delivered on saturated filter papers (Blakeslee and Fox 1932). As threshold techniques became dominant, the filter paper method faded from use until it was revived as a rough screening tool for use at group functions (Bartoshuk et al. 1996). Today, PROP papers are made by soaking laboratory-grade filter papers in a supersaturated solution of PROP heated to just below boiling. When dry, each paper contains ~1.6 mg (Bartoshuk et al. 1996). (By comparison, patients with hyperthyroidism are prescribed 100–300 mg PROP daily [Cooper 2005].) Variants of this method have been described (e.g., Tepper et al. 2001; Zhao et al. 2003), but all share the common goal of introducing a small amount of crystalline PROP to the tongue surface.

Intended as a rough estimate of PROP taster status, the filter paper technique shows promise because of its simplicity, but its technical limitations warrant careful consideration. To produce a taste, the paper must be completely moistened with saliva, which requires both healthy salivary function and a sufficient period of contact with the tongue. Some studies have reported high false-positive and false-negative responses to PTC/PROP filter papers, but these response rates may reflect minor variations in protocol that confer bias (Azevedo et al. 1965; Lawless 1980). Filter paper testing shows only moderate concordance with threshold sensitivity (Hartmann 1939), but this finding probably reflects the dissociation between threshold and suprathreshold measures of PROP bitterness that occurs under proper scaling conditions (e.g., Bartoshuk 1989).

Consistent with this view, filter paper ratings and laboratory assessments of suprathreshold PROP bitterness show significant agreement (Bartoshuk et al. 1996; Kaminski et al. 2000; Zhao et al. 2003) and high test–retest reliability (Ly and Drewnowski 2001; Zhao et al. 2003). One of the reasons that filter paper delivery functions so well may be that the exact concentration of PROP on each paper is trivial provided that it is high. Comparisons of PROP bitterness produced by filter papers vs. solution suggest that the concentration of PROP dissolved from the paper into saliva approaches the solubility limit of PROP. Thus, papers made with saturated PROP (Bartoshuk et al. 1996) produce comparable results to those made from defined concentrations approaching saturation (Zhao et al. 2003).

5.3.2 VIDEOMICROSCOPY OF THE TONGUE

Several findings indicate that taste sensation varies with the number of taste buds stimulated. One particularly clear example of this relationship is that threshold and suprathreshold taste function increase with the size of the area stimulated on the tongue, presumably because a larger stimulus area captures more taste buds (Hara 1955; Smith 1971; Linschoten and Kroeze 1991; Doty et al. 2001). Clinical data paint a similar picture, as patients with lingual nerve damage show parallel losses of fungiform papillae and taste perception (Bull 1965; Ogden 1989; Cowan 1990) that recover partially with nerve regeneration (Robinson et al. 2000; Zuniga et al. 1997). Finally, inbred mouse strains expressing differences in bitter avoidance (Harder et al. 1984) show corresponding differences in taste bud density (Miller and Whitney 1989) and gustatory nerve activity (Shingai and Beidler 1985).

To examine variation in human oral anatomy, Miller and Reedy (1990a,b) developed a method for visualizing the tongue in vivo. The anterior surface of the human tongue is covered with two types of papillae; fungiform papillae are larger and hold taste buds, but smaller filiform papillae do not (e.g., Miller and Bartoshuk 1991). When blue food coloring is applied to the tongue, it fails to stain fungiform papillae, which appear as pink circles against a blue background. Fungiform papillae can be counted with a magnifying glass and a flashlight, with still photography, or with videomicroscopy at higher resolution (Shahbake et al. 2005). At sufficiently high magnification, videomicroscopy reveals small blue dots on the surfaces of fungiform papillae, which are pores that serve as conduits to the apical tips of taste buds.

Visualization of lingual anatomy has revealed robust positive associations among PROP intensity, fungiform papilla density, and taste bud density (Miller and Reedy 1990b; Zuniga et al. 1993; Bartoshuk et al. 1994a; Delwiche et al. 2001). Fungiform papillae are innervated by both CT and V (Gairns 1953), which accounts for the elevated taste and oral tactile sensations experienced by supertasters (e.g., Prutkin et al. 2000; Essick et al. 2003). Videomicroscopy of the tongue has also revealed some forms of oral sensory pathology. Human fungiform papillae and taste buds degenerate with lingual nerve damage (Zuniga et al. 1994, 1997), but CT damage alone sacrifices taste buds while leaving fungiform papillae intact (Schwartz 1998). In individuals with taster genotypes and nontaster PROP ratings, high fungiform papilla counts signal anterior taste damage (e.g., Bartoshuk et al. 2004a).

5.3.3 Spatial Taste Testing

Because different nerves innervate different regions of the oral cavity, oral sensation can be absent in one area but remain intact in others. Nevertheless, individuals with significant taste damage are often unaware of it unless it is accompanied by tactile loss (House 1963; Moon and Pullen 1963; Rice 1963; Bull 1965; Pfaffmann and Bartoshuk 1989, 1990). This phenomenon occurs because taste cues are referred perceptually to sites in the mouth that are touched whether or not taste receptors at those sites are present or functional (Todrank and Bartoshuk 1991; Delwiche et al. 2000; Green 2002). Because of this *tactile referral*, regional taste loss rarely produces whole mouth taste loss, but it remains clinically significant as a precursor to altered, heightened, and phantom oral sensations. Measures of regional taste function are an important tool for identifying the source of these complaints.

The integrity of specific taste nerves is assessed via spatial testing in which suprathreshold concentrations of sweet, sour, salty, and bitter stimuli are applied to the anterior tongue tip, foliate papillae (i.e., posterolateral edges of tongue), circumvallate papillae (i.e., raised circular structures on the posterior tongue), and soft palate (Bartoshuk 1989; Mueller et al. 2003). Stimuli are presented on the right and left sides at each site, and subjects make quality and intensity judgments using magnitude matching or the gLMS/GIS. Special care must be taken to avoid stimulating both sides of the mouth at the same time (which impedes localization), triggering a gag reflex during circumvallate stimulation, or allowing palate stimuli to reach the tongue surface (which leads to inflated palate ratings). Following regional testing, subjects swallow a small volume of each solution and rate its intensity, which enables comparisons of regional and whole mouth sensation. Psychophysical functions across oral loci indicate that taste cues are perceived at similar intensity on all tongue areas holding taste buds but less so on the palate (Bartoshuk 1988). As such, oral sensory loss can be identified as significant local variations from otherwise stable perception across the tongue surface.

For several decades, virtually the only feature of taste perception mentioned in textbooks was a map showing areas on the tongue sensitive to each of the four basic tastes: sweet on the tip, salty and sour on the edges, and bitter at the rear. Spatial taste testing demonstrates that this *tongue map* is inaccurate, and further study reveals that it was based on a misinterpretation of data. Hänig (1901) showed that thresholds for the basic tastes show slight variation across various tongue loci, but he never proposed that individual taste qualities are limited to specific regions of the tongue. Later, Boring (1942) plotted the reciprocal of Hänig's threshold values as a measure of the sensitivity of each tongue area—but he did not include numbers on his graph, so subsequent readers failed to realize that his data actually represented very small threshold differences. Thus, a myth was born.

5.3.3.1 Clinical Correlates of Localized Taste Loss

Disorders of oral sensation are widespread and variable, yet appropriate resources and treatment are frustratingly sparse (e.g., Deems et al. 1991; Hoffman et al. 1998). Because taste cues influence nutritional health, metabolism, and affect, their loss can be devastating (e.g., Giduck et al. 1987; Tennen et al. 1991; Mattes and Cowart

1994); yet in many cases, the absence is hardly noticed (e.g., Bull 1965; Goto et al. 1983; Tomita et al. 1986). Moreover, taste disturbances are often associated with specific disorders and interventions, but just as often they are unpredictable and idiosyncratic (e.g., Bromley and Doty 2003). As a result of this complexity, a full oral sensory evaluation requires thorough examination of physical (e.g., oral anatomy, oral and salivary pathology, nongustatory neurological damage), sensory (e.g., taste, oral somatosensation, retronasal olfaction), and emotional aspects of chemosensation (e.g., psychopathology, quality of life).

Spatial taste testing is especially powerful when used in combination with genetic and anatomical data, as it reveals discordance between heredity and experience that arises via pathology (e.g., Snyder et al. 2006). Sophisticated chemosensory psychophysics, in particular the development of measures permitting valid across-group comparisons, has revealed a great deal about the consequences of localized oral sensory damage, which is implicated in an ever-growing array of health conditions. While these relationships do not wholly validate the methods used to discover them, their parallel relationship to measures of oral anatomy suggests that improved psychophysical methods yield meaningful differences in human experience.

5.3.3.1.1   Oral Disinhibition

Dysgeusia refers to a chronic taste sensation that occurs in the absence of obvious stimulation (Snow et al. 1991). Many clinical complaints of dysgeusia result from taste stimuli that are not readily apparent to the patient, such as medications tasted in saliva, crevicular fluid, or blood (Bradley 1973; Alfano 1974; Stephen et al. 1980; Fetting et al. 1985). However, some chronic taste sensations, known as phantoms, appear to arise from altered interactions in the central nervous system.

While some neurological disorders can generate taste phantoms (Hausser-Hauw and Bancaud 1987; El-Deiry and McCabe 1990), CT damage presents as a primary factor in clinical accounts (Bull 1965; Jones and Fry 1984; Yamada and Tomita 1989). Supporting this view, electrophysiological recordings from rodents and dogs show that blocking CT input produces elevated activity in brain regions receiving input from IX (Halpern and Nelson 1965; Norgren and Pfaffmann 1975; Ninomiya and Funakoshi 1982; Ogawa and Hayama 1984; Sweazey and Smith 1987). Together, these data imply that CT inhibits IX normally, so CT loss should disinhibit IX. Human psychophysical data support this model: in patient cohorts (e.g., head injury, craniofacial tumors, ear infections) and healthy subjects under anesthesia, unilateral CT loss leads to increased whole mouth perceived bitterness via increased contralateral taste sensation at IX (Catalanotto et al. 1993; Kveton and Bartoshuk 1994; Lehman et al. 1995; Yanagisawa et al. 1998), an effect that appears to occur preferentially in PROP supertasters (Snyder 2010). Most oral sensory input rises ipsilaterally into the central nervous system (Norgren 1990), so these contralateral effects strongly implicate central modulation.

During CT anesthesia, approximately 40% of healthy subjects experience contralateral taste phantoms at IX that vary in quality and intensity, fading with the anesthetic (Yanagisawa et al. 1998). Topical anesthesia at the site of sensation abolishes these *release-of-inhibition* phantoms (Yanagisawa et al. 1998) presumably by suppressing spontaneous neural activity at their source (Norgren and Pfaffmann 1975).

Also, in one case report (Bartoshuk et al. 1994b), a bitter phantom arose bilaterally at IX following tonsillectomy. Spatial testing indicated complete IX loss, yet the phantom intensified with whole mouth topical anesthesia. This *nerve-stimulation* phantom was probably caused by surgical damage to IX and further disinhibited by CT anesthesia. In both of these examples, the common theme is lateral disinhibition subsequent to nerve damage.

In addition to its interaction with IX, CT input also appears to inhibit trigeminal cues. Functionally, this interaction may suppress oral pain during intake, and it may guide tactile referral of taste cues following localized taste damage. However, because supertasters have the most extensive taste and trigeminal input, CT damage may carry adverse sensory consequences due to extreme trigeminal disinhibition: following unilateral CT anesthesia, PROP supertasters show increased ratings for the burn of capsaicin on the contralateral anterior tongue (Tie et al. 1999). In addition, severe childhood ear infections are thought to compromise CT (e.g., Bartoshuk et al. 1996; Gedikli et al. 2001), which leads to augmented tactile sensations from dietary fat that may drive sweet–fat food acceptance and long-term weight gain (e.g., Snyder et al. 2003; Kim et al. 2007; Catalanotto et al. 2009; Ventura et al. 2009; Bartoshuk et al. 2012).

Oral pain phantoms are another serious consequence of trigeminal disinhibition. Burning mouth syndrome (BMS), a condition found mainly in postmenopausal women, is characterized by severe oral pain in the absence of visible pathology (Grushka and Sessle 1987). BMS is often described as psychogenic, but chemosensory testing suggests otherwise. Patients with BMS show significantly reduced bitterness for quinine on the anterior tongue, which is consistent with CT damage (Bartoshuk et al. 1999; Grushka and Bartoshuk 2000). Nearly 50% of BMS patients experience taste phantoms at IX (Grushka et al. 1986), and topical anesthesia usually intensifies BMS-related taste phantoms and oral pain (Ship et al. 1995). Finally, BMS pain is correlated with high fungiform papillae density, indicating that BMS is especially prevalent among supertasters. Together, these data strongly suggest that BMS is an oral pain phantom generated by CT damage. Further supporting this view, agonists to the inhibitory neurotransmitter γ-aminobutyric acid (GABA) suppress BMS pain (Grushka et al. 1998) presumably by restoring lost inhibition from absent taste cues.

5.3.3.1.2 Oral Anesthesia in Clinical Evaluation

Laboratory and clinical data support the use of topical anesthesia in the mouth to determine the locus of oral sensory dysfunction. However, interpretations of topical anesthesia must be made with care, as incomplete anesthesia will hinder differential diagnosis. In a typical protocol, patients hold ~5 mL of 0.5% dyclone in the mouth for 60 s, rest for 60 s, rinse with water, and describe any oral sensation experienced for the duration of the sensory block (Bartoshuk et al. 1994b). Anesthesia should always be accompanied by a thorough medical history, physical examination, and thorough evaluation of spatial and whole mouth oral sensation.

If a taste or oral pain complaint becomes more intense following oral anesthesia, then it does not arise from normal stimulation of oral sensory receptors. Venous taste sensations and other dysgeusias may be caused by intake of certain therapeutic agents (Bradley 1973; Stephen et al. 1980; Fetting et al. 1985), so a patient's use of medications and supplements should be reviewed. Another possibility is that the nerve innervating the region of sensory disturbance has sustained physical damage. If damage is peripheral to ganglion cell bodies, the resulting neuroma may produce a nerve-stimulation phantom; topical anesthesia exacerbates nerve-stimulation phantoms via central disinhibition (Bartoshuk et al. 1994b). Conclusions involving nerve damage should be confirmed by further neurological examination.

When local anesthesia abolishes a taste or oral pain complaint, an actual stimulus may be present in the mouth. To test for the presence of such a stimulus, the patient should attempt to rinse it from the mouth; if the offending sensation subsides at all, an actual stimulus should be considered. Alternatively, nerve damage unrelated to the altered sensation may have disinhibited input related to it, resulting in a central release-of-inhibition phantom; topical anesthesia further intensifies these phantoms (Bartoshuk et al. 1994b). Spatial testing should reveal localized taste loss at a site distant from the phantom.

5.3.4 RETRONASAL OLFACTION

Odorants reach receptors in the nasal mucosa by two different routes: orthonasal olfaction refers to odorants that enter the nostrils during sniffing, whereas retronasal olfaction refers to odors that are emitted by foods and forced behind the palate into the nasal cavity during chewing and swallowing (Rozin 1982). This distinction is not merely conceptual, as orthonasal and retronasal olfaction are processed in different brain regions (e.g., Small et al. 1997, 2005). Perceptually, retronasal odor cues fuse with taste and oral tactile sensations, culminating in a unitary sensation of flavor that is localized to the mouth. For many years, this process was thought to involve oral touch alone (Hollingworth and Poffenberger 1917), but mounting data indicate that taste input plays a significant role: taste and retronasal odor cues enhance one another when mixed (e.g., Kuo et al. 1993; Murphy et al. 1977; Frank et al. 1989); PROP supertasters experience stronger retronasal odor sensations than do nontasters (Bartoshuk et al. 2002a; Snyder et al. 2007); and regional taste loss suppresses retronasal olfaction and whole mouth taste in parallel (Snyder 2010; Bartoshuk et al. 2012). Clinical accounts of chemosensory disturbance often begin with reports of flavor loss, and industrial applications of oral sensory testing typically involve the impact of altered food composition or manufacturing on flavor; thus, retronasal olfactory testing has emerged as a useful element of oral sensory evaluation.

Methods for the presentation of retronasal odor stimuli vary considerably, including odors infused into a water or tastant solution, vapor-phase odorants released into the mouth, and sampled food items. All of these methods are confounded to varying degrees by enhancement or *dumping* effects arising from odor–taste integration (e.g., Frank and Byram 1988; Stevenson et al. 1999), which undermines the validity of retronasal intensity ratings. As a result, consistent procedures for retronasal olfactory evaluation have not been established, although there is general agreement that an oral stimulus must be present to induce sufficient levels of retronasal sensation. One approach used recently involves the spatial and temporal dissection of flavor components: foods are sniffed (orthonasal olfaction) and then sampled with the nose plugged (taste and oral somatosensation), and the nose is released to elicit a distinct retronasal cue (Snyder 2010). Testing in this manner permits evaluation of flavor loss induced by oral sensory insult vs. other factors (e.g., olfactory deficits, nasal blockade).

The capacity to evaluate distinct components of flavor experience holds great potential for food industry efforts to enhance food palatability. For economic reasons, food manufacturers have long added taste stimuli to food to enhance its flavor, as commodities like sugar and salt are generally less costly than flavor extracts (e.g., Noble 1996). However, rising consumer awareness of health risks associated with added sugar and salt has raised interest in alternative strategies for flavor enhancement. Recent data offer an intriguing possibility: chemical and sensory measurements from tomatoes reveal that some flavor volatiles enhance sweetness independently of sugar (Tieman et al. 2012). In other words, some of the sweetness perceived in fruits and vegetables arises from sugars, and some of it arises from retronasal odor cues associated with sweetness. Thus, the addition of volatiles to food may represent a novel way to enhance sweetness, flavor, and palatability without adding sugar.

5.4 CONCLUSION

Human psychophysical evaluation is an essential tool in clinical, basic, and consumer science, offering rich insight into neurobehavioral processes that are often inaccessible by other means. In the chemical senses, significant efforts have been made to develop and optimize measurement tools that reflect individual differences accurately and allow flexible use in clinical, research, industrial, and field settings. Conservative approaches to this task emphasize threshold measures, but contemporary suprathreshold scaling has emerged as a sophisticated means of measuring and comparing biologically relevant experiences at real-world levels. When performed correctly, these methods have facilitated the study of oral sensory variation in health and disease, and the systematic use of techniques from psychophysics, anatomy, neurology, and genetics has revealed complex relationships among oral sensation, affect, behavior, nutrition, and health. In short, ongoing refinements in chemosensory assessment have strong implications for long-term health outcomes, as they yield highly predictive and highly comparable measures of sensory and hedonic experience.

REFERENCES

Adler, J. 1972. Chemoreception in bacteria. In *Olfaction and Taste IV*, ed. D. Schneider, pp. 70–80. Stuttgart: Wissenschaftliche Verlagsgesellschaft MBH.

Aitken, R.C.B., H.M. Ferres, and J.L. Gedye. 1963. Distraction from flashing lights. *Aerosp Med* 34:302–306.

Alfano, M. 1974. The origin of gingival fluid. *J Theoret Biol* 47:127–136.

Algom, D. 1992. Memory psychophysics: An examination of its perceptual and cognitive prospects. In *Psychophysical Approaches to Cognition*, ed. D. Algom, pp. 441–513. New York: North-Holland.

Azevedo, E., H. Krieger, M.P. Mi, and N.E. Morton. 1965. PTC taste sensitivity and endemic goiter in Brazil. *Am J Hum Genet* 17:87–90.

Barnicot, N.A., H. Harris, and H. Kalmus. 1951. Taste thresholds of further eighteen compounds and their correlation with P.T.C. thresholds. *Ann Eugen* 16:119–128.

Bartoshuk, L.M. 1974. NaCl thresholds in man: Thresholds for water taste or NaCl taste? *J Com Physiol Psychol* 87:310–325.

Bartoshuk, L.M. 1978. The psychophysics of taste. *Am J Clin Nutr* 31:1068–1077.

Bartoshuk, L.M. 1979. Bitter taste of saccharin: Related to the genetic ability to taste the bitter substance 6-*n*-propylthiouracil (PROP). *Science* 205:34–935.

Bartoshuk, L.M. 1988. Clinical psychophysics of taste. *Gerodontics* 4:249–255.

Bartoshuk, L.M. 1989. Clinical evaluation of the sense of taste. *Ear Nose Throat J* 68:331–337.

Bartoshuk, L.M. 2000. Comparing sensory experiences across individuals: Recent psychophysical advances illuminate genetic variation in taste perception. *Chem Senses* 25:447–460.

Bartoshuk, L.M., and V.B. Duffy. 1994. Supertasting and earaches: Genetics and pathology alter our taste worlds. *Appetite* 23:292–293.

Bartoshuk, L.M., and D.J. Snyder. 2004. Psychophysical measurement of human taste experience. In *Handbook of Behavioral Neurobiology Vol. 14: Neurobiology of Food and Fluid Intake, 2nd ed.*, eds. E.M. Stricker and S.C. Woods, pp. 89–107. New York: Plenum Press.

Bartoshuk, L.M., B. Rifkin, L.E. Marks, and P. Bars. 1986. Taste and aging. *J Gerontol* 41:51–57.

Bartoshuk, L.M., S. Desnoyers, C.A. Hudson et al. 1987. Tasting on localized areas. *Ann NY Acad Sci* 510:166–168.

Bartoshuk, L.M., V.B. Duffy, and I.J. Miller. 1994a. PTC/PROP tasting: Anatomy, psychophysics, and sex effects. *Physiol Behav* 56:1165–1171.

Bartoshuk, L.M., J.F. Kveton, K. Yanagisawa, and F.A. Catalanotto. 1994b. Taste loss and taste phantoms: A role of inhibition in taste. In *Olfaction and Taste XI*, eds. K. Kurihara, N. Suzuki, and H. Ogawa, pp. 557–560. New York: Springer-Verlag.

Bartoshuk, L.M., V.B. Duffy, D.R. Reed, and A.L. Williams. 1996. Supertasting, earaches, and head injury: Genetics and pathology alter our taste worlds. *Neurosci Biobehav Rev* 20:79–87.

Bartoshuk, L.M., V.B. Duffy, L.A. Lucchina, J.M. Prutkin, and K. Fast. 1998. PROP (6-*n*-propylthiouracil) supertasters and the saltiness of NaCl. *Ann NY Acad Sci* 855:793–796.

Bartoshuk, L.M., M. Grushka, V.B. Duffy et al. 1999. Burning mouth syndrome: Damage to CN VII and pain phantoms in CN V. *Chem Senses* 24:609.

Bartoshuk, L.M., V.B. Duffy, K. Fast et al. 2001. What makes a supertaster? *Chem Senses* 26:1074.

Bartoshuk, L.M., A.K. Chapo, V.B. Duffy et al. 2002a. Oral phantoms: Evidence for central inhibition produced by taste. *Chem Senses* 27:A52.

Bartoshuk, L.M., V.B. Duffy, K. Fast, B.G. Green, J.M. Prutkin, and D.J. Snyder. 2002b. Labeled scales (e.g., category, Likert, VAS) and invalid across-group comparisons: What we have learned from genetic variation in taste. *Food Qual Pref* 14:125–138.

Bartoshuk, L.M., V.B. Duffy, A.K. Chapo et al. 2004a. From psychophysics to the clinic: Missteps and advances. *Food Qual Pref* 15:617–632.

Bartoshuk, L.M., V.B. Duffy, B.G. Green et al. 2004b. Valid across-group comparisons with labeled scales: The gLMS vs. magnitude matching. *Physiol Behav* 82:109–114.

Bartoshuk, L.M., V.B. Duffy, K. Fast, and D.J. Snyder. 2004c. Genetic differences in human oral perception: Advanced methods reveal basic problems in intensity scaling. In *Genetic Variation in Taste Sensitivity: Measurement, Significance, and Implications*, eds. J. Prescott and B.J. Tepper, pp. 1–42. New York: Marcel Dekker.

Bartoshuk, L.M., K. Fast, and D.J. Snyder. 2005. Differences in our sensory worlds: Invalid comparisons with labeled scales. *Cur Dir Psycho Sci* 14:122–125.

Bartoshuk, L.M., V.B. Duffy, J.E. Hayes, H. Moskowitz, and D.J. Snyder. 2006. Psychophysics of sweet and fat perception in obesity: Problems, solutions, and new perspectives. *Philo Trans R Soc B* 361:1137–1148.

Bartoshuk, L.M., J.J. Kalva, L.A. Puentes, D.J. Snyder, and C.A. Sims. 2010. Valid comparisons of food preferences. *Chem Senses* 35:A20.

Bartoshuk, L.M., F.A. Catalanotto, H. Hoffman, H.N. Logan, and D.J. Snyder. 2012. Taste damage (otitis media, tonsillectomy, and head and neck cancer), oral sensations, and BMI. *Physiol Behav.* 107:516–526.

Basson, M.D., L.M. Bartoshuk, S.Z. Dichello, L. Panzini, J. Weiffenbach, and V.B. Duffy. 2005. Association between 6-n-propylthiouracil (PROP) bitterness and colonic neoplasms. *Dig Dis Sci* 50:483–489.

Berry, H., and E.C. Huskisson. 1972. Treatment of rheumatoid arthritis. *Clin Trials J* 9:13–14.

Biernat, M., and M. Manis. 1994. Shifting standards and stereotype-based judgments. *J Pers Soc Psychol* 66:5–20.

Birnbaum, M.H. 1999. How to show that 9 > 221: Collect judgments in a between-subjects design. *Psychol Methods* 4:243–249.

Blakeslee, A.F. 1932. Genetics of sensory thresholds: Taste for phenyl thio carbamide. *Proc Natl Acad Sci* 18:120–130.

Blakeslee, A.F., and A.L. Fox. 1932. Our different taste worlds. *J Hered* 23:97–107.

Borg, G. 1970. Perceived exertion as an indicator of somatic stress. *Scand J Rehab Med* 2:92–98.

Borg, G. 1982. A category scale with ratio properties for intermodal and interindividual comparisons. In *Psychophysical Judgment and the Process of Perception*, eds. H.G. Geissler and P. Petzold, pp. 25–34. Berlin: VEB Deutscher Verlag der Wissenschaften.

Borg, G. 1990. Psychophysical scaling with applications in physical work and the perception of exertion. *Scand J Work Environ Health* 16:1:55–58.

Boring, E.G. 1942. *Sensation and Perception in the History of Experimental Psychology.* New York: Appleton.

Bradley, R.M. 1973. Electrophysiological investigations of intravascular taste using perfused rat tongue. *Am J Psychol* 224:300–304.

Brindley, G.S. 1960. *Physiology of the Retina and the Visual Pathway.* London: Edward Arnold.

Bromley, S.M., and R.L. Doty. 2003. Clinical disorders affecting taste: Evaluation and management. In *Handbook of Olfaction and Gustation*, ed. R.L. Doty, pp. 935–957. New York: Marcel Dekker.

Bufe, B., P.A.S. Breslin, C. Kuhn et al. 2005. The molecular basis of individual differences in phenylthiocarbamide and propylthiouracil bitterness perception. *Curr Biol* 15:322–327.

Bujas, Z. 1971. Electrical taste. In *Handbook of Sensory Physiology, Vol. 4, Part 2: Chemical Senses—Taste*, ed. L.M. Beidler, pp. 180–199. Berlin: Springer.

Bull, T.R. 1965. Taste and the chorda tympani. *J Laryngol Otol* 79:479–493.

Cain, W.S., and J.C. Stevens. 1989. Uniformity of olfactory loss in aging. *Ann NY Acad Sci* 561:29–38.

Calò, C., A. Padiglia, A. Zonza et al. 2011. Polymorphisms in TAS2R38 and the taste bud trophic factor gustin gene co-operate in modulating PROP taste phenotype. *Physiol Behav* 104:1065–1071.

Catalanotto, F.A., L.M. Bartoshuk, K.M. Östrom, J.F. Gent, and K. Fast. 1993. Effects of anesthesia of the facial nerve on taste. *Chem Senses* 18:461–470.

Catalanotto, F.A., E.T. Broe, L.M. Bartoshuk, V.D. Mayo, and D.J. Snyder. 2009. Otitis media and intensification of non-taste oral sensations. *Chem Senses* 34:A120.

Collings, V.B. 1974. Human taste response as a function of locus of stimulation on the tongue and soft palate. *Percept Psychophys* 16:169–174.

Cooper, D.S. 2005. Antithyroid drugs. *New Engl J Med* 352:905.

Cornsweet, T.M. 1962. The staircase method in psychophysics. *Am J Psychol* 75:485–491.

Cowan, P.W. 1990. Atrophy of fungiform papillae following lingual nerve damage—A suggested mechanism. *Br Dent J* 168:95.

Cowart, B.J. 1989. Relationships between taste and smell across the adult life span. *Ann NY Acad Sci* 561:39–55.

Deems, R.O., M.I. Friedman, L.S. Friedman, and W.C. Maddrey. 1991. Clinical manifestations of olfactory and gustatory disorders associated with hepatic and renal disease. In *Smell and Taste in Health and Disease*, eds. T.V. Getchell, R.L. Doty, L.M. Bartoshuk, and J.B. Snow, Jr., pp. 805–816. New York: Raven Press.

Delwiche, J.F., M.F. Lera, and P.A.S Breslin. 2000. Selective removal of a target stimulus localized by taste in humans. *Chem Senses* 25:181–187.

Delwiche, J.F., Z. Buletic, and P.A.S. Breslin. 2001. Relationship of papillae number to bitter intensity of quinine and PROP within and between individuals. *Physiol Behav* 74:329–337.

Desai, H., G. Smutzer, S.E. Coldwell, and J.W. Griffith. 2011. Validation of edible taste strips for identifying PROP taste recognition thresholds. *Laryngoscope* 121:1177–1183.

DeSimone, J.A., G.L. Heck, and L.M. Bartoshuk. 1980. Surface active taste modifiers: A comparison of the physical and psychophysical properties of gymnemic acid and sodium lauryl sulfate. *Chem Senses* 5:317–330.

DeSimone, J.A., G.L. Heck, and S.K. DeSimone. 1981. Active ion transport in dog tongue: A possible role in taste. *Science* 214:1039–1041.

DeSimone, J.A., G.L. Heck, S. Mierson, and S.K. DeSimone. 1984. The active ion transport properties of canine lingual epithelia in vitro: Implications for gustatory transduction. *J. Gen Physiol* 83:633–656.

Dinehart, M.E., J.E. Hayes, L.M. Bartoshuk, S.L. Lanier, and V.B. Duffy. 2006. Bitter taste markers explain variability in vegetable sweetness, bitterness, and intake. *Physiol Behav* 87:304–313.

Doty, R.L., R. Bagla, M. Morgenson, and N. Mirza. 2001. NaCl thresholds: Relationship to anterior tongue locus, area of stimulation, and number of fungiform papillae. *Physiol Behav* 72:373–378.

Drayna, D., H. Coon, U.-K. Kim et al. 2003. Genetic analysis of a complex trait in the Utah Genetic Reference Project: A major locus for PTC taste ability on chromosome 7q and a secondary locus on chromosome 16p. *Hum Genet* 112:567–572.

Drewnowski, A. 2003. Genetics of human taste perception. In *Handbook of Olfaction and Gustation, 2nd ed.*, ed. R.L. Doty, pp. 847–860. New York: Marcel Dekker.

Drewnowski, A., S.A. Henderson, C.S. Hann, W.A. Berg, and M.T. Ruffin. 2000. Genetic taste markers and preferences for vegetables and fruit of female breast care patients. *J Am Diet Assoc* 100:191–197.

Duffy, V.B. 2004. Associations between oral sensation, dietary behaviors, and risk of cardiovascular disease (CVD). *Appetite* 43:5–9.

Duffy, V.B. 2007. Variation in oral sensation: Implications for diet and health. *Curr Opin Gastroenterol* 23:171–177.

Duffy, V.B., M.N. Phillips, J.M. Peterson, and L.M. Bartoshuk. 2001. Bitterness of 6-*n*-propylthiouracil (PROP) associates with bitter sensations and intake of vegetables. *Appetite* 37:137–138.

El-Deiry, A., and B.F. McCabe. 1990. Temporal lobe tumor manifested by localized dysgeusia. *Ann Otol Rhinol Laryngol* 99:586–587.

Engen, T. 1972. Psychophysics. I. Discrimination and detection. In *Woodworth & Schlosberg's Experimental Psychology (Vol. 1: Sensation and Perception)*, eds. J.W. Kling and L.A. Riggs, pp. 11–46. New York: Holt, Rinehart and Winston.

Essick, G.K., A. Chopra, S. Guest, and F. McGlone. 2003. Lingual tactile acuity, taste perception, and the density and diameter of fungiform papillae in female subjects. *Physiol Behav* 80:289–302.

Fast, K., B.G. Green, D.J. Snyder, and L.M. Bartoshuk. 2001. Remembered intensities of taste and oral burn correlate with PROP bitterness. *Chem Senses* 26:1069.

Fast, K., B.G. Green, and L.M. Bartoshuk. 2002. Developing a scale to measure just about anything: Comparisons across groups and individuals. *Appetite* 39:75.

Fay, T. 1927. Observations and results from intracranial section of the glossopharyngeus and vagus nerves in man. *J Neurol Psychopathol* 8:110–123.

Fechner, G. 1860/1966. *Elements of Psychophysics*, trans. H.E. Adler, D.H. Howes, and E.G. Boring. New York: Holt, Rinehart and Winston.

Fetting, J.H., P.M. Wilcox, V.R. Sheidler, J.P. Enterline, R.C. Donehower, and L.B. Grochow. 1985. Tastes associated with parenteral chemotherapy for breast cancer. *Cancer Treat Rep* 69:1249–1251.

Fischer, R. 1967. Genetics and gustatory chemoreception in man and other primates. In *The Chemical Senses and Nutrition*, eds. M.R. Kare and O. Maller, pp. 621–681. Baltimore: Johns Hopkins University Press.

Fischer, R., F. Griffin, S. England, and S. Garn. 1961. Taste thresholds and food dislikes. *Nature* 191:1328.

Fischer, R., F. Griffin, and A.R. Kaplan. 1963. Taste thresholds, cigarette smoking, and food dislikes. *Med Exp* 9:151–167.

Fox, A.L. 1931. Six in ten "taste blind" to bitter chemical. *Sci News Lett* 9:249.

Fox, A.L. 1932. The relationship between chemical constitution and taste. *Proc Natl Acad Sci* 18:115–120.

Frank, M.E., and D.V. Smith. 1991. Electrogustometry: A simple way to test taste. In *Smell and Taste in Health and Disease*, eds. T.V. Getchell, R.L. Doty, L.M. Bartoshuk, & J.B. Snow, Jr., pp. 503–514. New York: Raven Press.

Frank, M.E., T.P. Hettinger, and M.A. Barry. 2003. Contemporary measurement of human gustatory function. In *Handbook of Olfaction and Gustation*, 2nd ed., ed. R.L. Doty, pp. 783–804. New York: Marcel Dekker.

Frank, R.A., and J. Byram. 1988. Taste–smell interactions are tastant and odorant dependent. *Chem Senses* 13:445–455.

Frank, R.A., K. Ducheny, and S.J.S. Mize. 1989. Strawberry odor, but not red color, enhances the sweetness of sucrose solutions. *Chem Senses* 14:371–377.

Fushan, A.A., C.T. Simons, J.P. Slack, and D. Drayna. 2010. Association between common variation in genes encoding sweet taste signaling components and human sucrose perception. *Chem Senses* 35:579–592.

Gairns, F.W. 1953. Sensory endings other than taste buds in the human tongue. *J Physiol* 121:33P–34P.

Galindo-Cuspinera, V., T. Waeber, N. Antille, C. Hartmann, N. Stead, and N. Martin. 2009. Reliability of threshold and suprathreshold methods for taste phenotyping: Characterization with PROP and sodium chloride. *Chemosens Percept* 2:214–228.

Gedikli, O., H. Doğru, G. Aydin, M. Tüz, K. Uygur, and A. Sari. 2001. Histopathological changes of chorda tympani in chronic otitis media. *Laryngoscope* 111:724–727.

Giduck, S.A., R.M. Threatte, and M.R. Kare. 1987. Cephalic reflexes: Their role in digestion and possible roles in absorption and metabolism. *J Nutr* 117:1191–1196.

Goto, N., T. Yamamoto, M. Kaneko, and H. Tomita. 1983. Primary pontine hemorrhage and gustatory disturbance: Clinicoanatomic study. *Stroke* 14:507–511.

Gracely, R.H., P. McGrath, and R. Dubner. 1978. Validity and sensitivity of ratio scales of sensory and affective verbal pain descriptors: Manipulation of affect by diazepam. *Pain* 5:19–29.

Grant, R., M.M. Ferguson, R. Strang, J.W. Turner, and I. Bone. 1987. Evoked taste thresholds in a normal population and the application of electrogustometry to trigeminal nerve disease. *J Neurol Neurosurg Psychiatry* 50:12–21.

Green, B.G. 2002. Studying taste as a cutaneous sense. *Food Qual Pref* 14:99–109.

Green, B.G., and P. George. 2004. "Thermal taste" predicts higher responsiveness to chemical taste and flavor. *Chem Senses* 29:617–628.

Green, B.G., and J.E. Hayes. 2004. Individual differences in perception of bitterness from capsaicin, piperine, and zingerone. *Chem Senses* 29:53–60.

Green, B.G., G.S. Shaffer, and M.M. Gilmore. 1993. A semantically-labeled magnitude scale of oral sensation with apparent ratio properties. *Chem Senses* 18:683–702.

Green, D.M., and J.A. Swets. 1966. *Signal Detection Theory and Psychophysics.* New York: John Wiley & Sons.

Groves, J., and W.P. Gibson. 1974. Significance of taste and electrogustometry in assessing the prognosis of Bell's (idiopathic) facial palsy. *J Laryngol Otol* 88:855–861.

Grushka, M., and L.M. Bartoshuk. 2000. Burning mouth syndrome and oral dysesthesias. *Can J Diagn* 17:99–109.

Grushka, M., and B.J. Sessle. 1987. Burning mouth syndrome: A historical review. *Clin J Pain* 2:245–252.

Grushka, M., B.J. Sessle, and T.P. Howley. 1986. Psychophysical evidence of taste dysfunction in burning mouth syndrome. *Chem Senses* 11:485–498.

Grushka, M., J. Epstein, and A. Mott. 1998. An open-label, dose escalation pilot study of the effect of clonazepam in burning mouth syndrome. *Oral Surg Oral Med Oral Pathol Oral Radiol Endod* 86:557–561.

Hall, M.J., L.M. Bartoshuk, W.S. Cain, and J.C. Stevens. 1975. PTC taste blindness and the taste of caffeine. *Nature* 253:442–443.

Halpern, B.P., and L.M. Nelson. 1965. Bulbar gustatory responses to anterior and to posterior tongue stimulation in the rat. *Am J Physiol* 209:105–110.

Hänig, D.P. 1901. Zur Psychophysik des Geschmackssinnes. *Philos Stud* 17:576–623.

Hara, S. 1955. Interrelationship among stimulus intensity, stimulated area, and reaction time in the human gustatory sensation. *Bull Tokyo Med Dent Univ* 2:147–158.

Harder, D.B., G. Whitney, P. Frye, J.C. Smith, and M.E. Rashotte. 1984. Strain differences among mice in taste psychophysics of sucrose octaacetate. *Chem Senses* 9:311–323.

Harris, H., and H. Kalmus. 1949a. The measurement of taste sensitivity to phenylthiourea (P.T.C.). *Ann Eugen* 15:24–31.

Harris, H., and H. Kalmus. 1949b. Chemical sensitivity in genetical differences of taste sensitivity. *Ann Eugen* 15:32–45.

Hartmann, G. 1939. Application of individual taste difference towards phenyl-thio-carbamide in genetic investigations. *Ann Eugen* 9:123–135.

Hausser-Hauw, C., and J. Bancaud. 1987. Gustatory hallucinations in epileptic seizures. *Brain* 110:339–359.

Hayes, J.E., and R.S.J. Keast. 2011. Two decades of supertasting: Where do we stand? *Physiol Behav* 104:1072–1074.

Hayes, J.E., L.M. Bartoshuk, J.R. Kidd, and V.B. Duffy. 2008. Supertasting and PROP bitterness depends on more than the TAS2R38 gene. *Chem Senses* 33:255–265.

Heath, T.P., J.K. Melichar, D.J. Nutt, and L.F. Donaldson. 2006. Human taste thresholds are modulated by serotonin and noradrenaline. *J Neurosci* 26:12664–12671.

Henkin, R.I., J.R. Gill, and F.C. Bartter. 1963. Studies on taste thresholds in normal man and in patients with adrenal cortical insufficiency: The role of adrenal cortical steroids and of serum sodium concentration. *J Clin Invest* 42:727–735.

Herness, M.S. 1985. Neurophysiological and biophysical evidence on the mechanism of electric taste. *J Gen Physiol* 86:59–87.

Hertz, J., W.S. Cain, L.M. Bartoshuk, and T.F. Dolan. 1975. Olfactory and taste sensitivity in children with cystic fibrosis. *Physiol Behav* 14:89–94.

Hetherington, M.M., and B.J. Rolls. 1987. Methods of investigating human eating behavior. In *Feeding and Drinking*, eds. F.M. Toates, and N.E. Rowland, pp. 77–109. New York: Elsevier.

Hoffman, H.J., E.K. Ishii, and R.H. Macturk. 1998. Age-related changes in the prevalence of smell/taste problems among the United States adult population: Results of the 1994 Disability Supplement to the National Health Interview Survey (NHIS). *Ann NY Acad Sci* 855:716–722.

Hollingworth, H.L., and A.T. Poffenberger. 1917. *The Sense of Taste*. New York: Moffat, Yard and Company.

House, H.P. 1963. Early and late complications of stapes surgery. *Arch Otolaryngol* 78:606–613.

Hummel, T., A. Erras, and G. Kobal. 1997. A test for screening of taste function. *Rhinology* 35:146–148.

Ileri-Gurel, E., B. Pehlivanoglu, and M. Dogan. 2013. Effect of acute stress on taste perception: In relation with baseline anxiety level and body weight. *Chem Senses* 38:27–34.

Jesteadt, W. 1980. An adaptive procedure for subjective judgments. *Percept Psychophys* 28:1:85–88.

Jones, L.V., D.R. Peryam, and L.L. Thurstone. 1955. Development of a scale for measuring soldier's food preferences. *Food Res* 20:512–520.

Jones, R.O., and T.L. Fry. 1984. A new complication of prosthetic ossicular reconstruction. *Arch Otolaryngol* 110:757–758.

Kalmus, H., and D. Farnsworth. 1959. Impairment and recovery of taste following irradiation of the oropharynx. *J Laryngol Otol* 73:180–182.

Kamen, J.M., F.J. Pilgrim, N.J. Gutman, and B.J. Kroll. 1961. Interactions of suprathreshold taste stimuli. *J Exp Psychol* 62:348–356.

Kaminski, L.C., S.A. Henderson, and A. Drewnowski. 2000. Young women's food preferences and taste responsiveness to 6-*n*-propylthiouracil (PROP). *Physiol Behav* 68:691–697.

Kanagasuntheram, R., W.C. Wong, and H.K. Chan. 1969. Some observations of the innervation of the human nasopharynx. *J Anat* 104:361–376.

Kashiwayanagi, M., K. Yoshii, Y. Kobatake, and K. Kurihara. 1981. Taste transduction mechanism: Similar effects of various modifications of gustatory receptors on neural responses to chemical and electrical stimulation in the frog. *J Gen Physiol* 78:259–265.

Keller, K.L., L.C. Liang, J. Sakimura et al. 2012. Common variants in the CD36 gene are associated with oral fat perception, fat preferences, and obesity in African Americans. *Obesity* 20:1066–1073.

Kim, J.B., D.C. Park, C.I. Cha, and S.G. Yeo. 2007. Relationship between pediatric obesity and otitis media with effusion. *Arch Otolaryngol Head Neck Surg* 133:379–382.

Kim, U.-K., E. Jorgenson, H. Coon, M. Leppert, N. Risch, and D. Drayna. 2003. Positional cloning of the human quantitative trait locus underlying taste sensitivity to phenylthiocarbamide. *Science* 299:1221–1225.

Kranzler, H.R., K. Skipsey, and V. Modesto-Lowe. 1998. PROP taster status and parental history of alcohol dependence. *Drug Alcohol Depend* 52:109–113.

Krarup, B. 1958. Taste reactions of patients with Bell's palsy. *Acta Oto-Laryngol* 49:389–399.

Kuo, Y-L., R.M. Pangborn, and A.C. Noble. 1993. Temporal patterns of nasal, oral, and retronasal perception of citral and vanillin and interaction of these odorants with selected tastants. *Int J Food Sci Tech* 28:127–137.

Kveton, J.F., and L.M. Bartoshuk. 1994. The effect of unilateral chorda tympani damage on taste. *Laryngoscope* 104:25–29.

Laming, D. 1997. *The Measurement of Sensation*. New York: Oxford University Press.

Lasagna, L. 1960. The clinical measurement of pain. *Ann NY Acad Sci* 86:28–37.

Lawless, H.T. 1980. A comparison of different methods used to assess sensitivity to the taste of phenylthiocarbamide (PTC). *Chem Senses* 5:247–256.

Lawless, H.T., and H. Heymann. 2010. *Sensory Evaluation of Food: Principles and Practices, 2nd ed.* New York: Springer.

Lawless, H.T., C.J.C. Thomas, and M. Johnston. 1995. Variation in odor thresholds for l-carvone and cineole and correlations with suprathreshold intensity ratings. *Chem Senses* 20:9–17.

Le Floch, J.P., G. Le Lievre, J. Verroust, C. Phillippon, R. Peynegre, and L. Perlemuter. 1990. Factors related to the electric taste threshold in type 1 diabetic patients. *Diabet Med* 7:526–531.

Lehman, C.D., L.M. Bartoshuk, F.A. Catalanotto, J.F. Kveton, and R.A. Lowlicht. 1995. The effect of anesthesia of the chorda tympani nerve on taste perception in humans. *Physiol Behav* 57:943–951.

Lewis, D., and W.E. Dandy. 1930. The course of the nerve fibers transmitting sensation of taste. *Arch Surg* 21:249–288.

Likert, R. 1932. A technique for the measurement of attitudes. *Arch Psychol* 140:5–55.

Lim, J., L. Urban, and B.G. Green. 2008. Measures of individual differences in taste and creaminess perception. *Chem Senses* 33:493–501.

Lim, J., A. Wood, and B.G. Green. 2009. Derivation and evaluation of a labeled hedonic scale. *Chem Senses* 34:739–751.

Linschoten, M.R., and J.H.A. Kroeze. 1991. Spatial summation in taste: NaCl thresholds and stimulated area on the anterior tongue. *Chem Senses* 16:219–224.

Linschoten, M.R., L.O. Harvey, P.A. Eller, and B.W. Jafek. 1996. Rapid and accurate measurement of taste and smell thresholds using an adaptive maximum-likelihood staircase procedure. *Chem Senses* 21:633–634.

Liu, H.-X., A.M. Staubach-Grosse, K.D. Walton, D.A. Saims, D.L. Gumucio, and C.M. Mistretta. 2009. WNT5a in tongue and fungiform papilla development. *Ann NY Acad Sci* 1170:11–17.

Lucchina, L.A., O.F. Curtis, P. Putnam, A. Drewnowski, J.M. Prutkin, and L.M. Bartoshuk. 1998. Psychophysical measurement of 6-*n*-propylthiouracil (PROP) taste perception. *Ann NY Acad Sci* 855:817–822.

Ly, A., and A. Drewnowski. 2001. PROP (6-*n*-propylthiouracil) tasting and sensory responses to caffeine, sucrose, neohesperidin dihydrochalcone, and chocolate. *Chem Senses* 26:41–47.

Mackenzie, I.C.K. 1955. A simple method of testing taste. *Lancet* 265:377–378.

Manis, M., M. Biernat, and T.F. Nelson. 1991. Comparison and expectancy processes in human judgment. *J Pers Soc Psychol* 61:203–211.

Marks, L.E. 1974. *Sensory Processes: The New Psychophysics*. New York: Academic Press.

Marks, L.E., and J.C. Stevens. 1980. Measuring sensation in the aged. In *Aging in the 1980s: Psychological Issues*, ed. L.W. Poon, pp. 592–598. Washington, DC: American Psychological Association.

Marks, L.E., J.C. Stevens, L.M. Bartoshuk, J.G. Gent, B. Rifkin, and V.K. Stone. 1988. Magnitude matching: The measurement of taste and smell. *Chem Senses* 13:63–87.

Mattes, R.D., and B.J. Cowart. 1994. Dietary assessment of patients with chemosensory disorders. *J Am Diet Assoc* 94:50–56.

McBurney, D.H. 1966. Magnitude estimation of the taste of sodium chloride after adaptation to sodium chloride. *J Exp Psychol* 72:869–873.

McBurney, D.H. 1986. Taste, smell, and flavor terminology: Taking the confusion out of fusion. In *Clinical Measurement of Taste and Smell*, eds. H.L. Meiselman and R.S. Rivlin, pp. 117–125. New York: Macmillan.

McBurney, D.H., and L.M. Bartoshuk. 1973. Interactions between stimuli with different taste qualities. *Physiol Behav* 10:1101–1106.

McBurney, D.H., and V.B. Collings. 1977. *Introduction to Sensation/Perception*. Englewood Cliffs, NJ: Prentice-Hall.

McBurney, D.H., and C. Pfaffmann. 1963. Gustatory adaptation to saliva and sodium chloride. *J Exp Psychol* 65:523–529.

McMahon, D.B.T., H. Shikata, and P.A.S. Breslin. 2001. Are human taste thresholds similar on the right and left sides of the tongue? *Chem Senses* 26:875–883.

Miller, I.J., and L.M. Bartoshuk. 1991. Taste perception, taste bud distribution, and spatial relationships. In *Smell and Taste in Health and Disease*, eds. T.V. Getchell, R.L. Doty, L.M. Bartoshuk, and J.B. Snow, pp. 205–233. New York: Raven Press.

Miller, I.J., and F.E. Reedy. 1990a. Quantification of fungiform papillae and taste pores in living human subjects. *Chem Senses* 15:281–294.

Miller, I.J., and F.E. Reedy. 1990b. Variations in human taste bud density and taste intensity perception. *Physiol Behav* 47:1213–1219.

Miller, I.J., and G. Whitney. 1989. Sucrose octaacetate-taster mice have more vallate taste buds than non-tasters. *Neurosci Lett* 100:271–275.

Mojet, J., E. Christ-Hazelhof, and J. Heidema. 2001. Taste perception with age: Generic or specific losses in threshold sensitivity to the five basic tastes? *Chem Senses* 26: 845–860.

Moon, C.N., and E.W. Pullen. 1963. Effects of chorda tympani section during middle ear surgery. *Laryngoscope* 73:392–405.

Moskowitz, H.R. 1977a. Magnitude estimation: Notes on what, how, when, and why to use it. *J Food Qual* 1:195–227.

Moskowitz, H.R. 1977b. Psychophysical and psychometric approaches to sensory evaluation. *CRC Crit Rev Food Sci Nutr* 9:41–79.

Mueller, C., S. Kallert, B. Renner et al. 2003. Quantitative assessment of gustatory function in a clinical context using impregnated "taste strips". *Rhinology* 41:2–6.

Murphy, C., W.S. Cain, and L.M. Bartoshuk. 1977. Mutual action of taste and olfaction. *Sens Proc* 1:204–211.

Murphy, C., C. Quinonez, and S. Nordin. 1995. Reliability and validity of electrogustometry and its application to young and elderly persons. *Chem Senses* 20:499–503.

Nakazato, M., S. Endo, I. Yoshimura, and H. Tomita. 2002. Influence of aging on electrogustometry thresholds. *Acta Otolaryngol* 546:16–26.

Narens, L., and R.D. Luce. 1983. How we may have been misled into believing in the interpersonal comparability of utility. *Theory Decis* 15:247–260.

Ninomiya, Y., and M. Funakoshi. 1982. Responsiveness of dog thalamic neurons to taste stimulation of various tongue regions. *Physiol Behav* 29:741–745.

Noble, A.C. 1996. Taste–aroma interactions. *Trends Food Sci Tech* 7:439–444.

Norgren, R. 1984. Central neural mechanisms of taste. In *Handbook of Physiology (Section 1, Vol. III: The Nervous System—Sensory Processes)*, eds. J.M. Brookhart and V.B. Mountcastle, pp. 1087–1128. Washington, DC: American Physiological Society.

Norgren, R. 1990. Gustatory system. In *The Human Nervous System*, ed. G. Paxinos, pp. 845–861. New York: Academic Press.

Norgren, R., and C. Pfaffmann. 1975. The pontine taste area in the rat. *Brain Res* 91:99–117.

Ogawa, H., and T. Hayama. 1984. Receptive fields of solitario-parabrachial relay neurons responsive to natural stimulation of the oral cavity in rats. *Exp Brain Res* 54:359–366.

Ogden, G.R. 1989. Atrophy of fungiform papillae following lingual nerve damage—A poor prognosis? *Br Dent J* 167:332.

Olson, J.M., M. Boehnke, K. Neiswanger, A.F. Roche, and R.M. Siervogel. 1989. Alternative genetic models for the inheritance of the phenylthiocarbamide taste deficiency. *Genet Epidemiol* 6:423–434.

Ovesen, L., M. Sorensen, J. Hannibal, and L. Allingstrup. 1991. Electrical taste detection thresholds and chemical smell detection thresholds in patients with cancer. *Cancer* 10:2260–2265.

Pangborn, R.M., H.W. Berg, E.B. Roessler, and A.D. Webb. 1964. Influence of methodology on olfactory response. *Percept Mot Skills* 18:91–103.

Parr, L.W. 1934. Taste blindness and race. *J Hered* 25:187–190.

Pavlidis, P., H. Gouveris, A. Anogeianaki, D. Koutsonikolas, G. Anogianakis, and G. Kekes. 2013. Age-related changes in electrogustometry thresholds, tongue tip vascularization, density, and form of the fungiform papillae in humans. *Chem Senses* 38:35–43.

Peryam, D.R., and N.F. Girardot. 1952. Advanced taste test method. *Food Eng* 24:58–61:194.

Pfaffmann, C., and L.M. Bartoshuk. 1989. Psychophysical mapping of a human case of left unilateral ageusia. *Chem Senses* 14:738.

Pfaffmann, C., and L.M. Bartoshuk. 1990. Taste loss due to herpes zoster oticus: An update after 19 months. *Chem Senses* 15:657–658.

Prescott, J., L.M. Bartoshuk, and J.M. Prutkin. 2004. 6-*n*-propylthiouracil tasting and the perception of non-taste oral sensations. In *Genetic Variation in Taste Sensitivity: Measurement, Significance, and Implications*, eds. J. Prescott and B.J. Tepper, pp. 89–104. New York: Marcel Dekker.

Pritchard, T.C., and R. Norgren. 2004. Gustatory system. In *The Human Nervous System, 2nd ed.*, eds. G. Paxinos and J.K. Mai, pp. 1171–1196. San Diego, CA: Elsevier Academic Press.

Prutkin, J.M., V.B. Duffy, L. Etter et al. 2000. Genetic variation and inferences about perceived taste intensity in mice and men. *Physiol Behav* 69:161–173.

Raliou, M., A. Wiencis., A.M. Pillias et al. 2009. Nonsynonymous single nucleotide polymorphisms in human tas1r1, tas1r3, and mGluR1 and individual taste sensitivity to glutamate. *Am J Clin Nutr* 90:789S–799S.

Rankin, K.M., N. Godinot, C.M. Christensen, B.J. Tepper, and S.V. Kirkmeyer. 2004. Assessment of different methods for 6-*n*-propylthiouracil status classification. In *Genetic Variation in Taste Sensitivity: Measurement, Significance, and Implications*, eds. J. Prescott and B.J. Tepper, pp. 63–88. New York: Marcel Dekker.

Reed, D.R. 2008. Birth of a new breed of supertaster. *Chem Senses* 33:489–491.

Reed, D.R., L.M. Bartoshuk, V.B. Duffy, S. Marino, and R.A. Price. 1995. Propylthiouracil tasting: Determination of underlying threshold distributions using maximum likelihood. *Chem Senses* 20:529–533.

Reed, D.R., E. Nanthakumar, M. North, C. Bell, L.M. Bartoshuk, and R.A. Price. 1999. Localization of a gene for bitter taste perception to human chromosome 5p15. *Am J Hum Genet* 64:1478–1480.

Reichert, F.L. 1934. Neuralgias of the glossopharyngeal nerve: With particular reference to the sensory, gustatory, and secretory functions of the nerve. *Arch Neurol Psychiatry* 32:1030–1037.

Rice, J.C. 1963. The chorda tympani in stapedectomy. *J Laryngol Otol* 77:943–944.

Robinson, P.P., A.R. Loescher, and K.G. Smith. 2000. A prospective, quantitative study on the clinical outcome of lingual nerve repair. *Br J Oral Maxillofac Surg* 38:255–263.

Rozin, P. 1982. "Taste–smell confusions" and the duality of the olfactory sense. *Percept Psychophys* 31:397–401.

Salata, J.A., J.M. Raj, and R.L. Doty. 1991. Differential sensitivity of tongue areas and palate to chemical stimulation: A suprathreshold cross-modal matching study. *Chem Senses* 16:483–489.

Schiffman, S.S. 1997. Taste and smell losses in normal aging and disease. *JAMA* 278:1357–1362.

Schutz, H.G., and A.V. Cardello. 2001. A labeled affective magnitude (LAM) scale for assessing food liking/disliking. *J Sens Stud* 16:117–159.

Schwartz, S.R. 1998. *The Effects of Chorda Tympani Nerve Transection on the Human Tongue: Anatomic and Somatosensory Alterations.* MD thesis, Yale University School of Medicine, New Haven, CT.

Shahbake, M., I. Hutchinson, D.G. Laing, and A.L. Jinks. 2005. Rapid quantitative assessment of fungiform papillae density in the human tongue. *Brain Res* 1052:196–201.

Shigemura, N., S. Shirosaki, K. Sanematsu, R. Yoshida, and Y. Ninomiya. 2009. Genetic and molecular basis of individual differences in human umami taste perception. *PLoS One* 4:e6717.

Shingai, T., and L.M. Beidler. 1985. Inter-strain differences in bitter taste responses in mice. *Chem Senses* 10:51–55.

Ship, J.A., M. Grushka, J.A. Lipton, A.E. Mott, B.J. Sessle, and R.A. Dionne. 1995. Burning mouth syndrome: An update. *J Am Dent Assoc* 126:842–853.

Small, D.M., M. Jones-Gotman, R.J. Zatorre, M. Petrides, and A.C. Evans. 1997. Flavor processing: More than the sum of its parts. *NeuroReport* 8:3913–3917.

Small, D.M., J.C. Gerber, Y.E. Mak, and T. Hummel. 2005. Differential neural responses evoked by orthonasal versus retronasal odorant perception in humans. *Neuron* 47:593–605.

Smith, D.V. 1971. Taste intensity as a function of area and concentration: Differentiation between compounds. *J Exp Psychol* 87:163–171.

Smutzer, G., S. Lam, L. Hastings et al. 2008. A test for measuring gustatory function. *Laryngoscope* 118:1411–1416.

Snow, J.B., R.L. Doty, L.M. Bartoshuk, and T.V. Getchell. 1991. Categorization of chemosensory disorders. In *Smell and Taste in Health and Disease*, eds. T.V. Getchell, R.L. Doty, L.M. Bartoshuk, and J.B. Snow, pp. 445–447. New York: Raven Press.

Snyder, D.J. 2010. *Multimodal Interactions Supporting Oral Sensory Capture and Referral.* PhD thesis, Yale University, New Haven, CT.

Snyder, D.J., V.B. Duffy, A.K. Chapo, H.J. Hoffman, and L.M. Bartoshuk. 2003. Food preferences mediate relationships between otitis media and body mass index. *Appetite* 40:360.

Snyder, D.J., J. Prescott, and L.M. Bartoshuk. 2006. Modern psychophysics and the assessment of human oral sensation. *Adv Otorhinolaryngol* 63:221–241.

Snyder, D.J., C.J. Clark, F.A. Catalanotto, and L.M. Bartoshuk. 2007. Oral anesthesia specifically impairs retronasal olfaction. *Chem Senses* 32:A15.

Snyder, D.J., V.B. Duffy, S.E. Marino, and L.M. Bartoshuk. 2008a. We are what we eat, but why? Relationships between oral sensation, genetics, pathology, and diet. In *Sweetness and Sweeteners: Biology, Chemistry, and Psychophysics*, eds. D.K. Weerasinghe and G.E. DuBois, pp. 258–284. Washington, DC: American Chemical Society.

Snyder, D.J., L.A. Puentes, C.A. Sims, and L.M. Bartoshuk. 2008b. Building a better intensity scale: Which labels are essential? *Chem Senses* 33:S142.

Snyder, L.H. 1931. Inherited taste deficiency. *Science* 74:151–152.

Stephen, K.W., J. McCrossan, D. Mackenzie, C.B. Macfarlane, and C.F. Speirs. 1980. Factors determining the passage of drugs from blood into saliva. *Br J Clin Pharmacol* 9:51–55.

Stevens, J.C. 1959. Cross-modality validation of subjective scales for loudness, vibration, and electric shock. *J Exp Psychol* 57:201–209.

Stevens, J.C., and L.E. Marks. 1965. Cross-modality matching of brightness and loudness. *Proc Natl Acad Sci* 54:407–411.

Stevens, J.C., and L.E. Marks. 1980. Cross-modality matching functions generated by magnitude estimation. *Percept Psychophys* 27:379–389.

Stevens, J.C., L.A. Cruz, J.M. Hoffman, and M.Q. Patterson. 1995. Taste sensitivity and aging: High incidence of decline revealed by repeated threshold measures. *Chem Senses* 20:451–459.

Stevens, S.S. 1946. On the theory of scales of measurement. *Science* 103:677–680.

Stevens, S.S. 1956. The direct estimation of sensory magnitudes—Loudness. *Am J Psychol* 69:1–25.

Stevens, S.S. 1958. Adaptation-level vs. the relativity of judgment. *Am J Psychol* 71:633–646.

Stevens, S.S. 1961. To honor Fechner and repeal his law. *Science* 133:80–86.

Stevens, S.S. 1962. The surprising simplicity of sensory metrics. *Am Psychol* 17:29–39.

Stevens, S.S., and E.H. Galanter. 1957. Ratio scales and category scales for a dozen perceptual continua. *J Exp Psychol* 54:377–411.

Stevenson, R.J., and J. Prescott. 1997. Judgments of chemosensory mixtures in memory. *Acta Psychol* 95:195–214.

Stevenson, R.J., J. Prescott, and R.A. Boakes. 1999. Confusing tastes and smells: How odours can influence the perception of sweet and sour tastes. *Chem Senses* 24:627–635.

Stillman, J.A., R.P. Morton, K.D. Hay, Z. Ahmad, and D. Goldsmith. 2003. Electrogustometry: Strengths, weaknesses, and clinical evidence of stimulus boundaries. *Clin Otolaryngol Allied Sci* 28:406–410.

Sunderland, E., and R.A. Cartwright. 1968. Iodine estimations, endemic goitre, and phenyl-thiocarbamide (PTC) tasting ability. *Acta Genet Stat Med* 18:593–598.

Sweazey, R.D., and D.V. Smith. 1987. Convergence onto hamster medullary taste neurons. *Brain Res* 408:173–184.

Teghtsoonian, R. 1973. Range effects in psychophysical scaling and a revision of Stevens' law. *Am J Psychol* 86:3–27.

Tennen, H., G. Affleck, and R. Mendola. 1991. Coping with smell and taste disorders. In *Smell and Taste in Health and Disease*, eds. T.V. Getchell, R.L. Doty, L.M. Bartoshuk, and J.B. Snow, pp. 787–802. New York: Raven Press.

Tepper, B.J., and N.V. Ullrich. 2002. Influence of genetic taste sensitivity to 6-*n*-propylthio-uracil (PROP), dietary restraint, and disinhibition on body mass index in middle-aged women. *Physiol Behav* 75:305–312.

Tepper, B.J., C.M. Christensen, and J. Cao. 2001. Development of brief methods to classify individuals by PROP taster status. *Physiol Behav* 73:571–577.

Tepper, B.J., E.A. White, Y. Koelliker, C. Lanzara, P. d'Adamo, and P. Gasparini. 2009. Genetic variation in taste sensitivity to 6-*n*-propylthiouracil and its relationship to taste perception and food selection. *Ann NY Acad Sci* 1170:126–139.

Tie, K., K. Fast, J.F. Kveton et al. 1999. Anesthesia of chorda tympani nerve and effect on oral pain. *Chem Senses* 24:609.

Tieman, D., P. Bliss, L.M. McIntyre et al. 2012. The chemical interactions underlying tomato flavor preferences. *Curr Biol* 22:1035–1039.

Todrank, J., and L.M. Bartoshuk. 1991. A taste illusion: Taste sensation localized by touch. *Physiol Behav* 50:1027–1031.

Tomita, H., M. Ikeda, and Y. Okuda. 1986. Basis and practice of clinical taste examinations. *Auris Nasus Larynx* 13:S1–S15.

Ventura, A.K., D.R. Reed, and J.A. Mennella. 2009. Chronic otitis media is associated with a marker of taste damage and higher weight status in children. *Chem Senses* 34:A37.

Weiffenbach, J.M. 1983. Taste quality recognition and forced-choice response. *Percept Psychophys* 33:251–254.

Wetherill, G.B., and H. Levitt. 1965. Sequential estimation of points on a psychometric function. *B J Math Stat Psychol* 18:1–10.

Wheatcroft, P.E.J., and C.C. Thornburn. 1972. Toxicity of the taste testing compound phenyl-thiocarbamide. *Nature New Biol* 235:93–94.

Whissell-Buechy, D. 1990. Genetic basis of the phenylthiocarbamide polymorphism. *Chem Senses* 15:27–37.

Whissell-Buechy, D., and C. Wills. 1989. Male and female correlations for taster (P.T.C.) phenotypes and rate of adolescent development. *Ann Hum Biol* 16:131–146.

Wooding, S., U.-K. Kim, M.J. Bamshad, L. Larsen, L.B. Jorde, and D. Drayna. 2004. Natural selection and molecular evolution in PTC, a bitter-taste receptor gene. *Am J Hum Genet* 74:637–646.

Yamada, Y., and H. Tomita. 1989. Influences on taste in the area of chorda tympani nerve after transtympanic injection of local anesthetic (4% lidocaine). *Auris Nasus Larynx* 16:S41–S46.

Yanagisawa, K., L.M. Bartoshuk, F.A. Catalanotto, T.A. Karrer, and J.F. Kveton. 1998. Anesthesia of the chorda tympani nerve and taste phantoms. *Physiol Behav* 63:329–335.

Zahm, D.S., and B.L. Munger. 1985. The innervation of the primate fungiform papilla—Development, distribution, and changes following selective ablation. *Brain Res Rev* 9:147–186.

Zhao, L., S.V. Kirkmeyer, and B.J. Tepper. 2003. A paper screening test to assess genetic taste sensitivity to 6-*n*-propylthiouracil. *Physiol Behav* 78:625–633.

Zuniga, J.R., S.H. Davis, R.A. Englehardt, I.J. Miller, S.S. Schiffman, and C. Phillips. 1993. Taste performance on the anterior tongue varies with fungiform taste bud density. *Chem Senses* 18:449–460.

Zuniga, J.R., N. Chen, and I.J. Miller. 1994. Effects of chorda-lingual nerve injury and repair on human taste. *Chem Senses* 19:657–665.

Zuniga, J.R., N. Chen, and C.L. Phillips. 1997. Chemosensory and somatosensory regeneration after lingual nerve repair in humans. *J Oral Maxillofac Surg* 55:2–13.

6 Color Correspondences in Chemosensation
The Case of Food and Drinks

Betina Piqueras-Fiszman and Charles Spence

CONTENTS

6.1 Introduction to Multisensory Perception: On the Fundamental
Importance of Color 139
    6.1.1 Cross-Modal Correspondences... 141
6.2 Basics of Color Perception... 142
6.3 On the Color of Food or Beverage... 143
    6.3.1 Color as a Cue to Flavor–Aroma Identity.. 144
    6.3.2 Color as a Cue to Flavor–Aroma Intensity 144
    6.3.3 Color as a Cue to Other Sensations 146
6.4 On the Color of the Packaging... 147
6.5 Interim Summary 148
6.6 On the Color of the Tableware... 149
6.7 Color of the Surroundings/Environment 151
6.8 Individual Differences in Color Correspondences 151
6.9 Conclusions and Directions for Future Research 152
References... 153

6.1 INTRODUCTION TO MULTISENSORY PERCEPTION: ON THE FUNDAMENTAL IMPORTANCE OF COLOR

Over the last three decades or so, a great deal of published research has demonstrated that the visual appearance of a variety of different food and drink products can have a profound effect not only on our perception of their sensory properties but also on how much food a person ultimately ends up consuming. While there are multiple aspects to visual appearance, including a foodstuff's opacity and texture, the majority of the research that has been conducted to date has tended to focus on color, and it is on this aspect of visual appearance that we too intend to concentrate here. Importantly, since color (along with orthonasal olfaction) is among the only sensory cues that are available to consumers before they purchase and then finally taste a product, it can provide a number of powerful cues about the food or beverage's likely sensory properties. This information can then set up expectations in the mind of the consumer about the likely taste, aroma, flavor, and even oral–somatosensory qualities of the product. Furthermore, depending on whether they are confirmed or disconfirmed (Schifferstein 2001; Spence 2012), such expectations may actually bias a consumer's subsequent perception of the stimulus in a variety of different ways (Yeomans et al. 2008). But it is not just that vision has temporal precedence over the majority of other food-related cues; it also tends to be the dominant sense when it comes to flavor identification.

The impact of color on a consumer's perception of a given food or drink item has been widely investigated both in terms of the *identification* of a certain taste or flavor (DuBose et al. 1980; Zampini et al. 2007, 2008; Levitan et al. 2008) and the *intensity* of the taste, aroma, or flavor (Johnson and Clydesdale 1982; Johnson et al. 1982, 1983; Spence et al. 2010). The influence of color on both orthonasal and retronasal odor identification and enhancement has also been extensively studied (Zellner and Kautz 1990; Zellner et al. 1991; Gilbert et al. 1996; Kemp and Gilbert 1997; Zellner and Whitten 1999; Morrot et al. 2001; Österbauer et al. 2005). Finally, several researchers have attempted to assess the existence of a number of simple color–odor associations within representative groups of consumers (Schifferstein and Tanudjaja 2004; Demattè et al. 2006; Zellner et al. 2008; Maric and Jacquot 2013). What this literature demonstrates is that the relationship between the dimensions that color and flavor, aroma, taste, etc., share in common (e.g., stimulus intensity) is not always linearly correlated and that the brain uses much more information in order to establish the meaning of the correspondence between the stimuli.

In addition, a growing number of studies have also started to demonstrate the impact that color cues can have on an observer's perception of a variety of other sensory attributes such as nasal temperature (Michael and Rolhion 2008), not to mention influencing more complex sensations such as how refreshing (Lee and O'Mahony 2005; Fenko et al. 2009) or thirst-quenching, as in the case of drinks (Clydesdale et al. 1992; Zellner and Durlach 2002, 2003), a product is rated as being.* Furthermore, it is important to note that color cues constitute an important sensorial attribute that can provide consumers with basic quality information and has close associations with qualities such as freshness, maturity, variety, desirability, and food safety (Clydesdale 1991; Wu and Sun 2012).

Looking beyond the color of the food or beverage product itself, it turns out that the color of the packaging (or container) in which the product happens to be presented and/or consumed[†] has also attracted a growing body of research interest over the last few years from researchers working in the fields of sensory science and nutrition. For instance, packaging color has been shown to influence both the expectations of consumers (Deliza et al. 2003) and, in many cases, their actual perception of the high-level sensory qualities associated with the product (e.g., its *premiumness*; see Garber et al. 2008; Becker et al. 2011; Esterl 2011 for examples demonstrating the impact of product packaging; for results demonstrating the impact of the color of a plastic cup on consumers' taste/flavor perception, see Guéguen 2003; Schifferstein 2009; Piqueras-Fiszman and Spence 2012).

---

* It should be noted that there are different sensory, physiological, and cognitive factors that contribute to the perception of oral freshness (Martin et al. 2005).

† According to Wansink (1996), people consume around 30% of their food direct from the packaging.

Finally, recent evidence has demonstrated that the presence of certain colors on food-related contexts may also influence our choices or, more directly, our approach (or avoidance) motivation toward products (in the food context, this would be translated, for instance, into the intake of a product; Genschow et al. 2012). These correspondences can influence our behavior not only as a result of expectancy effects but potentially also by means of priming effects. However, on occasion, one mechanism implies the presence of the other, and being able to separate them (or quantify the impact of each individually) is quite complex. Although the literature on this topic as it applies to the world of food science is still in its infancy, in Section 6.6, we present the current thinking around this issue.

The aim of the present review, then, is to bring together the latest findings from a variety of different research fields that help to demonstrate the importance of the cross-modal correspondences that exist between the color of the food or beverage, not to mention the color of the packaging (or container), and other sensory attributes (smell, texture, flavor, taste) of the food. An overview of the latest techniques that have been used to investigate these correspondences will be given in order to gain a better insight into how color can exert such a profound effect on our (sensory and hedonic) perception of foods.

6.1.1 Cross-Modal Correspondences

On one hand, part of the diverse body of research that is included in this chapter (which is analyzed in greater detail from Section 6.3) deals directly with the topic of cross-modal correspondences (or associations) between the color of the food (or container/packaging) and other of its sensory properties. These correspondences are most likely learned from pre-exposure to certain combination of stimuli and as a result lead to the creation of specific expectations. On the other hand, another part of the research that will be reviewed here deals with the color correspondences that exist between certain colors and other nonsensory (e.g., conceptual or emotional) related meanings that may indirectly affect how we perceive (or respond to) food and/or how much we eat due to generalized priming effects. What both parts of the literature reviewed here have in common is the fact that the effects are driven by color correspondences, some of which are conscious and others that may operate below the level of awareness. However, what is important to highlight is that the literature on color correspondences is somewhat inconsistent and inconclusive (that is, not all studies show the same effect of color on people's perception or flavor/aroma) and that, in many cases, the robustness or validity of the effects that have been demonstrated depends to a great extent on the characteristics of the particular product that happens to have been studied (Fenko et al. 2009; Piqueras-Fiszman and Spence 2011) and on individual differences (be they cultural [Shankar et al. 2010a; Wan et al. 2014] or physiological in origin [Small 2009; Felsted et al. 2010]).

The question here is how are these color correspondences established in the first place? According to Garber et al. (2000), sensory stimuli have a dual nature: (1) On one hand, there is a direct effect of the sensory experience itself; and (2) on the other is any underlying meaning that a consumer may happen to associate with that sensory experience, which he or she refers to as its cognitive component. This assertion is rooted in a model of color and psychological functioning that was originally proposed by Elliot and Maier (Elliot et al. 2007). These authors have put forward the view that colors do not simply carry esthetic value (Clydesdale 1993); rather, they suggest that colors also convey very specific types of semantic information (as, for example, when certain food colors come to signify particular brands or when they provide a semantic cue as to the identity of a food or a beverage item; Stevenson et al. 2012). Elliot and Maier argue that these meanings can be derived by means of learned associations developed as a result of the repeated co-occurrence of specific colors with specific semantic/semiotic information.* Such meanings then have the potential to dominate an observer's direct sensory experience and to mediate the influence of color (Garber et al. 2000). According to the cognitive-based approach to color correspondences (Shankar et al. 2010a), prior experience plays a crucial role in terms of shaping consumers' expectations (which might then bias their perception of a food or beverage item) and their approach or avoidance motivation (which might then bias their willingness to try a food or affect their intake).

Summarizing these notions, as a result of the repeated exposure or co-occurrence of specific colors with other sensory attributes (i.e., flavors, textures, smells, etc.), people may learn to associate the elements of those stimulus combinations and hence to attach different semantic meanings to the colors (e.g., sweetness, vanilla, softness) regardless of whether the origin of that association is in some sense natural (as in the case of a fruit's color; Maga 1974) or artificial (as when imposed by marketing strategies; Garber et al. 2008; Piqueras-Fiszman and Spence 2011).† Hence, due to the consumer's experience with natural and processed (and branded/packaged) foods, and due to the fact that color contributes to the consumer's (first) visual assessment of many products, color correspondences (not only within the food/beverage itself but also involving the packaging/container color) should be studied from a more holistic standpoint in order to determine their impact on the overall acceptability of a product. This should be done both at the point of sale (where the first impression is made) and at the point of consumption (where the first sensory/hedonic impression is either going to be confirmed or disconfirmed).

6.2 BASICS OF COLOR PERCEPTION

Before we go any further, it is important to introduce some basic concepts from the field of color perception research. Color is defined as a perceptual response to the visible spectrum of light (the distribution of light power as a function of the wavelength) reflected or emitted by the surface of an object. This signal interacts in the eye with the L, M, and S cones in the retina; these names refer to the long-, middle-, and short-wavelength sensitive cones, respectively. These signals are then ultimately transmitted to the visual cortex by the optic nerve (Zeki 1993). Eventually, the human

---

* There might be another route in here in terms of cross-modal associations that are innate (i.e., which do not have to be learned). However, although sometimes postulated, there is no really solid evidence to support their existence as yet.
† See Schaefer and Schmidt (2013) for evidence concerning the interesting coevolution of color signaling and what is being signaled. Such developments can be applied both in nature and to the environment of the supermarket.

observer assigns a color to this signal. Such arguments have led some researchers to suggest that color is not an intrinsic property of the surface of an object, since if the light source changes, so too does the color of its surface (Melendez-Martinez et al. 2005; Shepherd 2012). The perception of color, then, is a complex phenomenon that depends on the properties of an object in a given illumination environment, the characteristics of the perceiving eye and brain, and the angle of illumination and viewing.

Color can be specified using models that produce a color space that is based on actual measurements of human color perception (these give rise to what are known as human-oriented color spaces). These correspond to the concepts of tint, shade, and tone, which are grounded on the intuitive characteristics of color. In general, human-oriented spaces can be represented using their hue and saturation, such as the hue, saturation, intensity; the hue, saturation, value; the hue, saturation, lightness; and the hue, saturation, brightness spaces. Hue is defined as the attribute of a visual sensation according to which an area appears to be similar to one of the perceived colors of the spectrum. Saturation is defined as the colorfulness of an area judged in proportion to its brightness. On the other hand, brightness is defined as the attribute of a visual sensation by means of which an observer is able to distinguish differences in luminance. Lightness is defined as the brightness of an area judged relative to the brightness of a similarly illuminated area that appears to be white (Fairchild 2005).

One way in which to model and simulate the human-oriented space (and hence predict how an observer will perceive a patch of illumination that he or she then ascribes a color to) is by using the CIELAB space. The CIELAB color space (CIE 2004) is a perceptually uniform color space composed of three orthogonal dimensions: L*, a*, and b*. L* stands for the axis of lightness, while a* and b* represent scales of opponent color pairs (i.e., redness–greenness and yellowness–blueness, respectively). Chroma and hue, two of the perceptual attributes of color, are defined by converting the orthogonal a* and b* axes into polar coordinates C* and h. More recently, research on visual judgments (presented on digital displays) of certain foods or drinks has been carried out simply by modifying the CIELAB color space systematically (e.g., Wei et al. 2012). This technique allows researchers to easily test expectations of specific sensory attributes by modulating a food's/drink's color digitally. In food analysis, these color parameters are normally measured using spectrophotometers.

6.3 ON THE COLOR OF FOOD OR BEVERAGE

Color has been the main parameter that has been investigated by researchers when studying the effect of visual cues on people's taste, aroma, and flavor perception. In fact, to date, more than 200 studies have been published on the topic over the last 80 years or so (Moir 1936; Masurovsky 1939). Color cues have been shown to exert a significant effect on people's perception of many different foods, including chocolate (Duncker 1939), sherbets (Hall 1958), cake (experiment 4; DuBose et al. 1980), cheese and jelly (Christensen 1985), wine gums (Teerling 1992), butter (Rohm et al. 1997), and beer (Guinard et al. 1998). However, the majority of the research that has been conducted to date has primarily been concerned with assessing people's perception of flavored drinks (Delwiche 2003; Spence et al. 2010). This is presumably because this is the format that is simply easier to create/manipulate and allows one to focus on the color cue, having the influence of other visual cues (such as a food's shape, texture, etc.) minimized.

6.3.1 Color as a Cue to Flavor–Aroma Identity

The effect of color on a consumer's ability to identify specific flavors has proven to be quite robust: when food or beverage items have been colored in a manner that is appropriate* to the specific flavors being tested (that is, the characteristic color of their natural ingredient or of the product that they have been pre-exposed to for longer, think of the brown color associated with cola-flavored drinks), the number of correct flavor responses was higher than when consumers had to identify the color of an inappropriately colored (or clear) solution (Zampini et al. 2007, 2008). Up to this point, then, there is nothing surprising: most of us would likely associate the red color of a drink with a red berry fruit, an orange liquid with an orange-flavored drink, and yellow with lemon. The same pattern of results has also been observed with odors, that is, people exhibit an impaired ability to identify odors correctly when they are presented in inappropriately colored formats (as when dissolved in solution).

In their now classic study, Morrot et al. (2001) provided support for such a conclusion using a more complex stimulus, namely, wine. These researchers concluded that certain white wines, when artificially colored red using an odorless food dye, are often described (by experts—French students on a university enology course) using more red wine odor terms than the same wines that are naturally colored (Parr et al. 2003; Spence 2010a,b). In addition, the results of an fMRI study by Österbauer et al. (2005) documented increased activity in the olfactory parts of the brain when the cross-modal congruency between simultaneously presented colors and aromas was increased (e.g., when a strawberry odor was paired with a simultaneously presented red color as compared to with, say, a turquoise color).

6.3.2 Color as a Cue to Flavor–Aroma Intensity

As soon as it comes to measuring the effect of color on flavor or odor intensity, the results that have been published to date tend to be more diverse and, on occasion, somewhat more complex. So, for example, some researchers have reported the existence of a correlation between the intensity of the color and the intensity of the flavor perceived. However, the magnitude of such effects would appear to depend on the particular color–flavor combination that is under consideration (DuBose et al. 1980). With regard to odors, significant effects of color cues on an observer's judgments of odor intensity have frequently been observed (Zellner and Kautz 1990; Blackwell 1995; Zellner and Whitten 1999; Morrot et al. 2001; Parr et al. 2003). However, once again, the results are not necessarily altogether consistent; that is, while certain studies have documented a positive correlation between color intensity and odor intensity, others have reported a negative one (Zellner and Kautz 1990). For instance, Zellner and Whitten (1999) reported that the correlation between color intensity and odor

---

* What exactly *appropriateness* means is not altogether clear (Shankar et al. 2010a).

intensity was not necessarily linear for all the odors that they tested. Interestingly, however, it was not important which specific color it was that happened to be added. That is, the ability of participants to indicate the odor intensity of benzaldehyde (the main note of cherry and almond aromas) was equally enhanced regardless of the intensity of the red colorant added when the participants were told that the odor was almond (putatively incongruent). However, the appropriateness ratings were negatively correlated with the color intensity in this condition. On the other hand, when the participants were told that the red solutions were cherry (supposedly congruent), a slight increase in participants' intensity ratings was observed as the red intensity increased, and the appropriateness ratings increased significantly. In brief, color intensity might not always be correlated with odor intensity, but when it is, appropriateness does not seem to be the only factor that affects a person's performance.

What is more, and to complicate matters still further, the method of delivery of the flavor (or odor) has been shown to exert a significant influence over the color–flavor/odor effects observed in at least one study. In particular, Koza et al. (2005) reported that when odorants were smelled orthonasally, the presence of color enhanced their participants' odor intensity ratings, but when they were smelled retronasally, color suppressed intensity ratings instead. The authors explained these results in terms of assimilation vs. contrast effects. In both conditions, the participants' expectation may have been that the colored solution would have a more intense odor than the colorless one. However, since the two solutions actually had the same intensity, there could have been some violation of expectation. In the retronasal olfaction condition, the discrepancy is more likely to be noticed because the olfactory input is both reliable and salient and thus will give rise to a lower intensity rating. On the other hand, in the orthonasal condition, the discrepancy is less likely to be noticed and thus may result in a higher intensity rating.

In terms of the effect of color on taste (sweetness, sourness, saltiness, bitterness, and umami) intensity ratings, the results of the research that has been published to date are much more complex. While some studies have demonstrated that certain colors, when added to foods (mostly solutions), are expected to be sweeter or sourer and do actually taste as expected once tasted, others have failed to replicate such effects (see Spence et al. 2010). Increasing the intensity of red coloring added to a solution has certainly been shown to enhance the rated sweetness intensity of aqueous solutions (Johnson and Clydesdale 1982), strawberry- and cherry-flavored beverages, and fruit punch (Johnson et al. 1982, 1983; Clydesdale et al. 1992). This is as expected, since in these cases, the red color is congruent with the fruit color associated with the flavor. Studies that have investigated the effect of the intensity of other colors on the perception of sweetness (Roth et al. 1988; Fletcher et al. 1991) and saltiness (Gifford and Clydesdale 1986; Gifford et al. 1987) have reported results that are not so clear-cut. Null findings have also been reported (Frank et al. 1989).

It should certainly be noted that the majority of the stimuli that have been used in these studies consisted of fruit flavors or odors. Fruit juices typically have their own natural color, and hence, it is easy to build on such associations when seeing a color or tasting/smelling a fruit-based stimulus. Researchers often find that those colors that happen to be associated with the ripening of fruits are particularly effective in terms of modulating perceived sweetness, whereas foods and drinks that have a green hue are often judged to be sourer (presumably because they are associated with unripe fruits; Maga 1974). As yet, though, food science researchers have found it rather more challenging to modulate people's perception of saltiness using changes in a food's coloration (Gifford and Clydesdale 1986; Gifford et al. 1987). Here, one suggestion has been that since salty foods come in all manner of colors, there is no natural (or predominant) color–taste association on which to build or for the consumer to pick up on.

Increasing the level of color in a solution has been shown to increase taste and flavor intensity ratings (DuBose et al. 1980; Johnson and Clydesdale 1982; Hyman 1983; Zampini et al. 2007). This might provide a means of enhancing the perception of saltiness in foods. For instance, one might hypothesize that the perception of saltiness in a soy sauce could be increased simply by making the solution a darker brown color.

6.3.3 Color as a Cue to Other Sensations

Color may also influence the perception of refreshment that can result from the consumption of foods and beverages. So, for example, Zellner and Durlach (2003) conducted a study in which they prepared three differently flavored beverages (mint, lemon, and vanilla) in eight colors (clear, red, blue, green, yellow, purple, orange, and brown). Three groups of American students each tasted one set of eight colored beverages and had to rate the perceived freshness intensity on a scale (where a score of 0 was used to indicate *not at all*, 50 *moderately*, and 100 *the most refreshing imaginable*). The color significantly influenced ratings of perceived refreshment of the lemon- and mint-flavored sets of drinks. For lemon, the participants rated the brown beverage as less refreshing than the clear, purple, and yellow versions; for mint, the brown and red drinks received the lowest refreshing intensity scores; while for vanilla, all of the colors were rated as being about equally refreshing (with all ratings falling at a score of around 40 on the scale). Zellner and Durlach suggested that the clear beverages were often rated as being most refreshing because of the association between clearness/transparency and water, while the less refreshing ratings given to the brown-colored lemon or mint-flavored drinks may have resulted from the fact that the color was inappropriate to the flavor.

Another example of how consumer insights may be used in marketing communications around color correspondences was illustrated in a study in which the expected refreshing properties of toothpastes were explored as a function of their color (Lee and O'Mahony 2005). The refreshing appearance of 20 commercial toothpastes having different colors was rated by more than 70 North Americans. The results revealed that these consumers expected transparent blue toothpaste to be the most refreshing and off-white the least. One can certainly speculate that transparent blue may be associated with a specific brand of toothpaste that participants had already experienced as *refreshing* in the marketplace. Alternatively, however, it may also have been the appearance that is most closely associated with water and therefore to notions of refreshing liquids. The latter suggestion is supported by the results of a study by Guéguen (2003) in which it was shown that the same beverage evaluated in four differently colored glasses (blue, red, green, and yellow) was perceived as most thirst-quenching when evaluated in a clear blue glass.

Zellner and Durlach (2002) reported that 92% of their sample of 86 American students associated a refreshing food or beverage to temperature-related sensory characteristics, and 50% expected that sweetness should be a characteristic of a thirst-quenching beverage. Meanwhile, Clydesdale and colleagues gave a questionnaire to a group of 75 American students in which the four colors that were most frequently associated with thirst-quenching were clear (36% of respondents), brown (24%), red (17%), and orange (12%). These findings contrast with sensory studies showing that brown and sweetness (McEwan and Colwill 1996; Guinard et al. 1998; Labbe et al. 2009) seem to be the negative drivers of the perception of refreshment. Part of the difference here may be explained by the fact that, in certain circumstances, associating brown color and sweetness with refreshing may result from previous experiences of drinking cola beverages in order to quench one's thirst (Clydesdale et al. 1992). In addition, it is possible that frequently seeing advertising claims that a major brand of cola is refreshing may further influence such perceptions (or ratings).

6.4 ON THE COLOR OF THE PACKAGING

Compared to the influence of the color of the food, the impact of the color of the packaging on the perception of food and drink is a topic that has hardly been studied from a food science perspective. On the other hand, numerous studies have been published over the years that have documented the role that packaging color plays in driving consumer expectations concerning the sensory qualities of the contents of that packaging (Cheskin 1957; Deliza et al. 2003; Marshall et al. 2006; Ares and Deliza 2010; Esterl 2011; Piqueras-Fiszman and Spence 2011; Piqueras-Fiszman et al. 2011). The reality is that people are affected by packaging, specifically by its color, in ways that they do not necessarily understand at a conscious level. Since color is perhaps the one feature of a product's packaging that triggers the fastest response (Swientek 2001), it is essential to consider the associations and expectations that consumers may have in the design process in order to ensure effectiveness and the successful communication of specific sensory qualities that happen to be associated with a brand. For instance, Ares and Deliza (2010) conducted a study showing that yoghurt tasted from cream-colored yoghurt pots was expected to taste of vanilla, whereas a brown-colored pot was associated with chocolate flavor. Meanwhile, Becker et al. (2011) demonstrated that the more saturated the yellow color in lemon-flavored yoghurt pots becomes, the more intense the taste was expected to be (although it should be remembered here that the results only achieved significance in those participants who had a sensitivity for design).

In terms of understanding the effects of these extrinsic elements on the consumer's perception and evaluation of food, a number of potentially relevant psychological and physiological explanations have been documented. Given that these cues do not come from the food itself, they could presumably be considered as being nondiagnostic (i.e., they objectively should not identify or prompt any effect in our perception of food). Therefore, the cross-modal correspondences that have been observed between the intrinsic and extrinsic elements of a food product could be regarded as giving rise to sensation transference (Cheskin 1957; Schifferstein 2009). Cognitive neuroscience researchers have recently started to provide an explanation for why sensation transference effects may occur.

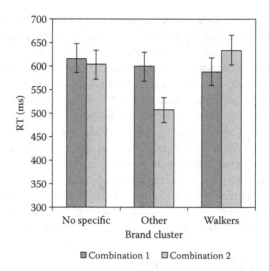

FIGURE 6.1 Representation of the mean reaction times (RTs) per brand cluster of consumers and type of combination, measured in an Implicit Association task. Combination 1 represents the color–flavor match present in crisps (and snack) brands in the United Kingdom that are not Walkers; combination 2 represents the color–flavor match present in Walkers crisps. Vertical bars represent Tukey's significant differences at $p < .05$.

Cross-modal correspondences between tastes/flavors/oral–somatosensory attributes and colors can be used on product packaging in order to set up expectations (often unconscious) concerning the sensory qualities of the contents contained within that packaging. Piqueras-Fiszman and Spence (2011) conducted one of the few studies to have shown that not do only consumers implicitly associate specific packaging colors with the flavor of the contents (in this case, potato crisps) but also that this affects the actual flavor that is perceived, due to the strong associations that consumers (of a brand) hold between a particular color of packaging and the expected flavor of the contents (see Figure 6.1).

6.5 INTERIM SUMMARY

As we have seen up to this point, our previous exposure to a food product (or a product category), and our knowledge about it, can set up expectations about its likely sensory properties (flavor, taste, aroma, etc.) when we come across that product (or a similar one). One might think that such cues should not necessarily affect the consumer's judgment of the food in question. However, on certain occasions, as we have reviewed above, these expectations are so strong that even if the color of the stimuli (say, a drink) is not correctly matched with its corresponding flavor or aroma, color information can nevertheless still override a consumer's experience of the product (at least when the discrepancy between the information received from the two modalities is not too large; Shankar et al. 2010a,c). In the following, we discuss the effect of the color of the surface against which the food is served and the color of the environment on the consumer's perception of food and drink. Here, other mechanisms, which do not necessarily have anything to do with expectations per se and which may influence our perception of food, are activated. A number of researchers have argued that color contrast effects between the food and the background can modulate how it is that a consumer will perceive the color of food and hence its sensory properties too. In addition, the literature hints at the possibility that color affects our mood/ emotions and by doing so could also potentially affect our judgments concerning any food or drink item that we happen to be assessing. Alternatively, however, color cues may simply just prime us about the associations that we have with specific colors regardless of whether or not they set up particular expectations.

6.6   ON THE COLOR OF THE TABLEWARE

Lyman (1989), in his book on the psychology of food, suggested that purple grapes do not look as appetizing when served from a blue plate. He argued that foods can be arranged in combinations such that their colors may be subtly enhanced, subdued, or otherwise modified due to the well-known simultaneous color contrast illusion (Ekroll et al. 2004). This is where a foreground object appears to have a different color (or contrast) depending on the color of the background against which it is seen (Leibowitz et al. 1955; Hutchings 1994). For example, Lyman (1989) suggested that yellow scrambled eggs eaten from a yellow plate will look paler because of lack of color contrast. Meanwhile, broccoli served together with a red fish will likely make the fish look redder, and slices of lime surrounding a grape mousse will apparently enhance the color of both (Lyman 1989).

It is, however, only over the last couple of years or so that such anecdotal claims (specifically that the color of the plateware might exert a significant impact on the taste/flavor of whatever happens to be served from it) have been assessed empirically. For example, in one laboratory study, Harrar et al. (2011) had people sample sweet or salty popcorn from four differently colored bowls: white, blue, green, and red. The salty popcorn was rated as tasting significantly sweeter when taken from either a blue or a red bowl, whereas the sweet popcorn was rated as tasting significantly saltier when lifted from the blue bowl instead. Although the magnitudes of these effects were pretty small (averaging only a 4% change in participants' responses for the food taken from the colored bowl as compared to that from the white bowl), they were nevertheless statistically reliable.

In another study, Piqueras-Fiszman et al. (2012a) compared the taste of a strawberry-flavored mousse (of a homogeneous texture and color) that was served on either a black or a white plate (though it should be noted that, strictly speaking, these are not colors). The dessert served from the white plate was perceived as being 15% more intense and 10% sweeter, and was 10% more liked than exactly the same mousse when served from a black (otherwise identical) plate instead.

In this case, the color of the plate may have affected the perceived color of the food by means of the simultaneous color contrast illusion mentioned above (Ekroll et al. 2004). According to such a low-level perceptual interpretation of their findings, the color of the mousse served in the study of Piqueras-Fiszman et al. (2012a) may have appeared more salient when set against the background of the white plate than when served from the black plate. Thus, the rated intensity of the food's taste/flavor will presumably have been influenced by its perceived color saturation, which, in turn, may have been influenced by the color saturation (or brightness, in this case) of the plate itself.

More recently, Piqueras-Fiszman et al. (2013) tested the extent to which the color of the plateware (again, black and white plates were used) would influence the gustatory and hedonic experiences of a complex food (desserts with layers and decorations having different colors, textures, and tastes/flavors). Importantly, the study was performed in an entirely naturalistic setting (in one of the restaurants at the Institut Paul Bocuse in Lyon, France), under conditions that were as ecologically valid as possible (i.e., using a between-participants experimental design and with the participants/diners being able to interact and consume the three-course meal at their own pace; Spence and Piqueras-Fiszman 2014). Over the course of the 2 weeks that the experiment was conducted, three different desserts were served to diners. The results revealed that the color of the plateware exerted a significant influence on the diners' perception of the food (i.e., how appetizing it was, its appearance, color intensity, flavor intensity, and the participants' overall liking) and that this effect varied as a function of the type of dessert that happened to be being served. Interestingly, however, these results could not be accounted for solely in terms of contrast effects, since it was the dessert that had a darker-brownish hue that the participants rated more highly when served from the black plate (while the other two desserts, which were red and creamy in color, were rated as looking more delicious when served from the white plate instead). It could be that the desserts simply looked better (that is, more visually appealing) on a plate of a certain color and that this visual appraisal of the overall product offering was what produced a halo effect on the other scores that the diners made (Asch 1946).

That said, color contrast cannot so easily be used to explain the complex effects of the colored bowls on the perception of popcorn reported by Harrar et al. (2011). A possible explanation here is that these effects demonstrate another example of sensation transference, given that red is typically associated with sweetness, whereas blue may more often be associated with saltiness in some product categories such as popcorn, as mentioned earlier (Maga 1974; Spence et al. 2010), and for similar effects with cutlery (Harrar and Spence 2013).

Regarding the effect of color on people's intake, and considering that red has been shown to elicit avoidance motivation across a variety of contexts* (Birren 1963; Mehta and Zhu 2009), several studies have investigated the effect that the color red has on snack food and soft drink consumption (e.g., Genschow et al. 2012). The participants in Genschow et al.'s study drank less from a cup with a red label than from a cup with a blue label and ate less snack food from a red plate than from a blue or white one. The authors concluded that red might function as a subtle stop signal that works even outside of a person's focused awareness and may thereby reduce incidental food and drink intake. Meanwhile, Bruno et al. (2013) extended this line of research looking further into this intriguing effect. Independent groups of participants were presented with a given amount of popcorn, chocolate chips, or moisturizing cream on red, blue, or white plates. The participants were asked to sample the foods (by tasting them) or the cream (by rubbing it on their hand and forearm) as

---

* Mostly originating from nonfood-related contexts (e.g., danger signs, traffic lights, etc.).

they desired and to complete some mock questionnaires. The results confirmed that red plates reduced the consumption of food and the use of cream products, while, interestingly, the samples of all the containers were rated as being similarly liked. In addition, Bruno et al.'s study suggested that these results were not dependent on the Michelson (luminance) contrast nor on the color contrast.

In conclusion, although explanations for the fact that the color of the plate can impact on taste/flavor perception have not yet been fully worked out, the results of a growing number of empirical studies show that the color of the plate really does matter in one way or the other. It will be a challenge for those working in this area in the coming years to replicate these findings and work out a coherent theoretical account for these increasingly oft-documented effects.

6.7 COLOR OF THE SURROUNDINGS/ENVIRONMENT

The majority of research on the effect of environmental lighting on taste and flavor perception has involved participants drinking liquids from black tasting glasses (Sauvageot and Struillou 1997; Oberfeld et al. 2009). By presenting the stimuli in this way, it has been possible for researchers to ensure that they were assessing the effect of the lighting itself rather than, say, the effect of the lighting on the appearance properties of the food. A number of early studies in this area have suggested that changes to the ambient illumination could impact on an observer's ability to discriminate the taste (e.g., the sourness) of a drink (Gregson 1964; Wilson and Gregson 1967; Sauvageot and Struillou 1997). There is also some laboratory-based evidence to suggest that people who like their coffee strong (in other words, bitter) drink more of the beverage under brighter ambient lighting conditions, whereas those who like their coffee weaker drink more under dim illumination (Gal et al. 2007).

More interesting, though, are those studies that have shown that people may be willing to pay as much as 50% more for a bottle of wine at a wine tasting under certain room illumination colors as compared to others (Oberfeld et al. 2009). In a study conducted in a winery on the Rhine, tourists said that they would have been willing to pay one-third more for the wine that they were sampling when the normal white lighting was replaced by red.

6.8 INDIVIDUAL DIFFERENCES IN COLOR CORRESPONDENCES

Of course, color correspondences may vary at an individual level depending on the nature of the association under investigation. As mentioned already, different colors can carry different semantic meanings depending on the specific color–flavor pairings that individuals have been systematically exposed to in their environments (Elliot et al. 2007). Regarding the color correspondences that have been observed in the world of food and beverage product packaging, researchers (or marketers) often tend to explain differences in observed color correspondences in terms of culture when the underlying factor is uniquely brand acquaintance (see Piqueras-Fiszman et al. 2012b). Having said that, when asking people from various cultures about the global meaning of color, many studies have documented cross-cultural differences (Jacobs et al. 1991; Madden et al. 2000; Singh 2006). There are also studies controlling for other population dimensions such as age. For instance, Lavin and Lawless (1998) demonstrated that the effect of color on sweetness perception is not as large in children as it is in adults, the argument being that children will simply have had less exposure to specific color–flavor combinations. For a review of developmental changes in the influence of color on taste/flavor perception, see Spence (2012).

Of course, how an individual perceives color (for instance, if he/she has a color-related visual impairment) is another important factor that should be considered when it comes to thinking about color correspondences (Broackes 2010). In most cases, color blindness and tetrachromacy (McCrone 2002) are visual impairments to avoid when participants are being recruited for studies involving the assessment of color associations.

Finally, it is important to note that there can also be individual differences in the impact of the color correspondences on the perception of food due to the taster status of the participant. Zampini et al. (2008) reported that supertasters (Reed 2008) were relatively unaffected by the color of dyed solutions when trying to identify their flavor, whereas medium tasters were moderately affected; and nontasters were profoundly affected.

6.9   CONCLUSIONS AND DIRECTIONS FOR FUTURE RESEARCH

In this chapter, we have attempted to provide a quick overview of color correspondences in chemosensation (in particular, as they relate to the perception of food and drink) in terms of the color of the food itself, the color of the packaging, and the color of the surroundings in which that food or beverage is consumed. Most of the research that has been published to date in this area has tended to focus on the effects of correspondences between specific colors and particular flavors, tastes, aromas, or sensations of refreshment on people's perception of food or drinks. Whether the results of such studies reflect a genuine perceptual effect, a predominantly decisional effect, or some unknown combination of the two, will likely only be unequivocally resolved by future research. What is evident already, though, is that previous experiences involving certain combinations of color and flavor/aroma will lead us to generate specific expectations regarding the likely flavor of future food products, expectations that might actually have a strong influence on our final sensory perception. However, the elimination of visual input (with the eyes closed or with a blindfold) does not significantly alter flavor from that of a colorless solution (Delwiche 2004), indicating that while color can alter perceived taste, smell, and flavor ratings, the elimination of visual input certainly does not eliminate the perception of flavor. In the case of color correspondences in product packaging, which is an area of research that has been little explored to date, the possible explanations are more clearly grounded in terms of the consumer's previous exposure to a specific brand or marketing campaign. It could also be the case that color may just prime the associations that we have with a particular color regardless of whether or not it sets up any particular expectations (Elliot and Maier 2012). Finally, with regard to the color of the plateware or of the environment, other mechanisms might be responsible for modulating our perception of the product, namely, contrast effects, conceptual associations, or indirect emotion-related effects, respectively.

Having demonstrated that food coloring does indeed influence flavor identification, the question of how best to unravel the various mechanisms that underlie such cross-modal effects, at both the behavioral and neural levels, clearly represents an important and challenging area for study in the years to come. It seems that techniques such as neuroimaging, in which a participant does not necessarily have to process the associations cognitively and report them, may reveal promising results that will help unpick various theoretical accounts about the origins and development of color correspondences (Österbauer et al. 2005; Skrandies and Reuther 2008). In addition, we believe that food science researchers would be well advised to move closer to the marketplace, and rather than using arbitrary colors in the laboratory for the experiments, they should consider taking their inspiration increasingly from the color–flavor associations that rule in the marketplace.

REFERENCES

Ares, G., and R. Deliza. 2010. Studying the influence of package shape and colour on consumer expectations of milk desserts using word association and conjoint analysis. *Food Quality and Preference* 21:930–937.

Asch, S.E. 1946. Forming impressions of personality. *Journal of Abnormal and Social Psychology* 41:258–290.

Becker, L., T.J.L. van Rompay, H.N.J. Schifferstein, and M. Galetzka. 2011. Tough package, strong taste: The influence of packaging design on taste impressions and product evaluations. *Food Quality and Preference* 22:17–23.

Birren, F. 1963. Color and human appetite. *Food Technology* 17:45–47.

Blackwell, L. 1995. Visual clues and their effects on odour assessment. *Nutrition and Food Science* 5:24–28.

Broackes, J. 2010. What do the color-blind see? In *Color Ontology and Color Science*, eds. J. Cohen and M. Matthen, pp. 291–389. Cambridge, MA: MIT Press.

Bruno, N., M. Martani, C. Corsini, and C. Oleari. 2013. The effect of the color red on consuming food does not depend on achromatic (Michelson) contrast and extends to rubbing cream on the skin. *Appetite* 71:307–313.

Cheskin, L. 1957. *How to Predict What People Will Buy*. New York: Liveright.

Christensen, C. 1985. Effect of color on judgments of food aroma and food intensity in young and elderly adults. *Perception* 14:755–762.

CIE. 2004. *Colorimetry, 3rd Ed.* Vienna: CIE Central Bureau.

Clydesdale, F.M. 1991. Colour perception and food quality. *Journal of Food Quality* 14:61–74.

Clydesdale, F.M. 1993. Color as a factor in food choice. *Critical Reviews in Food Science and Nutrition* 33:1:83–101.

Clydesdale, F.M., R. Gover, D. Philipsen, and C. Fugardi. 1992. The effect of color on thirst quenching, sweetness, acceptability and flavor intensity in fruit punch flavored beverages. *Journal of Food Quality* 15:19–38.

Deliza, R., H. MacFie, and D. Hedderley. 2003. Use of computer-generated images and conjoint analysis to investigate sensory expectations. *Journal of Sensory Studies* 18:465–486.

Delwiche, J.F. 2003. Attributes believed to impact flavor: An opinion survey. *Journal of Sensory Studies* 18:437–444.

Delwiche, J. 2004. The impact of perceptual interactions on perceived flavor. *Food Quality and Preference* 15:137–146.

Demattè, M.L., D. Sanabria, and C. Spence. 2006. Cross-modal associations between odors and colors. *Chemical Senses* 31:531–538.

DuBose, C.N., A.V. Cardello, and O. Maller. 1980. Effects of colourants and flavourants on identification, perceived flavour intensity, and hedonic quality of fruit-flavoured beverages and cake. *Journal of Food Science* 45:1393–1399, 1415.

Duncker, K. 1939. The influence of past experience upon perceptual properties. *American Journal of Psychology* 52:255–265.

Ekroll, V., F. Faul, and R. Niederée. 2004. The peculiar nature of simultaneous colour contrast in uniform surrounds. *Vision Research* 44:1765–1786.

Elliot, A.J., and M.A. Maier. 2012. Color-in-context theory. *Advances in Experimental Social Psychology* 45:63–125.

Elliot, A.J., M.A. Maier, A.C. Moller, R. Friedman, and J. Meinhardt. 2007. Color and psychological functioning: The effect of red on performance attainment. *Journal of Experimental Psychology: General* 136:154–168.

Esterl, M. 2011. A frosty reception for Coca-Cola's white Christmas cans. *The Wall Street Journal* (December 1). Available at http://online.wsj.com/article/SB100014240529702 04012004577070521211375302.html (accessed October 28, 2012).

Evans, D. 2002. *Emotion: The Science of Sentiment.* Oxford: Oxford University Press.

Fairchild, M.D. 2005. *Color Appearance Models.* Chichester: John Wiley & Sons.

Felsted, J., X. Ren, and D.M. Small. 2010. Genetically determined differences in brain response to a primary food reward. *Journal of Neuroscience* 30:2428–2432.

Fenko, A., H.N. Schifferstein, T.C. Huang, and P. Hekkert. 2009. What makes products fresh: The smell or the colour? *Food Quality and Preference* 20:372–379.

Fletcher, L., H. Heymann, and M. Ellersieck. 1991. Effects of visual masking techniques on the intensity rating of sweetness of gelatins and lemonades. *Journal of Sensory Studies* 6:179–191.

Frank, R.A., K, Ducheny, and S.J.S. Mize. 1989. Strawberry odor, but not red color, enhances the sweetness of sucrose solutions. *Chemical Senses* 14:371–377.

Gal, D., S.C. Wheeler, and B. Shiv. 2007. Cross-modal influences on gustatory perception. Working paper. Abstract available at http://ssrn.com/abstract=1030197.

Garber, L., E. Hyatt, and R. Starr. 2000. The effect of food colour on perceived flavour. *Journal of Marketing Theory and Practice* 8:59–72.

Garber, Jr., L.L., E.M. Hyatt, and Ü.Ö. Boya. 2008. The mediating effects of the appearance of nondurable consumer goods and their packaging on consumer behavior. In *Product Experience*, eds. H.N.J. Schifferstein and P. Hekkert, pp. 581–602. London: Elsevier.

Genschow, O., L. Reutner, and M. Wanke. 2012. The color red reduces snack food and soft drink intake. *Appetite* 58:699–702.

Gifford, S.R., and F.M. Clydesdale. 1986. The psychophysical relationship between color and sodium chloride concentrations in model systems. *Journal of Food Protection* 49:977–982.

Gifford, S.R., F.M. Clydesdale, and R.A. Damon, Jr. 1987. The psychophysical relationship between color and salt concentrations in chicken-flavored broths. *Journal of Sensory Studies* 2:137–147.

Gilbert, A.N., R. Martin, and S.E. Kemp. 1996. Cross-modal correspondence between vision and olfaction: The color of smells. *American Journal of Psychology* 109:335–351.

Gregson, R.A.M. 1964. Modification of perceived relative intensities of acid tastes by ambient illumination changes. *Australian Journal of Psychology* 16:190–199.

Guéguen, N. 2003. The effect of glass colour on the evaluation of a beverage's thirst-quenching quality. *Current Psychology Letters* 11:1–6.

Guinard, J.X., A. Souchard, M. Picot, M. Rogeaux, and J.M. Siefferman. 1998. Sensory determinants of the thirst-quenching character of beer. *Appetite* 31:101–115.

Hall, R.L. 1958. Flavor study approaches at McCormick and Company, Inc. In *Flavor Research and Food Acceptance: A Survey of the Scope of Flavor and Associated Research, Compiled from Papers Presented in a Series of Symposia Given in 1956–1957*, ed. A.D. Little Inc., pp. 224–240. New York: Reinhold.

Harrar, V., and C. Spence. 2013. The taste of cutlery. *Flavour* 2:21.

Harrar, V., B. Piqueras-Fiszman, and C. Spence. 2011. There's more to taste in a coloured bowl. *Perception* 40:880–882.

Hutchings, J.B. 1994. *Food Colour and Appearance*. London: Blackie Academic and Professional.

Hyman, A. 1983. The influence of color on the taste perception of carbonated water preparations. *Bulletin of the Psychonomic Society* 21:145–148.

Jacobs, L., C. Keown, R. Worthley, and K.I. Ghymn. 1991. Cross-cultural colour comparisons: Global marketers beware! *International Marketing Review* 8:3:21–31.

Johnson, J., and F.M. Clydesdale. 1982. Perceived sweetness and redness in colored sucrose solutions. *Journal of Food Science* 47:747–752.

Johnson, J.L., E. Dzendolet, R. Damon, M. Sawyer, and F.M. Clydesdale. 1982. Psychophysical relationships between perceived sweetness and color in cherry-flavored beverages. *Journal of Food Protection* 45:601–606.

Johnson, J.L., E. Dzendolet, and F.M. Clydesdale. 1983. Psychophysical relationships between perceived sweetness and redness in strawberry-flavored beverages. *Journal of Food Protection* 46:21–25, 28.

Kemp, S.E., and A.N. Gilbert. 1997. Odor intensity and color lightness are correlated sensory dimensions. *American Journal of Psychology* 11:35–46.

Koza, B.J., A. Cilmi, M. Dolese, and D.A. Zellner. 2005. Color enhances orthonasal olfactory intensity and reduces retronasal olfactory intensity. *Chemical Senses* 30:643–649.

Labbe, D., F. Gilbert, N. Antille, and N. Martin. 2009. Sensory determinants of refreshing. *Food Quality and Preference* 20:100–109.

Lavin, J., and H. Lawless. 1998. Effects of color and odor on judgments of sweetness among children and adults. *Food Quality and Preference* 9:283–289.

Lee, H.S., and M. O'Mahony. 2005. Sensory evaluation and marketing: Measurement of a consumer concept. *Food Quality and Preference* 16:227–235.

Leibowitz, H., N.A. Myers, and P. Chinetti. 1955. The role of simultaneous contrast in brightness constancy. *Journal of Experimental Psychology* 50:15–18.

Levitan, C., M. Zampini, R. Li, and C. Spence. 2008. Assessing the role of colour cues and people's beliefs about colour–flavour associations on the discrimination of the flavour of sugar-coated chocolates. *Chemical Senses* 33:415–423.

Lyman, B. 1989. *A Psychology of Food, More Than a Matter of Taste*. New York: Avi, van Nostrand Reinhold.

Madden, T.J., K. Hewett, and M.S. Roth. 2000. Managing images in different cultures: A cross-national study of color meanings and preferences. *Journal of International Marketing* 8:4:90–107.

Maga, J.A. 1974. Influence of color on taste thresholds. *Chemical Senses and Flavor* 1:115–119.

Maric, Y., and M. Jacquot. 2013. Contribution to understanding odour–colour associations. *Food Quality and Preference* 27:191–195.

Marshall, D., M. Stuart, and R. Bell. 2006. Examining the relationship between product package colour and product selection in preschoolers. *Food Quality and Preference* 17: 615–621.

Martin, N., K. Gartenmann, R. Cartier, C. Vaccher, P. Callier, L. Engelen, and E. Belin. 2005. Olfactory cues modulate sensory expectations and actual perceptions of texture and complex sensory attributes. In *Abstract Book of the Sixth Pangborn Sensory Symposium*, p. 9. Oxford: Elsevier.

Masurovsky, B.I. 1939. How to obtain the right food color. *Food Engineering* 11(13):55–56.

McCrone, J. 2002. Tetrachromats. *The Lancet Neurology* 1:136.

McEwan, J.A., and J.S. Colwill. 1996. The sensory assessment of the thirst-quenching characteristics of drinks. *Food Quality and Preference* 7:101–111.

Mehta, R., and R. Zhu. 2009. Blue or red? Exploring the effect of color on cognitive task performances. *Science* 323:1226–1229.

Melendez-Martinez, A.J., I.M. Vicario, and F.J. Heredia. 2005. Instrumental measurement of orange juice colour: A review. *Journal of the Science of Food and Agriculture* 85: 894–901.

Michael, G.A., and P. Rolhion. 2008. Cool colors: Color-induced nasal thermal sensations. *Neuroscience Letters* 436:2:141–144.

Moir, H.C. 1936. Some observations on the appreciation of flavour in foodstuffs. *Journal of the Society of Chemical Industry: Chemistry & Industry Review* 14:145–148.

Morrot, G., F. Brochet, and D. Dubourdieu. 2001. The color of odors. *Brain and Language* 79:309–320.

Oberfeld, D., H. Hecht, U. Allendorf, and F. Wickelmaier. 2009. Ambient lighting modifies the flavor of wine. *Journal of Sensory Studies* 24:797–832.

Österbauer, R.A., P.M. Matthews, M. Jenkinson, C.F. Beckmann, P.C. Hanse, and G.A. Calvert. 2005. The colour of scents: Chromatic stimuli modulate odor responses in the human brain. *Journal of Neurophysiology* 93:3434–3441.

Parr, W.V., K.G. White, and D. Heatherbell. 2003. The nose knows: Influence of colour on perception of wine aroma. *Journal of Wine Research* 14:79–101.

Piqueras-Fiszman, B., and C. Spence. 2011. Cross-modal correspondences in product packaging: Assessing color–flavor correspondences for potato chips (crisps). *Appetite* 57:753–757.

Piqueras-Fiszman, B., and C. Spence. 2012. The influence of the colour of the cup on consumers' perception of a hot beverage. *Journal of Sensory Studies* 27:324–331.

Piqueras-Fiszman, B., G. Ares, and P. Varela. 2011. Semiotics and perception: Do labels convey the same message to older and younger consumers? *Journal of Sensory Studies* 26:3:197–208.

Piqueras-Fiszman, B., J. Alcaide, E. Roura, and C. Spence. 2012a. Is it the plate or is it the food? The influence of the color and shape of the plate on the perception of the food placed on it. *Food Quality and Preference* 24:205–208.

Piqueras-Fiszman, B., C. Velasco, and C. Spence. 2012b. Exploring implicit and explicit cross-modal colour–flavour correspondences in product packaging. *Food Quality and Preference* 25:148–155.

Piqueras-Fiszman, B., A. Giboreau, and C. Spence. 2013. Assessing the influence of the colour/finish of the plate on the perception of the food in a test in a restaurant setting. *Flavor* 2:24.

Reed, D.R. 2008. Birth of a new breed of supertaster. *Chemical Senses* 33:489–491.

Rohm, H., M. Strobi, and D. Jaros. 1997. Butter colour affects sensory perception of spreadability. *Z Lebensm Unters Forsch* A205:108–110.

Roth, H., L. Radle, S. Gifford, and F. Clydesdale. 1988. Psychophysical relationships between perceived sweetness and color in lemon- and lime-flavored drinks. *Journal of Food Science* 53:1116–1119.

Sauvageot, F., and A. Struillou. 1997. Effet d'une modification de la couleur des échantillons et de l'éclairage sur la flaveur de vins évaluée sur une échelle de similarité (Effect of the modification of wine color and lighting conditions on the perceived flavour of wine, as measured by a similarity scale). *Science des Aliments* 17:45–67.

Schifferstein, H.N.J. 2001. Effects of product beliefs on product perception and liking. In *Food, People and Society: A European Perspective of Consumers' Food Choices*, eds. L. Frewer, E. Risvik, and H. Schifferstein, pp. 73–96. Berlin: Springer Verlag.

Schifferstein, H.N.J. 2009. The drinking experience: Cup or content? *Food Quality and Preference* 20:268–276.

Schifferstein, H.N.J., and I. Tanudjaja. 2004. Visualising fragrances through colours: The mediating role of emotions. *Perception* 33:1249–1266.

Shankar, M.U., C. Levitan, and C. Spence. 2010a. Grape expectations: The role of cognitive influences in color–flavor interactions. *Consciousness & Cognition* 19:380–390.

Shankar, M., C. Simons, C. Levitan, B. Shiv, S. McClure, and C. Spence. 2010b. An expectations-based approach to explaining the cross-modal influence of color on odor identification: The influence of temporal and spatial factors. *Journal of Sensory Studies* 25:791–803.

Shankar, M., C. Simons, B. Shiv, C. Levitan, S. McClure, and C. Spence. 2010c. An expectations-based approach to explaining the influence of color on odor identification: The influence of degree of discrepancy. *Attention, Perception, & Psychophysics* 72:1981–1993.

Shepherd, G.M. 2012. *Neurogastronomy: How the Brain Creates Flavor and Why It Matters.* New York: Columbia University Press.

Singh, S. 2006. Impact of color on marketing. *Management Decision* 44:783–789.

Skrandies, W., and N. Reuther. 2008. Match and mismatch of taste, odor, and color are reflected by electrical activity in the human brain. *Journal of Psychophysiology* 22:175–184.

Small, D.M. 2009. Individual differences in the neurophysiology of reward and the obesity epidemic. *International Journal of Obesity* 33:S44–S48.

Spence, C. 2010a. The color of wine—Part 1. *The World of Fine Wine* 28:122–129.

Spence, C. 2010b. The color of wine—Part 2. *The World of Fine Wine* 29:112–119.

Spence, C. 2012. The development and decline of multisensory flavour perception. In *Multisensory Development*, eds. A.J. Bremner, D. Lewkowicz, and C. Spence, pp. 63–87. Oxford: Oxford University Press.

Spence, C., and B. Piqueras-Fiszman. 2014. *The Perfect Meal: The Multisensory Science of Food and Dining.* Oxford: Wiley-Blackwell.

Spence, C., C.A. Levitan, M.U. Shankar, and M. Zampini. 2010. Does food colour influence taste and flavour perception in humans? *Chemosensory Perception* 3:68–84.

Stevenson, R.J., A. Rich, and A. Russell. 2012. The nature and origin of cross-modal associations to odours. *Perception* 41:606–619.

Swientek, B. 2001. Uncanny developments: Food and beverage cans evolve to deliver greater convenience and shelf impact. *Beverage Industry* 92:12:38–39.

Teerling, A. 1992. The colour of taste. *Chemical Senses* 17:886.

Wan, X., C. Velasco, C. Michel, B. Mu, A.T. Woods, and C. Spence. 2014. Does the type of receptacle influence the cross-modal association between colour and flavour? A cross-cultural comparison. *Flavor* 3:3.

Wei, S.T., L.C. Ou, M.R. Luo, and J.B. Hutchings. 2012. Optimisation of food expectations using product colour and appearance. *Food Quality and Preference* 23:49–62.

Wilson, G.D., and R.A.M. Gregson. 1967. Effects of illumination on perceived intensity of acid tastes. *Australian Journal of Psychology* 19:69–72.

Wu, D., and D.W. Sun. 2012. Colour measurements by computer vision for food quality control: A review. *Trends in Food Science & Technology* 29:5–20.

Yeomans, M., L. Chambers, H. Blumenthal, and A. Blake. 2008. The role of expectancy in sensory and hedonic evaluation: The case of smoked salmon ice cream. *Food Quality and Preference* 19:565–573.

Zampini, M., D. Sanabria, N. Phillips, and C. Spence. 2007. The multisensory perception of flavour: Assessing the influence of colour cues on flavour discrimination responses. *Food Quality and Preference* 18:975–984.

Zampini, M., E. Wantling, N. Phillips, and C. Spence. 2008. Multisensory flavour perception: Assessing the influence of fruit acids and colour cues on the perception of fruit-flavoured beverages. *Food Quality and Preference* 19:335–343.

Zeki, S. 1993. *A Vision of the Brain.* Oxford: Blackwell.

Zellner, D.A., and P. Durlach. 2002. What is refreshing? An investigation of the color and other sensory attributes of refreshing foods and beverages. *Appetite* 39:185–186.

Zellner, D.A., and P. Durlach. 2003. Effect of color on expected and experienced refreshment, intensity, and liking of beverages. *American Journal of Psychology* 116:633–647.

Zellner, D.A., and M.A. Kautz. 1990. Color affects perceived odor intensity. *Journal of Experimental Psychology: Human Perception and Performance* 16:391–397.

Zellner, D.A., and L.A. Whitten. 1999. The effect of color intensity and appropriateness on color-induced odor enhancement. *American Journal of Psychology* 112:585–604.

Zellner, D.A., A.M. Bartoli, and R. Eckard. 1991. Influence of color on odor identification and liking ratings. *American Journal of Psychology* 104:547–561.

Zellner, D.A., A. McGarry, R. Mattern-McClory, and D. Abreu. 2008. Masculinity/femininity of fine fragrances affects color–odor correspondences: A case for cognitions influencing cross-modal correspondences. *Chemical Senses* 33:211–222.

7 Effect of Visual Cues on Sensory and Hedonic Evaluation of Food

Debra A. Zellner

CONTENTS

7.1 Introduction 159
7.2 Color and Identification 160
7.3 Color and Liking.. 161
7.4 Color and Flavor Intensity 161
7.5 Color and Refreshment 163
7.6 Visual Cues for Freshness 164
7.7 Food Presentation 165
7.8 Mechanisms by Which These Effects Might Occur.............................. 167
7.9 Expectations... 167
7.10 Perceptual Learning 169
References... 171

7.1 INTRODUCTION

Eating a food is a multisensory experience. When we eat a food, we smell the food (olfaction), taste the food (gustation), experience the texture of the food in our mouths (tactile), and are aware of the food's temperature. We also can experience stimulation to the trigeminal nerve if, for example, the food contains chili pepper. Input from these many senses makes up what we call the flavor of the food (Delwiche 2004).

Other senses are also stimulated during the act of eating a food. For example, if the food is crunchy, we can experience the sound of the food (audition; for a review of the effects of audition on flavor, see Spence 2012). Vision is usually the first sense that is stimulated when eating a food (although at times, we smell a food before seeing it). Visual information usually arrives prior to the introduction of the food into the mouth. Seeing the food we are about to ingest provides a lot of information about the food. Through the pairing of certain visual cues with the flavor of the food in the past, we learn the associations between these visual cues and the flavor that we experience once we ingest the food. Thus, information from seeing the food can lead to expectations about both the sensory and hedonic experiences to come. How the food looks can also affect the perception of the sensory qualities of the food and our hedonic evaluation of the food.

This chapter will review what we know about how various visual characteristics of the food affect the sensory and hedonic perceptions of the food. It will also discuss how perceptual learning and expectations might contribute to these effects.

Although many characteristics of the food, including the shape, color, size, translucency, and texture of a food, provide information about the food that we are about to ingest, this chapter will focus on color, surface luminance, and aesthetic arrangement since most research has been done investigating those visual characteristics. Of those, color has been the most studied. For many foods, in the absence of labels (which are visual stimuli but not a property of the food itself), color provides the most information about the identity of the food that we are about to eat.

7.2   COLOR AND IDENTIFICATION

The importance of color in identifying a food depends on how strongly associated the color is with the food. Tanaka and Presnell (1999) included a lot of foods on their list of objects having what they call high color diagnosticity (highly associated with a color). For example, yellow is very highly associated with lemon, and green is very highly associated with lettuce. Therefore, if these objects are colored inappropriately, they are harder to recognize than are other objects in which color is less diagnostic. For example, peppers are a food item where color is less diagnostic than it is with lemons or lettuce. Peppers are now sold in many different colors (e.g., green, red, orange, yellow, and purple), so the color does not help much in identifying an object as a pepper.

The importance of color in flavor identification also depends upon what other cues are available, including the shape of the food item. If one views a whole fruit or vegetable (such as a banana), the shape is as, if not more, important than the color in identifying the food. On the other hand, if one views a scoop of sorbet or a glass of juice, the only visual clue as to its flavor is the color. Therefore, most studies on color's effect on flavor identification have used food items such as beverages where color is the most salient cue predicting the flavor of the food.

For example, DuBose et al. (1980) had subjects identify the flavor of appropriately colored, inappropriately colored, and colorless orange-, cherry-, and lime-flavored beverages. When the orange beverage was colored orange, the cherry colored red, and the lime colored green, the flavors were identified correctly 81.5%, 70.4%, and 48.2% of the time, respectively. However, the subjects were much less accurate in identifying the same beverages when they were colored inappropriately (28.4%) or when they were colorless (37%). The inappropriately colored beverages were often identified as flavors that were associated with the inappropriate color. So, for example, when the orange-flavored beverage was colored green, it was often identified as being lime-flavored. Similar results using beverages (Hyman 1983; Stillman 1993; Garber et al. 2000) and sherbet (Hall 1958) have been found by others.

Colors that are appropriate for the beverage appear to help the subjects identify the flavor, whereas inappropriate colors decrease accuracy, leading to incorrect identifications. However, Zampini et al. (2007) failed to see a facilitative effect of appropriate colors when they provided the subjects with a list of possible flavors to choose from. This suggests that if the list of possible flavors is already sufficiently narrowed, by providing the subjects with a list of flavors, the color helps the identification less than if the subjects have to choose a flavor from all the possibilities.

The facilitative effect of an appropriate color on flavor identification is probably a result of the color's activating odor search images and labels in memory that have been associated with that color in the past, in that context (e.g., brown color in a beverage). A different set of odor images might be activated by a color if the object being consumed is a beverage rather than an ice cream. So, for example, a brown beverage might be expected to be a cola or a root beer, whereas a brown ice cream might be expected to have a chocolate flavor (Zellner 2013).

That the more frequently associated flavors are the ones most strongly activated by a particular color is supported by a study by Zellner et al. (1991). Their subjects smelled 10 different fruit solutions (rather than consuming them) and were asked to identify the odor. They found that an appropriate color facilitated the identification of a fruit odor that was commonly associated with that color but not one that was less commonly associated. For example, the color red increased the accuracy of identification of the cherry solution but not the watermelon.

7.3   COLOR AND LIKING

In addition to helping us identify the flavor of a food, color might also influence how much we like it. Zellner et al. (1991) found that appropriately colored fruit-flavored solutions were rated as more pleasant than inappropriately colored ones when smelled orthonasally. For example, a yellow-colored grape solution (inappropriately colored) was judged as less pleasant-smelling than the same solution colored purple (appropriately colored). The same effect was obtained when the subjects ingested appropriately and inappropriately colored sherbets (Hall 1958). With both the sherbets and the orthonasal odors, this decrease in pleasantness of the inappropriately colored items seems to occur only when the color prevents the odor or food flavor from being correctly identified (Hall 1958; Zellner et al. 1991). If we can identify an odor or flavor, even if incorrectly colored, it is still pleasant.

It is not clear that what is true for odors is true for foods. One anecdotal report (Wheatley 1973) suggests that inappropriately colored foods are not liked as much as appropriately colored foods. Wheatley reports that people became nauseated when, after eating a meal under light-masking conditions that made the food look to be normally colored, the masking light was turned off; and the subjects saw that they had been eating blue steak, green French fries, and red peas. A more recent example is the marketing of Crystal Pepsi (Triplett 1994). This was a cola that was reported to be identical to regular Pepsi but without the brown cola color. People did not like the taste, and it was taken off the market.

7.4   COLOR AND FLAVOR INTENSITY

There is quite a lot of evidence showing that color increases the odor of a food (which is a large component of what we call flavor) presented orthonasally (inhaled through the nostrils) (Christensen 1983; Zellner and Kautz 1990; Zellner and Whitten 1999; Koza et al. 2005). However, when an odor is experienced retronasally (when put into the mouth), no color-induced increase (Christensen 1983; Zampini et al. 2007) or a decrease in odor intensity has been found (Zellner and Durlach 2003; Koza et al. 2005). Although we do not know for certain why orthonasal olfactory intensity is increased by color and retronasal olfactory intensity seems not to be, there are some possible explanations for these differences.

The odors judged in the above studies (with the exception of Christensen 1983) were odors presented in solutions with little else other than, in some cases, sugar. When actual foods, such as cake, have been used (DuBose et al. 1980), a color-induced increase in flavor intensity has been found. DuBose et al. (1980) found both an increase in the intensity of the lemon flavor in a cake with an increase in the yellow color of that cake, and an increase in the intensity of the orange flavor of a beverage when the intensity of the orange color was increased. Although Christensen's (1983) effects for flavor intensity ratings between the colored and colorless versions of her foods were not significantly different, they were higher in the colored than in the colorless solution for most of the foods (e.g., margarine, bacon, orange drink). The lack of significant effect in her study could have been the result of a small number of subjects ($n = 15$).

The complex foods used by DuBose et al. and Christensen (e.g., cake, bacon), unlike the simple flavors in water used in the studies finding retronasal odor suppression (e.g., Zellner and Durlach 2003; Koza et al. 2005), have more complex flavors, including numerous gustatory components, which might also become associated with the color resulting in a conditioned gustatory percept. When odor is the major component of the flavor (as in Zellner and Durlach 2003; Koza et al. 2005), the reduction of the retronasal odor might be the result of a contrast effect between the intensity of the initially experienced orthonasal odor as it is smelled before entering the mouth and that of the same odor experienced retronasally once in the mouth. The enhancement of orthonasal odor intensity by color is a robust phenomenon. Thus, the orthonasal odor intensity of a colored solution will be perceived as stronger than a colorless one. That will lead the subject to expect the colored solution to have a stronger flavor than the colorless one. Once the solution is in the mouth, the color is no longer seen. When the retronasal odor is experienced after smelling the strong color-enhanced orthonasal odor, the retronasal odor might be experienced as weaker than expected. This will result in intensity contrast when the solution is colored, thus the color-induced retronasal odor suppression.

Obviously, the effect of color on flavor intensity needs to be investigated further. Color might be influencing separate components of the flavor experience differently. For example, we know that while the effect of color on orthonasal olfaction is always enhancement, a similar effect does not occur with gustation. Sometimes, colors enhance the intensity of gustatory stimuli (e.g., Johnson and Clydesdale 1982; Johnson et al. 1982, 1983; Lavin and Lawless 1998), but the results of the effect of color on gustation have been inconsistent. For example, Maga (1974) found that green coloring decreased the taste threshold for sucrose in a solution, but Pangborn (1960) found that green pear nectar was perceived as less sweet than colorless pear nectar. However, in a second study using pear nectar, Pangborn and Hansen (1963) failed to replicate the effect of green coloring on the sweetness of pear nectar.

7.5 COLOR AND REFRESHMENT

In addition to helping us identify a food and affecting the pleasantness and perceived intensity of a food, color has been found to have an effect on judgments of expected and actual refreshment. Most studies examining the effect of color on refreshment have used beverages because a beverage is most often named as the most refreshing food or drink (Zellner and Durlach 2002). Thus, *refreshing* is very similar to *thirst-quenching*, and both terms have been used.

In questionnaire studies using the two terms (thirst-quenching in Clydesdale et al. 1992; refreshing in Zellner and Durlach 2002), the subjects indicated that clear is the most refreshing color for a beverage. However, these two studies differed in judgments of how refreshing a brown color is. Clydesdale et al.'s (1992) subjects reported brown as one of the most refreshing colors, whereas Zellner and Durlach's (2002) subjects reported it as being unrefreshing. The difference between the studies probably had to do with what items the subjects had in mind while answering the question. Zellner and Durlach asked the subjects to indicate the most refreshing color for a food or drink, whereas Clydesdale et al. asked the subjects about nonalcoholic beverages that would satisfy their thirst. If, in both cases, the subjects reported the color of the refreshing items that came to mind, it is much more likely in the Clydesdale et al. study than in Zellner and Durlach that the subjects were thinking of colas (as the authors suggest). Clydesdale et al. also suggest that the subjects reported clear because they were thinking about water. The idea that the subjects' answers about what colors are refreshing are based on what refreshing beverages come to mind is supported by the fact that in Zellner and Durlach, the subjects who listed brown as a refreshing color also reported a brown food or beverage as the most refreshing food or beverage, and those subjects who listed brown as an unrefreshing color did not.

So, how refreshing a colored food item is perceived as being probably depends upon the type of food item being evaluated. In the case of beverages, it is probably related to the flavor of the beverage. Evidence for this comes from studies where subjects judge the refreshment of differently colored beverages after tasting them. For example, Guinard et al. (1998) found that the more brown a beer, the less thirst-quenching it was judged to be. This is probably because the subjects expect a dark brown beer to be a stronger, more bitter-tasting beer, which is less refreshing than a pale, less flavorful beer.

Zellner and Durlach's (2003) results add further support for the idea that how refreshing a beverage of a particular color is tends to be flavor-dependent. Their study presented subjects with 24 different beverages. There were three differently flavored beverages (lemon, mint, and vanilla) colored seven different colors and colorless. The subjects rated how refreshing they expected the different beverages to be (prior to tasting them) and how refreshing the beverages were (after tasting them). Not surprisingly, the colorless versions of all three beverages were expected to be the most refreshing. When the subjects actually tasted the beverages, the colorless versions were still often judged as more refreshing than many of the colored beverages. The brown versions of the lemon and mint beverages were expected to be the least refreshing and were also rated as such when tasted. However, the brown vanilla beverage was not expected to be unrefreshing and was not rated as particularly unrefreshing compared to the other colors. This effect of brown vanilla was most likely the result of brown being an appropriate color for vanilla (since vanilla extract is dark brown) and was therefore a predictor of flavor rather than the refreshingness of the flavor, unlike the beer in Guinard et al. (1998) where the darkness of a beer is generally a predictor of degree of refreshment.

The effect that color has on perceived refreshment appears related to what we have learned about color's relationship to the degree of refreshment of a particular beverage in the past. In general, clear beverages are more refreshing because they are usually water. The lighter the color, the more watery the beverage (as in the case of beer), and thus the more refreshing it is. Colors that decrease the refreshingness of one flavor can increase the refreshingness of another flavor if that color is appropriate for that flavor.

7.6   VISUAL CUES FOR FRESHNESS

Another characteristic of food that is important when consumers are making food selections is the freshness of the food. Freshness is related to the age of the food. As foods age, there is decomposition. This decomposition can lead to changes in the texture, odor, and taste of a food. Visual changes also occur. In fact, studies have found that visual cues are extremely important in evaluating the freshness of fruits (Peneau et al. 2007; Arce-Lopera et al. 2012), vegetables (Peneau et al. 2007; Wada et al. 2010; Arce-Lopera et al. 2013), and fish (Murakoshi et al. 2013).

Although the color of some foods changes during decomposition, color changes seem not to be a very important attribute of freshness except in the case of meat (Issanchou 1996; Carpenter et al. 2001; Troy and Kerry 2010). While color is a good predictor of the degree of ripeness of some fruits and vegetables (e.g., strawberries but not carrots), it is not a good predictor of freshness. Instead, Peneau et al. (2007) found that the shininess of the surface of carrots and strawberries was an important characteristic in evaluating freshness, whereas a shriveled surface was a characteristic of carrots and strawberries that are not fresh.

Shininess is related to the luminance distribution of the surface of the food. Recently, the luminance distribution of the surface of a cabbage leaf has been found to be related to judged freshness (Wada et al. 2010). Subsequent studies using images of a section of cabbage leaf (Arce-Lopera et al. 2013) or strawberry (Arce-Lopera et al. 2012) in which color was held constant but the luminance information varied indicated that the surface luminance of these foods provides freshness information to subjects. Color change was not necessary for subjects to judge the freshness of these foods. Recently, a similar effect of the luminance distribution of fish eyes was shown to be related to the judged freshness of fish (Murakoshi et al. 2013). Since the luminance distribution changed with the freshness of the food, the fact that the subjects are able to judge freshness using this cue provides convincing evidence that visual cues, particularly the luminance distribution of the food surface, are a good guide for consumers to use to select fresh food. This relationship between surface luminance and freshness is one that has clearly been learned by the subjects in these studies.

7.7   FOOD PRESENTATION

The studies discussed up to this point have investigated the effect of visual cues, primarily color, on a single food item, mostly beverages. However, most of our food consumption occurs in meals that consist of more than one food item, often presented together on a plate. Culinary institutes put a lot of emphasis on presentation aesthetics (*plating*). Color and balance are two important factors that are thought to contribute to the visual appeal of food on a plate (Hutchings 1999; Spears and Gregoire 2004).

A presentation with some color variation should be seen as more appealing than a monochrome presentation, because adding color increases complexity. A moderate degree of visual complexity on a plate of food might be expected to increase the attractiveness of the presentation (Berlyne et al. 1968) and possibly, therefore, liking for the food if we have learned an association between visual attractiveness and hedonic value of the flavor of the food. This contribution of color to complexity and liking is supported by the discussion of a 1997 luncheon organized by the Colour Society of Australia (Hutchings 2003). The meal was composed entirely of white foods and was described as *boring* by the diners.

Balance is a visual feature that has been found to be important in the aesthetic evaluation of a painting (see Locher 1996 for a review). A painting canvas, or in the case of food, a plate, is considered to be balanced when the elements are arranged around the center of the painting or plate in such a manner that they appear anchored or stable. The more balanced an artwork, the greater the aesthetic appeal (Lega et al. 2003).

In the first empirical study (Zellner et al. 2010) testing the effects of these two variables on both the attractiveness of the plate of food and liking for the taste of the food, an interaction was seen between color and balance on attractiveness judgments. Using slices of water chestnuts, presented in either a balanced or unbalanced manner, with either colored (red and green) or naturally colored tahini decorations, the colored-balanced presentation was found to be more attractive than the colored-unbalanced presentation or the monochrome-balanced presentations. However, the increase in attractiveness of the colored-balanced presentation did not affect the liking for the taste of the water chestnuts. This study suggests that although color and balance do affect the visual aesthetics of a plate of food, they might not influence the liking for the taste of that food.

The lack of an effect of color and balance on liking in Zellner et al. (2010) might have been the result of the simplicity of the food and the presentation used. Most culinary presentations involve more complex food items and combinations and also more complex presentations. Therefore, in a subsequent study, subjects were presented with one of two plates (balanced and unbalanced) consisting of red pepper hummus presented on a romaine lettuce leaf with three baby carrots, three grape tomatoes, and four pita chips. The balanced and unbalanced versions of the plate were equally colorful. In this study, although the subjects did not find the balanced plate more attractive than the unbalanced plate, they did judge the hummus as tasting better when eaten from the balanced plate than from the unbalanced plate.

Further investigation (Zellner et al. 2011, Experiment 2) suggests that rather than balance affecting liking for the hummus in Experiment 1, it might have been the messiness of the presentation that did so. In addition to being unbalanced, the unbalanced hummus presentation also was quite messy, looking as though all of the food items had slid to the bottom of the plate. Therefore, in Experiment 2, balance was made the same for two presentations of chicken salad, but the neatness of the presentation was manipulated. The subjects in this second study judged the attractiveness and the liking for chicken salad presented on a romaine lettuce leaf either in a neat mound in the center of the leaf (Neat presentation) or spread out across the lettuce leaf in a messy but balanced manner (Messy presentation). Although the subjects did not find the Neat presentation to be more attractive than the Messy one, they did like the taste of the chicken salad more when eaten from the Neat plate than from the Messy plate.

These results suggest that although balance might be an important visual contributor to the attractiveness of visual art, it is less important than neatness when it comes to food presentation. In Experiment 3 of Zellner et al. (2011), the subjects looked at the pictures of the foods presented in Experiments 1 (hummus) and 2 (chicken salad) and made a variety of ratings of the plates of the food pictured. The amount of care taken by the preparer with the food was judged as greater in the Neat than in the Messy presentations. People also indicated that they were willing to pay more for the Neat than for the Messy foods and thought that the quality of the restaurant in which the meal was prepared was higher for the neatly presented food than for the messy food. Thus, seeing food neatly presented on a plate indicates that the food is of higher quality, and it is therefore judged to be better-tasting than the food that is not presented neatly on the plate.

However, while the degree of neatness of the presentations varied in Zellner et al. (2011), the attractiveness of the presentations did not. The question therefore still remains as to whether a more attractive presentation of food on the plate will increase liking for the food when both presentations are neat and vary only on attractiveness. In a recent study (Zellner et al. 2014), we presented diners in a restaurant with a meal consisting of a sautéed chicken breast with a *fines herbes* sauce, brown rice pilaf, and sautéed green beans with toasted almonds prepared, and arranged in two different ways, by a professional chef at the Culinary Institute of America in Hyde Park, New York. One presentation was a standard presentation with the chicken breast and sauce at the bottom of the plate and the rice and beans in the upper left and right quadrants, respectively. The other presentation was a more creative presentation with the rice in the center of the plate. Spiraling outward from the rice was the chicken breast and sauce with green beans arranged around the periphery. This second, more creative presentation was judged as significantly more attractive by the diners than was the more standard presentation. The diners also thought that the food preparer had taken more care with the food; however, unlike in the previous study, the subjects did not indicate that they would pay more for the attractive plate (possibly because they were frequent customers at the restaurant and did not want the food to be expensive even if they would have been willing to pay more).

The two different presentations were served to diners in the restaurant on two different nights. After eating the meal, the diners rated how much they liked the meal overall and then rated how much they liked the four components of the meal (chicken, sauce, rice, and beans). They liked the overall meal and the chicken, sauce, and rice more when presented in the more attractive presentation than the more standard presentation. This shows that both neatness of the food presented on the plate and the attractiveness of the presentation affect how much people like the taste of the food.

7.8 MECHANISMS BY WHICH THESE EFFECTS MIGHT OCCUR

The data discussed here support the idea that *the first taste is always with the eyes.* That *visual taste* occurs before a food is ingested. From vision, we receive a lot of information about the food, which helps us to identify the food. If we cannot identify the food, it is probably unfamiliar. If we can identify it, the food is most likely familiar. This information will enter into our decision to ingest the food. If it is unfamiliar, we will be less likely to consume it due to neophobia—the fear of new foods that is present in many of us (Pliner and Salvy 2006). If it is familiar, ingestion will in part be determined by whether we have liked the food in the past. Once we consume the food, visual characteristics influence the food's perceived flavor and how much we like it.

Visual cues will also help us evaluate whether the food is something that is liable to be refreshing and affect whether it is perceived as refreshing. These cues also tell us if a food is fresh. In addition, the quality of the food will be influenced by the neatness and attractiveness of its presentation.

It is clear that the visual characteristics of a food affect our evaluation of its other sensory characteristics and hedonic value. This occurs by at least two mechanisms. Both involve learning an association between the visual cue and the flavor through repeated experience. One mechanism involves learned associations in which the visual cues set up expectations about the sensory and hedonic aspects of the food that we eventually put in into our mouths. The other mechanism is perceptual learning where a visual cue, through pairing with a taste and/or odor (the two main components of flavor), elicits a conditioned flavor percept.

7.9 EXPECTATIONS

Color–flavor associations, as well as the association of other visual cues (e.g., shape, size) with flavor, will result in expectations about the sensory properties and hedonic value of the food. Usually, the visual cues provide accurate information about the flavor of the food. However, when expectations are violated, both the sensory and hedonic judgments of the food are affected in one of two ways.

In some cases, our judgments of a food can be assimilated to our expectations. For example, if a coffee is expected to be less bitter than it actually is, the coffee might be judged as less bitter by the subjects with that expectation than by the subjects without that expectation (Olson and Dover 1976). In other cases, our judgments of a food can be contrasted away from our expectations. For example, if the subjects expect a moderately intense orange juice to be intense, it will be judged as less intense than if the subjects expect it to be weak (Cardello et al. 1996). Similar assimilation and contrast effects have been found for hedonic judgments (e.g., assimilation—see Cardello and Sawyer 1992; contrast—see Cardello et al. 1996; Zellner et al. 2003).

In one study (Mace and Enzie 1970) in which color was used to produce expectations for either a hedonically positive beverage (7UP) or a hedonically negative beverage (quinine), contrast was seen when the color-induced hedonic expectations were violated. All subjects in the study first tasted two standard solutions: yellow 7UP and green quinine. These solutions were followed by either two yellow 7UP samples or two green quinine samples. These two samples were followed by a sample of the beverage not presented in the first two samples, which was colored inappropriately (i.e., green 7UP or yellow quinine). If the subjects received the green 7UP after the two green quinine samples, they had an expectation that the solution was going to be the unpleasant quinine. This expectation was violated, and the green 7UP was rated as better than it was when presented as the yellow standard. The opposite was also true. When people received the yellow quinine after the two samples of yellow 7UP, their expectation of another hedonically pleasant 7UP was violated, and they rated the quinine as worse than when it was presented as a standard. Unfortunately, in this study, color was not counterbalanced and so the effects might have been due to a direct effect of the color on liking, but this seems improbable.

Other studies induce expectations by presenting a series of context solutions prior to the presentation of a test solution or test solutions that are of a greater or lesser hedonic value than the context series. These procedures also produce hedonic contrast (Riskey et al. 1979; Riskey 1982; Cardello et al. 1996; Zellner et al. 2003). For example, Zellner et al. (2003) found that when subjects drank and rated how much they liked a series of eight, hedonically positive, fruit juices prior to drinking and rating two, less hedonically positive diluted fruit juices, they rated the diluted fruit juices as less hedonically positive than did the subjects who did not get the series of hedonically positive fruit juices first.

However, when expectations are caused by labeling (e.g., Allison and Uhl 1964; Cardello and Sawyer 1992; Wansink et al. 2007), the subjects show assimilation rather than contrast. For example, Wansink et al.'s subjects, who saw a wine labeled as coming from North Dakota, expected to like it less than did a second group who saw the same wine labeled as coming from California. After drinking the wine, the group who drank the wine with the North Dakota label rated the wine as tasting less good than did the group who drank the same wine with the California label.

Assimilation is also found when expectations are caused by telling the subjects how much others liked the food (e.g., Cardello and Sawyer 1992; Siegrist and Cousin 2009). Zellner et al. (2004) suggest that some of these assimilation effects are caused by social influence where subjects feel obligated to give certain ratings. Other cases of assimilation are the result of the food's expected and actual sensory or hedonic qualities not being very different. If the expected and actual sensory or hedonic experiences are close, subjects might pay attention to the sensory or hedonic quality that they are primed to pay attention to and therefore give ratings similar to what is suggested.

For example, Shankar et al. (2010) found, using orthonasal odors, that misidentifications of an odor based on color occurred when the expected odor was not very different from the actual odor. For example, purple cranberry and blueberry odors were misidentified as grape. However, if the expected and actual odors were highly discrepant, such misidentification did not occur. For example, a banana solution colored purple was not called a grape. Thinking about the cranberry odor as grape might have caused the subject to pay attention to certain components of the flavor that were similar to grape.

This same effect might occur with hedonics. If the subjects expect a food to taste good and it has good and bad aspects, the subjects might pay more attention to the good ones and less to the bad. This might lead to a higher hedonic rating than they would have given the food without that expectation. For example, when food is presented neatly (Zellner et al. 2011) or in a very attractive manner (Zellner et al. 2014), the subjects might expect the food to not only look good but also taste good. Those expectations might cause the higher hedonic ratings seen in neatly presented, attractive presentations.

These results suggest that visual cues produce expectations about the sensory and hedonic qualities of a food. If these expectations are close enough to the actual food's qualities (as in Zellner et al. 2011, 2014), sensory and hedonic assimilation will probably occur. However, if these expectations are different enough from the actual experience of the food, sensory and hedonic contrast should occur. There is evidence for such contrast as a result of more extreme violation of visual expectations, particularly for hedonic evaluations.

For example, Carlson (1930) describes his reaction to the taste of his first tomato that he thought was an apple (most likely because it was red and the size of an apple) as "the disgusting, disagreeable effect on me of that fluid, insipid, warm mass that filled my mouth was something very striking, and I have not forgotten it in forty years" (p. 89). Here, the visual cues led him to expect a flavor that was very different from the tomato that he actually ate, and hedonic contrast occurred. Others have demonstrated such hedonic contrast in experiments. For example, hedonic contrast occurred in Mace and Enzie (1970), and violations of expectations can also explain why inappropriately colored solutions that are not identified correctly are also disliked (Zellner et al. 1991).

However, this expectation-based approach to explaining the interactions of visual cues and flavor reviewed here has difficulty explaining the changes in intensity that have been found with color. If a color predicts a flavor and colorlessness predicts no flavor (e.g., water), we might expect colorless solutions to taste stronger than equally intense colored ones. This intensity contrast should occur if people expect the colorless solution to have no flavor and it actually has a fairly strong flavor once consumed, so that the expected and actual flavors are very different. However, intensity contrast is not always seen in this situation (Koza et al. 2005), and color often enhances flavor (DuBose et al. 1980; Christensen 1983; Koza et al. 2005). Although these effects might be explained by assimilation, given the obvious discrepancies between expected and actual flavor intensity in these studies, they are probably not that. Instead, these results suggest that expectations do not provide the only mechanism by which visual cues affect flavor. Another mechanism, perceptual learning, better explains the enhancement of flavor by the presence of color and might explain other findings as well.

7.10 PERCEPTUAL LEARNING

Expectations induced by visual stimuli are most likely the result of the retrieval of a food image with certain sensory properties and a particular hedonic value. The actual food might be compared to this image, and the sensory or hedonic evaluation of the food might then be contrasted away from the image if the two are dissimilar enough.

However, there is some reason to believe that the repeated pairings of the visual characteristics (such as color) and the food flavors are not just causing us to expect certain flavors when we see foods with certain visual properties (e.g., colors) but are, in addition, causing us to experience those flavors. Perceptual conditioning has been found by pairing odors with tastes (Stevenson et al. 1995a,b, 1998, 2000a,b; Yeomans et al. 2006) and by pairing odors with other odors (Stevenson 2001a,b, 2003; Case et al. 2004). For example, pairing a cherry odor with a smoky odor by repeatedly exposing the subjects to an odor mixture of the two resulted in the cherry odor smelling smokier when it was presented alone (Stevenson et al. 2001a).

It is possible that similar perceptual conditioning occurs when a color is paired with a flavor repeatedly, especially in the same context (such as a soda or yogurt). For example, after repeatedly eating a blue yogurt that has a blueberry flavor, a flavorless yogurt colored blue might elicit a conditioned blueberry percept. Evidence for such perceptual conditioning comes from a study in which subjects were given white wine that was colored red (Morrot et al. 2001). When asked to describe the flavor of the white wine when it was its natural color, they used descriptors of items having the color of white wine such as *honey*, *lemon*, and *almond*. When the white wine was colored red, the subjects used descriptors of items having a red color, such as *raspberry*, *blackcurrant*, and *cherry*. If the red color was causing a conditioned flavor percept, one would expect subjects to experience those *red wine* notes.

Of course, if color generates a flavor percept, the conditioned percept caused by the color would occur along with the still-present flavor. When a color is appropriate to the flavor, and the flavor is a common, easily identified one, the fusion of the color-induced conditioned flavor percept and the food-induced flavor might not noticeably affect the flavor quality of the food. This is true if the color-induced flavor percept is the same as, or similar to, the actual flavor. However, when the color is inappropriate and the color-induced flavor percept is different from the flavor of the food, a problem could arise. If the flavor induced by the color is not similar to the flavor of the food, the resultant experience could be an unpleasant combination flavor. This appears only to occur when the color prevents the flavor (or odor) from being correctly identified (Hall 1958; Zellner et al. 1991). If we can correctly identify a flavor (or odor), even if incorrectly colored, it is still pleasant.

This is also probably true for foods when color and other visual cues are inappropriate. If we can identify the food, even if these visual cues are wrong, the food will still be pleasant. For example, Chef Wyle Dufresne's *cyber-egg* is composed of a carrot–cardamom puree yolk and a hardened coconut milk egg white. It looks like a fried egg but does not taste like one. However, since the diners know it is not really an egg, it is not unpleasant. How pleasant a food with an inappropriate visual appearance is can obviously be influenced by other knowledge such as the flavor of the food or the fact that it is St. Patrick's Day so green beer is acceptable.

If visual cues such as color produce a conditioned flavor percept, not only would one predict that inappropriately colored foods would be unpleasant, but also the intensity of the flavor should be higher when the visual cues are present than when they are not. As was reviewed previously, the evidence for a conditioned flavor percept produced by color cues is mixed. There is strong evidence that color increases the perceived intensity of orthonasal odors prior to the introduction of a food into the mouth (Zellner and Kautz 1990; Zellner and Whitten 1999); however, the effect of such cues on flavor or retronasal odor is mixed (DuBose et al. 1980; Christensen 1983; Koza et al. 2005). Sometimes (e.g., Koza et al. 2005), the retronasal odor intensity is lower in the colored than in the colorless solutions.

This color-induced retronasal suppression has been explained above as an intensity contrast effect produced by the color enhancing the orthonasal odor of the food prior to it entering the mouth. The color-induced enhancement of the intensity of the orthonasal odor leads the subject to expect the flavor in the mouth to be stronger for the colored than for the colorless solutions. When the solution enters the mouth, the color of the solution is no longer visible. The retronasal odor experience might therefore be weaker than the orthonasal odor was, and intensity contrast will occur with the colored solutions.

A simple perceptual conditioning explanation also has difficulty explaining positive hedonic contrast in which expecting a hedonically bad food makes a moderately good food better, such as in the study by Mace and Enzie (1970). They found that subjects getting 7UP when expecting quinine judged the 7UP even better. Clearly expecting quinine would make a very bitter unpleasant conditioned flavor percept that would fuse with the 7UP, making it worse and not better.

The role of visually induced conditioned percepts in the perception of foods needs further study. Although they clearly influence both the sensory perception and hedonic evaluation of foods, the effect they have is impacted by sensory and hedonic expectations and other cognitive influences.

What we know is that visual cues produce expectations concerning the flavor, intensity, hedonic value, refreshingness, and freshness of foods as reviewed here. Those visual cues probably activate search images produced by prior associations to which the actual food, once tasted, is compared. In addition, there is also evidence that those search images can cause conditioned flavor percepts, which also play a role in the sensory and hedonic perception of food.

REFERENCES

Allison, R.I. and K.P. Uhl. 1964. Influence of beer brand identification on taste perception. *Journal of Marketing Research* 1:29–36.

Arce-Lopera, C., T. Masuda, A. Kimura, Y. Wada, and K. Okajima. 2012. Luminance distribution modifies the perceived freshness of strawberries. *i-Perception* 3:338–355.

Arce-Lopera, C., T. Masuda, A. Kimura, Y. Wada, and K. Okajima. 2013. Luminance distribution as a determinant for visual freshness perception: Evidence from image analysis of a cabbage leaf. *Food Quality and Preference* 27:202–207.

Berlyne, D.E., J.C. Ogilvie, and L.C.C. Parham. 1968. The dimensionality of visual complexity, interestingness, and pleasingness. *Canadian Journal of Psychology* 22:376–387.

Cardello, A.V. and F.M. Sawyer. 1992. Effects of disconfirmed consumer expectations on food acceptability. *Journal of Sensory Studies* 7:253–277.

Cardello, A.V., S.M. Melnick, and P.A. Rowan. 1996. Expectations as a mediating variable in context effects. In *Proceedings of the Food Preservation 2000 Conference*, eds. I. Taub and R. Bell. Hampton, VA: Science & Technology Corporation.

Carlson, A.J. 1930. Physiology of hunger and appetite in relation to the emotional life of the child. In *The Child's Emotions: Proceedings of the Mid-West Conference on Character Development*, pp. 81–90. Chicago: University of Chicago Press.

Carpenter, C.E., D.P. Cornforth, and D. Whittier. 2001. Consumer preferences for beef color and packaging did not affect eating satisfaction. *Meat Science* 57:359–363.

Case, T.I., R.J. Stevenson, and R.A. Dempsey. 2004. Reduced discriminability following perceptual learning with odours. *Perception* 33:113–119.

Christensen, C.M. 1983. Effects of color on aroma, flavor and texture judgments of foods. *Journal of Food Science* 48:787–790.

Clydesdale, F.M., R.R. Gover, D.H. Philipsen, and C. Fugardi. 1992. The effect of color on thirst quenching, sweetness, acceptability and flavor intensity in fruit punch flavored beverages. *Journal of Food Quality* 15:19–38.

Delwiche, J. 2004. The impact of perceptual interactions on perceived flavor. *Food Quality and Preference* 15:137–146.

DuBose, C.N., A.V. Cardello, and O. Maller. 1980. Effects of colorants and flavorants on identification, perceived flavor intensity, and hedonic quality of fruit-flavored beverages and cake. *Journal of Food Science* 45:1393–1399.

Garber, Jr., L.L., E.M. Hyatt, and R.G. Starr, Jr. 2000. Measuring consumer response to food products. *Food Quality and Preference* 14:3–15.

Guinard, J.X., A. Souchard, M. Picot, M. Rogeaux, and J.M. Sieffermann. 1998. Sensory determinants of the thirst-quenching character of beer. *Appetite* 31:101–115.

Hall, R.L. 1958. Flavor study approaches at McCormick & Company, Inc. In *Flavor Research and Food Acceptance*, ed. Arthur D. Little, Inc., pp. 224–240. New York: Reinhold Publishing.

Hutchings, J.B. 1999. *Food Color and Appearance, 2nd ed.* Gaithersburg, MD: Aspen Publishers.

Hutchings, J.B. 2003. *Expectations and the Food Industry: The Impact of Color and Appearance.* New York: Kluwer Academic/Plenum Publishers.

Hyman, A. 1983. The influence of color on the taste perception of carbonated water preparations. *Bulletin of the Psychonomic Society* 21:145–148.

Issanchou, S. 1996. Consumer expectations and perceptions of meat and meat product quality. *Meat Science* 43:S5–S19.

Johnson, J. and F.M. Clydesdale. 1982. Perceived sweetness and redness in colored sucrose solutions. *Journal of Food Science* 47:747–752.

Johnson, J., E. Dzendolet, R. Damon, M. Sawyer, and F.M. Clydesdale. 1982. Psychophysical relationships between perceived sweetness and color in cherry-flavored beverages. *Journal of Food Protection* 45:601–606.

Johnson, J., E. Dzendolet, and F.M. Clydesdale. 1983. Psychophysical relationships between perceived sweetness and color in strawberry-flavored drinks. *Journal of Food Protection* 46:21–25.

Koza, B.J., A. Cilmi, M. Dolese, and D.A. Zellner. 2005. Color enhances orthonasal olfactory intensity and reduces retronasal olfactory intensity. *Chemical Senses* 30:643–649.

Lavin, J.G. and H. Lawless. 1998. Effects of color and odor on judgments of sweetness among children and adults. *Food Quality and Preference* 9:283–289.

Lega, L., L. Paula-Pereira, D. Giron, D. Pastor, P. Locher, and G. Hoyos. 2003. A cross-cultural analysis of the visual rightness theory of picture perception. *Bulletin of Psychology and the Art* 4:86–89.

Locher, P. 1996. The contribution of eye-movement research to an understanding of the nature of pictorial balance perception: A review of the literature. *Empirical Studies of the Arts* 14:143–163.

Mace, K.C. and R.F. Enzie. 1970. Dissonance versus contrast in an ego-involved situation with disconfirmed expectancies. *The Journal of Psychology* 75:107–121.

Maga, J.A. 1974. Influence of color on taste thresholds. *Chemical Senses and Flavor* 1:115–119.

Morrot, G., F. Brochet, and D. Dubourdieu. 2001. The color of odors. *Brain and Language* 79:309–320.

Murakoshi, T., T. Masuda, K. Utsumi, K. Tsubota, and Y. Wada. 2013. Glossiness and perishable food quality: Visual freshness judgment of fish eyes based on luminance distribution. *PLOS ONE* 8:1–5.

Olson, J.C. and P. Dover. 1976. Effects of expectation creation and disconfirmation on belief elements of cognitive structure. In *Advances in Consumer Research, Vol. III*, ed. B.B. Anderson, pp. 168–175. Cincinnati, OH: Association for Consumer Research.

Pangborn, R.M. 1960. Influence of color on the discrimination of sweetness. *The American Journal of Psychology* 73:229–238.

Pangborn, R.M. and B. Hansen. 1963. The influence of color on discrimination of sweetness and sourness in pear-nectar. *The American Journal of Psychology* 76:315–317.

Peneau, S., P.B. Brockhoff, F. Escher, and J. Nuessli. 2007. A comprehensive approach to evaluate the freshness of strawberries and carrots. *Postharvest Biology and Technology* 45:20–29.

Pliner, P. and S.J. Salvy. 2006. Food neophobia in humans. In *The Psychology of Food Choice*, eds. R. Shepherd and M. Raats, pp. 75–92. Cambridge, MA: CABI.

Riskey, D.R. 1982. Effects of context and interstimulus procedures in judgments of saltiness and pleasantness. In *Selected Sensory Methods: Problems and Approaches to Measuring Hedonics*, eds. J.T. Kuznicki, R.A. Johnson, and A.F. Rutkiewic, pp. 71–83. Philadelphia, PA: American Society for Testing and Materials.

Riskey, D.R., A. Parducci, and G.K. Beauchamp. 1979. Effects of context in judgments of sweetness and pleasantness. *Perception & Psychophysics* 26:171–176.

Shankar, M., C. Simons, B. Shiv, S. McClure, C.A. Levitan, and C. Spence. 2010. An expectations-based approach to explaining the cross-modal influence of color on orthonasal olfactory identification: The influence of the degree of discrepancy. *Attention, Perception, & Psychophysics* 72:1981–1993.

Siegrist, M. and M.E. Cousin. 2009. Expectations influence sensory experience in a wine tasting. *Appetite* 52:762–765.

Spears, M.C. and M.B. Gregoire. 2004. *Foodservice Organizations: A Managerial and Systems Approach, 5th ed.* Upper Saddle River, NJ: Pearson/Prentice-Hall.

Spence, C. 2012. Auditory contributions to flavour perception and feeding behaviour. *Physiology & Behavior* 107:505–515.

Stevenson, R.J. 2001a. Associative learning and odor quality perception: How sniffing an odor mixture can alter the smell of its parts. *Learning and Motivation* 32:154–177.

Stevenson, R.J. 2001b. Perceptual learning with odors: Implications for psychological accounts of odor quality perception. *Psychonomic Bulletin & Review* 8:708–712.

Stevenson, R.J., J. Prescott, and R.A. Boakes. 1995. The acquisition of taste properties by odors. *Learning and Motivation* 26:433–455.

Stevenson, R.J., R.A. Boakes, and J. Prescott. 1998. Changes in odor sweetness resulting from implicit learning of a simultaneous odor–sweetness association: An example of learned synesthesia. *Learning and Motivation* 29:113–132.

Stevenson, R.J., R.A. Boakes, and J.P. Wilson. 2000a. Counter-conditioning following human odor–taste and color–taste learning. *Learning and Motivation* 31:114–127.

Stevenson, R.J., R.A. Boakes, and J.P. Wilson. 2000b. Resistance to extinction of conditioned odor perceptions: Evaluative conditioning is not unique. *Journal of Experimental Psychology: Learning, Memory, and Cognition* 26:423–440.

Stevenson, R.J., T.I. Case, and R.A. Boakes. 2003. Smelling what was there: Acquired olfactory percepts are resistant to further modification. *Learning and Motivation* 34:185–202.

Stillman, J.A. 1993. Color influences flavor identification in fruit-flavored beverages. *Journal of Food Science* 58:810–812.

Tanaka, J.M. and L.M. Presnell. 1999. Color diagnosticity in object recognition. *Perception & Psychophysics* 61:1140–1153.

Triplett, T. 1994. Consumers show little taste for clear beverages. *Marketing News* 28:1. Retrieved February 16, 2009 from ABI/INFORM Global database. (Document ID: 626238).

Troy, D.J. and J.P. Kerry. 2010. Consumer perception and the role of science in the meat industry. *Meat Science* 86:214–226.

Wada, Y., C. Arce-Lopera, T. Masuda et al. 2010. Influence of luminance distribution on the appetizingly fresh appearance of cabbage. *Appetite* 54:363–368.

Wansink, B., C.R. Payne, and J. North. 2007. Fine as North Dakota wine: Sensory expectations and the intake of companion foods. *Physiology & Behavior* 90:712–716.

Wheatley, J. 1973. Putting color into food. *Marketing* 67:26–29.

Yeomans, M.R., S. Mobini, T.D. Elliman, H.C. Walker, and R.J. Stevenson. 2006. Hedonic and sensory characteristics of odors conditioned by pairing with tastants in humans. *Journal of Experimental Psychology: Animal Behavior Processes* 32:215–228.

Zampini, M., D. Sanabria, N. Phillips, and C. Spence. 2007. The multisensory perception of flavor: Assessing the influence of color cues on flavor discrimination responses. *Food Quality and Preference* 18:975–984.

Zellner, D.A. 2013. Color–odor interactions: A review and model. *Chemosensory Perception* 6:155–169.

Zellner, D.A. and P. Durlach. 2002. What is refreshing? An investigation of the color and other sensory attributes of refreshing foods and beverages. *Appetite* 39:185–186.

Zellner, D.A. and P. Durlach. 2003. Effect of color on expected and experienced refreshment, intensity, and liking of beverages. *The American Journal of Psychology* 116:633–647.

Zellner, D.A. and M.A. Kautz. 1990. Color affects perceived odor intensity. *Journal of Experimental Psychology: Human Perception and Performance* 16:391–397.

Zellner, D.A. and L.A. Whitten. 1999. The effect of color intensity and appropriateness on color-induced odor enhancement. *The American Journal of Psychology* 112:585–604.

Zellner, D.A., A.M. Bartoli, and R. Eckard. 1991. Influence of color on odor identification and liking ratings. *The American Journal of Psychology* 104:547–561.

Zellner, D.A., E.A. Rohm, T.L. Bassetti, and S. Parker. 2003. Compared to what? Effects of categorization on hedonic contrast. *Psychonomic Bulletin & Review* 10:468–473.

Zellner, D.A., D. Strickhouser, and C.E. Tornow. 2004. Disconfirmed hedonic expectations produce perceptual contrast, not assimilation. *The American Journal of Psychology* 117:363–387.

Zellner, D.A., M. Lankford, L. Ambrose, and P. Locher. 2010. Art on the plate: Effect of balance and color on attractiveness of, willingness to try and liking for food. *Food Quality and Preference* 21:575–578.

Zellner, D.A., E. Siemers, V. Teran et al. 2011. Neatness counts. How plating affects liking for the taste of food. *Appetite* 57:642–648.

Zellner, D.A., C.R. Loss, J. Zearfoss, and S. Remolina. 2014. It tastes as good as it looks! The effect of food presentation on liking for the taste of food. *Appetite* 77:31–35.

8 Chemesthesis, Thermogenesis, and Nutrition

Hilton M. Hudson, Mary Beth Gallant-Shean, and Alan R. Hirsch

The holistic experience of eating is the integration of myriad senses. While the scientific zeitgeist has focused on the ultimate and penultimate sensations of retronasal olfaction and gustation, other less clearly defined sensations warrant heuristic exploration. These include visual, auditory, thermal, somesthetic, and nociceptive. The impact of visual sensation on nutrition has been delineated in Chapters 6 and 7 of this book, and of auditory sensation by Alan Hirsch in Chapter 10 of this book. Thus, not for *remplissage* but rather for the axiopisty of consumption, these other senses are presented in this chapter.

The concept of thermogenesis is that energy is required to digest food. In the process, an exothermic reaction occurs, burning calories in the production of heat. Thus, thermogenesis has been touted as a potential approach to weight loss. While such a method does not necessarily require sensory mechanisms, activation of sensory systems may be one of the means by which these thermogenic substances act to reduce weight, not in their thermogenic effects but rather through their trigeminal and chemesthetic influence. Trigeminally mediated pain, in and of itself, has been demonstrated to inhibit appetite (Malick et al. 2001).

A shared trait of traditional thermogenic foods is their ability to stimulate the common chemical sense in the mouth and throat—they taste hot (Alimohammadi and Silver 2002). Such sensation occurs as a result of small unmyelinated 1C nerve fibers firing through the trigeminal nerve, or irritant nerve, producing the sensation of heat, burning, and, in the extreme, pain (Szolcsanyi 1990). Activation of such pathways may interact with olfaction and enhance sensory-specific satiety and fullness, followed by reduction in appetite and consumption, culminating in weight loss (Sochtig et al. 2014).

Studies of thermogenic substances usually do not differentiate between their thermogenic and sensory properties as to their mechanism of weight loss, so it could be a combination of both factors to which their action may be attributed. It is even unclear whether thermogenic foods and flavorful spicy hot foods are necessarily the same. However, such a logical assumption—hot feeling in the mouth equals heating up the body—appears to have been the basis of the concept. With this as a proem, let us review some of the salient literature connecting the common chemical senses, thermogenesis, and nutrition.

In the realm of foods, this can be delineated in relation to mustard, red pepper, capsaicin, or piperine as present in chili pepper and curry (Lawless and Stevens 1990). Capsaicin can be recognized at very low concentrations: the median recognition threshold is approximately 1 nmol (Smutzer et al. 2014). The oral burn of capsaicin is mediated through the capsaicin receptor, which is the transient receptor potential vanilloid 1 (TRPV1) (Montell and Caterina 2007). The pungent component of mustard is allyl isothiocyanate, whereas for chili, it is capsaicin (Muraki 1989). Yellow curry, fresh chili pepper, and red hot pepper all have a common factor—they contain capsaicin. Red hot pepper can be considered a delivery device for capsaicin as can yellow curry. Each gram of red hot pepper contains 3 mg of capsaicin (Ku and Choi 1990).

The ingestion of these thermogenic agents in the form of capsules, where the chemesthetic sensory experience is not included, has been thoroughly evaluated. This literature, as a whole, will not be reviewed in this chapter but can be seen in Table 8.1 and has been thoroughly reviewed by Ludy et al. (2012).

In summary, nonchemosensory origins of thermogenic compounds can be demonstrated through bypassing the mouth—as when systemically administered or consumed in capsule form. The predominance of studies has demonstrated a thermogenic effect of hot chili peppers, or its key ingredient, capsaicin, when administered orally in capsule form (Shin and Moritani 2007). However, some have shown no significant effect (Manuela et al. 2003; Galgani and Ravussin 2010). The effect of an enteric-coated capsule implies that capsaicin's influence is on the gastric mucosa or elsewhere in the body rather than the oral chemosensory system (Belza and Jessen 2005). Nontrigeminally pungent capsaicin derivatives ingested in capsules also demonstrate thermogenesis and enhanced fat oxidation with reduction in hunger and increase in satiety, further lending doubt to the postulate that the mechanism of thermogenic compounds is through their irritative effects in the mouth (Inoue et al. 2007; Reinbach et al. 2009; Snitker et al. 2009; Lee et al. 2010).

Regarding the chemosensory effect of capsaicin, over 30 years ago, the physiologist, LeBlanc, first demonstrated diet-induced thermogenesis in rats (LeBlanc et al. 1981). Extending his work to humans, eight fasting normal weight men were provided a 755-kcal meal of a submarine sandwich, sugar pie, and soft drink. On another day, they were provided 755 kcal of a commercial liquid diet (Ensure) via a nasogastric (NG) tube and on another day, the control condition, isovolumic water through an NG tube. The resting metabolic rate was measured for 90 min. No change in the resting metabolic rate was noted during the control period. Actual meal consumption led to the increase of 400% in the resting metabolic rate, as measured by the respiratory quotient, an indicator of glucose oxidation, compared to the tube-feeding condition (LeBlanc et al. 1984). Thus, by circumventing the sensory and cognitive factors associated with eating, the thermogenic effect of food was markedly diminished. They concluded that as part of consumption, food palatability is essential for maximizing postprandial heat production and speculated whether highly palatable thermogenic diets would induce weight loss.

These findings were brought into question, however, when a replication was attempted of thermogenic response to ingestion, as opposed to the feeding of an identical meal (just blenderized) in six subjects (Hill et al. 1985). Contrary to LeBlanc's

TABLE 8.1
Studies on the Effect of Capsaicin on Thermogenesis and Appetite

References	Participants	Experimental Design/Intervention	Thermogenesis	Appetite
Ludy and Mattes (2011b)	14 ♂ and 11 ♀ in the United States (IN) Age 23.0 ± 0.5 years BMI 22.6 ± 0.3 kg/m² 13 regular spicy food users and 12 nonusers (mean ± SE)	Randomized crossover Lunch containing 1. 1 g RP (following high-FAT diet) 2. 1 g RP (following high-CHO diet) 3. 0 (control, following high-FAT diet) 4. 0 (control, following high-CHO diet) 5. Preferred dose RP orally (1.8 ± 0.3 g in users; 0.3 ± 0.1 g in nonusers) 6. Preferred dose RP in capsule form (1.8 ± 0.3 g in users; 0.3 ± 0.1 g in nonusers) RP: 1995 µg/g capsaicin, 247 µg/g nordihydrocapsaicin, and 1350 µg/g dihydrocapsaicin; 53 800 SHU (mean ± SE)	↑ EE, core body temperature, and FAT oxidation (when consumed orally compared with in capsule form) ↓ Skin temperature	↓ Preoccupation with food and desire to eat fatty/salty/sweet foods in nonusers, but not users ↓ EI in nonusers, but not users No effect on desire to eat in general, fullness, prospective food intake, thirst, or hunger
Reinbach et al. (2010)	17 ♂ and 23 ♀ in Denmark Age 24.6 ± 2.5 years BMI 22.5 ± 7 kg/m² Likers of hot spices (mean ± SD)	Randomized crossover (10 visits) *starter meal:* 1. With or without chili peppers (0.3 g RP; 0.375 mg capsaicin) 2. With or without ginger 3. With or without mustard 4. With or without horseradish 5. With or without wasabi Ad libitum dinner	n/a	↑ Desire to eat sweet foods ↓ Desire to eat hot foods No effect on EI, food intake (g), hunger, satiety, or desire to eat bitter/fatty/salty/sour (results for RP only)
Smeets and Westerterp-Plantenga (2009)	11 ♂ and 19 ♀ in the Netherlands Age 31 ± 14 years BMI 23.8 ± 2.8 kg/m² (mean ± SD)	Randomized crossover Lunch containing 1. Capsaicin (1.03 g RP; 80,000 SHU) 2. No capsaicin	No effect on EE or RQ	↑ GLP-1 Tended to ↓ ghrelin No effect on self-reported satiety or PYY

(Continued)

TABLE 8.1 (CONTINUED)

Studies on the Effect of Capsaicin on Thermogenesis and Appetite

References	Participants	Experimental Design/Intervention	Thermogenesis	Appetite
Shin and Moritani (2007)	10 sedentary ♂ in Japan Age 24.4 ± 1.9 years BMI 20.2 ± 1.7 kg/m² (mean ± SE)	Randomized crossover Supplement 1 h before exercise containing 1. Capsaicin (150 mg) (capsules) 2. Placebo 30 min on cycle	↑ FAT oxidation No effect on ANS activity	n/a
Ahuja et al. (2007)	14 ♂ and 22 ♀ in Australia Age 46 ± 12 years BMI 26.3 ± 4.6 kg/m² <daily chili (~90% naïve/infrequent consumers) (mean ± SD)	Randomized crossover 4-week dietary periods containing 1. Chili (30 g/day chili blend, 55% cayenne RP; 33 mg/day capsaicin) 2. Bland spice-free	No effect on RMR, RQ, FAT oxidation, BMI, FAT mass, or lean mass	No effect on total energy, PRO, FAT, or CHO intake
Ahuja et al. (2006)	14 ♂ and 22 ♀ in Australia Age 46 ± 12 years BMI 26.3 ± 4.6 kg/m² <daily chili (~90% naïve/infrequent consumers) (mean ± SD)	Randomized crossover 4-week dietary periods containing 1. Chili (30 g/day chili blend, 55% cayenne RP; 33 mg/day capsaicin) 2. Bland spice-free	↓ EE BMI > 26.3 kg/m² No effect on EE using all BMIs or BMI < 26.3 kg/m²	n/a
Westerterp-Plantenga et al. (2005)	12 Caucasian ♂ and 12 Caucasian ♀ in the Netherlands Age 25–45 years BMI 25 ± 2.4 kg/m² Used to eating spicy foods > 1 ×/week (mean ± SD)	Randomized crossover 2-day treatments 30 min before every meal containing 1. 0.9 g RP in tomato juice 2. 0.9 g RP in 2 capsules 3. Placebo in tomato juice 4. Placebo in 2 capsules RP (0.9 g): 2.25 mg capsaicin; 80,000 SHU	n/a	↓ EI (juice > capsules) ↑ Satiety and CHO intake ↓ Hunger, energy density, and FAT intake

Study	Subjects	Intervention		
Yoshioka et al. (2004)	16 ♂ in Japan Age 22.4 ± 3.2 years Wt 79.4 ± 19.4 kg Ht 176.1 ± 6.7 cm (mean ± SD)	Randomized crossover Soup (prelunch) containing 1. Self-perceived moderate RP soup (0.064 ± 0.046 g; 0.192 ± 0.138 mg capsaicin; 55,000 SHU) and capsule (placebo) 2. Self-perceived strong RP soup (0.923 ± 1.377 g; 2.769 ± 4.131 mg capsaicin; 55,000 SHU) and capsule (placebo) 3. Soup (placebo) and self-perceived strong RP capsules (0.923 ± 1.377 g; 2.769 ± 4.131 mg capsaicin; 55,000 SHU) 4. Soup (placebo) and capsule (placebo) ad libitum lunch until satiated (mean ± SD)	Biphasic effect on SNS:PSNS (moderate = maximum tolerable > strongest/excessive)	Dose-dependent ↓ EI (soup = capsules) Dose-dependent ↓ FAT intake (soup = capsules) Positive correlation between EI and FAT intake Negative correlation between change in EI and RP ingested
Chaiyata et al. (2003)	12 ♀ in Thailand Consumers of <10 g/day chili peppers	Glucose drink containing 5 g fresh chili pepper (*Capsicum frutescens*): 3.5 mg capsaicin	↑EE above RMR immediately after ingestion	n/a
Lejeune et al. (2003)	91 subjects in the Netherlands Capsaicin 12 ♂ and 30 ♀ Placebo: 11 ♂ and 38 ♀ Age 18–60 years BMI 25–35 kg/m² Not habitual capsaicin users	Randomized double blind 4-week very low energy diet intervention (mean ↓ 6.6 ± 2 kg or 7.8 ± 1.8% body wt) 3-month wt-maintenance period with supplements containing 1. 135 mg/day capsaicin (capsules with 3 meals) 2. 0 (placebo) (mean ± SD)	↑REE during wt maintenance ↑FAT oxidation No effect on percent or rate of regain	No effect on hunger or satiety

(Continued)

TABLE 8.1 (CONTINUED)
Studies on the Effect of Capsaicin on Thermogenesis and Appetite

References	Participants	Experimental Design/Intervention	Thermogenesis	Appetite
Matsumoto et al. (2000)	8 lean ♀ in Japan Age 19.6 ± 0.26 years BMI 21.0 ± 0.57 kg/m² 8 overweight/obese ♀ in Japan Age 20.1 ± 0.40 years BMI 28.8 ± 1.01 kg/m² No long-term history of eating spices (mean ± SE)	Randomized crossover Breakfast containing 1. 3 mg capsaicin 2. 0 (control)	↑ EE in lean but not overwt/obese ↑ Total, very low, low, and very low: total frequency heart waves (SNS activity) in lean but not overwt/obese Trend toward ↑ CHO oxidation in lean but no effect in entire group; no effect on high-frequency heart waves (PSNS activity) in either group	n/a
Yoshioka et al. (1999) (Study 1)	13 Japanese ♀ Age 25.8 ± 2.8 years Wt 54.2 ± 6.4 kg Ht 157 ± 4 cm Accustomed to eating spicy foods (mean ± SD)	Randomized crossover Breakfast containing 1. 10 g RP (high FAT, 30 mg capsaicin) 2. 10 g RP (high CHO, 30 mg capsaicin) 3. 0 (high FAT, control) 4. 0 (high CHO, control) Ad libitum lunch buffet until satiated	n/a	↓ Lunch intake 1. PRO (HF > HC) 2. FAT (HF > HC) Self-reported appetitive sensations 1. ↓ Prospective food consumption before lunch, but ↑ prospective food consumption after lunch 2. ↓ Desire to eat and hunger immediately after breakfast and before lunch

Reference	Subjects	Design	Outcomes	
Yoshioka et al. (1999) (Study 2)	10 Caucasian ♂ Age 32.9 ± 7.8 years Wt 72.5 ± 10.1 kg Ht 175 ± 6 cm (mean ± SD)	Randomized crossover Lunch appetizers containing 1. 6 g RP (18 mg capsaicin) 2. 0 (control) Ad libitum lunch and snack buffet until satiated	↑ SNS:PSNS Trend toward a negative correlation between SNS:PSNS and EI	↓ Total energy and CHO intakes during lunch and snack
Yoshioka et al. (1998)	13 Japanese ♀ Age 25.8 ± 2.8 years Wt 54.2 ± 6.4 kg Ht 157.3 ± 4.5 cm Hotness of habitual meals between RP and control meals (mean ± SD)	Randomized crossover Breakfast containing 1. 10 g RP (high FAT) 2. 10 g RP (high CHO) 3. 0 (control, high FAT) 4. 0 (control, high CHO)	↑ EE (VO_2) and FAT oxidation	↓ Appearance, taste, and smell ↑ Hot sensation
Lim et al. (1997)	8 ♂ long-distance runners in Korea Age 20.8 ± 0.5 years Wt 58.5 ± 2.1 kg Ht 169.5 ± 1.8 cm (mean ± SE)	Randomized crossover Breakfast containing 1. 10 g RP (30 mg capsaicin) 2. 0 (control) Followed by 2.5-h rest, then 1-h cycling	↑ CHO oxidation both at rest and during exercise ↑ Epinephrine and norepinephrine 30 min after meal No effect on VO_2	n/a
Yoshioka et al. (1995) (Study 1)	8 ♂ long-distance runners Age 20.5 ± 1 years Wt 58.5 ± 5.6 kg Ht 169.5 ± 4.7 cm (mean ± SD)	Randomized crossover Breakfast containing 1. 10 g RP (30 mg capsaicin) 2. 0 (control)	↑ CHO oxidation Tended to ↑ EE (VO_2)	n/a
Yoshioka et al. (1995) (Study 2)	7 ♂ long-distance runners Age 21.6 ± 0.7 years Wt 61.3 ± 11.6 kg Ht 170.9 ± 6.3 cm (mean ± SD)	Randomized crossover Breakfast containing 10 g RP (30 mg capsaicin) followed by 1. β-adrenergic blocker (propranolol) 2. Placebo	Propranolol inhibited the initial ↑ in EE caused by RP	n/a

Note: ANS: autonomic nervous system; CHO: carbohydrate; EI: energy intake; GLP-1: glucagon-like peptide 1; n/a: not applicable; PRO: protein; PSNS: parasympathetic nervous system; PYY: peptide YY; REE: resting energy expenditure; RMR: resting metabolic rate; RP: red pepper; SHU: Scoville Heat Unit; VO_2: oxygen consumption.

findings, no difference in respiratory quotient in thermogenesis was found. Hill concluded that sensory and cognitive factors in consumption of a meal contributed little, if any, to the thermogenic effects. The reason for such contradictory conclusions is unclear but may reflect methodological differences. LeBlanc used Ensure, whereas Hill gave the identical (but blenderized) meal through the NG tube. LeBlanc used a standard 755-kcal meal for each subject, whereas Hill varied the meal size for each subject to equal one-third of their daily caloric requirement.

LeBlanc went further and followed up his study with an evaluation of eight normal weight women who were provided a highly palatable meal of 2970 kJ composed of parmesan fondue, spaghetti and meatballs, a chocolate éclair, and soda (LeBlanc and Brondel 1985). In a randomized order, they were presented either with the above meal or a nonpalatable meal, *tasteless* formed from the same food, mixed and sculpted into the shape of a biscuit. He demonstrated an increase over 90 min of the resting metabolic rate as measured by the respiratory quotient with a palatable meal as opposed to the tasteless biscuit. This confirmed the earlier experiment that thermogenesis was directly related to food palatability.

One of the earliest experiments assessed the thermogenic effects of mustard and chili sauces. Food spiced with these led to a 44% increase in energy expenditure at 15 min postprandial as compared to a 15% increase in the control meal (Henry and Emery 1986).

Looking specifically at the effects of dietary red pepper on energy metabolism, eight male long-distance runners were served an identical breakfast, with or without 10 g of red pepper, and energy expenditure was assessed for 2.5 h (Yoshioka et al. 1995). For 30 min, energy expenditure was higher for the red pepper group (32% increase versus 9% increase in the non-red pepper control group). Indication of such increase in metabolism was demonstrated by change of the respiratory quotient and carbohydrate and lipid oxidation. Such increases were blocked by preloading with the beta blocker, propranolol. While this may be interpreted that systemic beta blockade occurred, thus inhibiting the thermogenic effect, it may have been through another mechanism altogether. Propranolol may have acted to reduce the common chemical sensation by inhibiting trigeminal discharge or central processes of such discharge (as occurs with its use as a prophylactic drug in migraines), thus reducing sensory stimulation and associated increased metabolism.

In 1997, in another study evaluating the influence of hot red pepper on energy expenditure at rest and during exercise, conflicting results emerged. In eight male long-distance runners, after eating a meal with 10 g red pepper, as compared to without the red pepper, no significant change in oxygen consumption or energy expenditure was seen at rest or during exercise (Lim et al. 1997). However, respiratory quotient was elevated both at rest and during exercise after hot red pepper consumption, suggesting increased carbohydrate oxidation.

In another study, 13 women were presented with a high-fat or high-carbohydrate meal. With the addition of red hot pepper, carbohydrate oxidation was decreased and lipid oxidation was increased, with an increase in thermogenesis. Consistent with this, red hot pepper had a greater efficacy in high-fat as opposed to high-carbohydrate meals (Yoshioka et al. 1998).

Further investigating the variability of effect based on concurrent food types, 13 women were provided 10 g of hot red pepper along with breakfast of high carbohydrate or high fat. High-carbohydrate breakfast and hot red pepper reduced the desire to eat and the hunger for lunch, and decreased protein and fat intake at lunch. Hot red pepper and high-fat breakfast decreased protein intake at lunch (Yoshioka et al. 1999).

Thermogenic effects are seen in men as well. As demonstrated in 10 men given a hot red pepper-laden appetizer at lunch, there was a decrease in carbohydrate and energy intake at lunch (Yoshioka et al. 1999). This suggests that hot red pepper as a preload (or part of an appetizer) may act to reduce food consumption at that meal.

In addition, the food may not even have to be solid or semisolid for hot chili pepper to have an effect. Ingestion by 10 subjects of capsaicin in the form of 5 g of ground chili pepper dissolved in 200 mL of glucose drink resulted in a 20% increase in metabolic rate with persistent thermogenesis for 1/2 h (Chaiyata et al. 2003).

However, body habits may impact thermogenesis. Ingestion of a meal with 3 mg of capsaicin in the form of yellow curry sauce in eight normal weight and obese women caused energy expenditure to increase in the normal weight, but not in the obese group, casting doubt as to the utility of thermogenic manipulation for weight loss (Matsumoto et al. 2000).

The evidence suggesting that it is not the hot common chemical sense sensory component of capsaicin that is the mediator of thermogenesis was elucidated by use of CH-19—a nonpungent cultivar of pepper that contains capsiate (a nonpungent capsaicin analog that does not activate the TRPV1 receptor in the mouth but still activates the sympathetic nervous system) (Ludy et al. 2012). After consumption of CH-19, at 0.1 g/kg of body weight, there was an increase in body temperature and oxygen consumption, demonstrating increased thermogenesis and energy expenditure in the absence of trigeminal stimulation (Ohnuki et al. 2001).

In an apparent death knoll of the trigeminal sensory mediation theory of thermogenic compounds, Yoshioka et al. (2004) had 16 men eat soup laden with different concentrations of red pepper or ingested red pepper capsules (0.923 g). After both soup and capsule ingestion, fat intake dropped 13%, demonstrating that the satiety effect was occurring independently of sensory fibers in the mouth. Others have similarly found increase in energy expenditure in response to ingestion of encapsulated capsaicin (see Table 8.1). It has even been demonstrated that 135 mg/day of capsaicin capsules ingested induced 119 kcal/day increase in energy expenditure (Lejeune et al. 2003).

However, resurrection of the sensory mechanisms was not long in forthcoming. Within a year, the impact on 12 men and women, normal weight to moderately overweight, who consumed 0.9 g of hot red pepper in tomato juice, was studied. There was a 16% reduction in average daily energy intake as opposed to a 10% reduction with hot red pepper in capsules (Westerterp-Plantenga et al. 2005). In the oral exposure condition, the decrease in energy intake and increase in satiety correlated with the perceived spiciness of the tomato juice. While previous investigators, as described previously, have demonstrated such an effect only in normal-weight individuals, both obese and people of normal weight were equally affected in this study (Matsumoto et al. 2000).

The use of the thermogenic effects of capsaicin in the management of obesity was considered. That capsaicin could potentially be utilized as part of a weight reduction program was explored in seven men. For 2 weeks, they consumed 0.4 g/kg body weight/day of CH-19 sweet, in three divided doses, prior to their main meals. Compared to the control group of five men given the identical foods without the CH-19, the body mass index, the visceral fat mass, and the fat-free mass decreased (Kawabata et al. 2006). This effect was postulated to be due to the activation of the sympathetic nervous system, which is relatively decreased in obesity. Since CH-19 sweet red pepper is not pungent, the mechanism of action may not be on a chemosensory basis.

Attempting to further delineate this mechanism, five men and seven women, after consuming breakfast, were provided CH-19 sweet red pepper (nonpungent) and hot red pepper (Cayenne Long Slim) at 0.1 g/kg of body weight. To maximize the sensory experience, they were instructed to chew 30 times prior to swallowing (Hachiya et al. 2007). Both equally increased thermogenesis as measured by tympanic, forehead, and neck temperatures. This suggests that the thermogenic component was either due to a nonpungent sensory component or based on nonsensory mechanisms.

Other studies have not demonstrated the positive effects of capsaicin on satiety or thermogenesis. For instance, in 15 subjects provided with 1030 mg of hot red pepper with lunch, compared to those without hot red pepper, no effect on satiety or energy expenditure was observed (Smeets and Westerterp-Plantenga 2009).

The effects of very low doses of capsaicin (0.9 mg) compared to 30 mg capsaicin in earlier studies (Yoshioka et al. 1998, 1999) were also evaluated. Forty subjects were served preload meals with and without chili pepper, horseradish, ginger, mustard, and wasabi (Reinbach et al. 2010). No effect on energy intake at a subsequent ad lib buffet was found. This negative study may reflect the low dose of capsaicin used—the dose that reflects the amount usually ingested in Western diets. This implies that a far greater amount of capsaicin must be considered to induce thermogenesis or satiety than is normally eaten by Westerners.

One hypothesis for the conflicting findings as to the importance of sensation in thermogenesis revolves around activation of the cephalic phase response (Mattes 1997). In this paradigm, the more palatable the food is, the greater the thermogenic response seen. This implies that the greatest effect would be seen when the capsaicin concentration is matched to the subjects' individual preferences. Such was the approach assessed by Ludy and Mattes (2011). Twenty-five normal-weight subjects chose the most palatable concentration of hot red pepper (from 0.1 to 3.5 g) mixed in 290 g of tomato soup. Consumption of the preferred red pepper dose caused a greater thermogenic effect than in the capsule form, demonstrating the importance of both hedonics and oral chemosensation on thermogenesis.

Part of the kippage in diversity of findings may be methodological. The sensory impact of the hot red pepper may be related to the type of liquid vehicle used to deliver the hot red pepper. In previous studies, mixed stock solutions of capsaicin and tomato juice have been used, whereas at other times, hot red pepper was mixed with fat-containing tomato soup, which used milk and cream as a base. This is important because capsaicin's trigeminal thermal sensory intensity is inversely related to the amount of fat in which it is dissolved (Carden et al. 1999). Capsaicin's hotness intensity rating decreases when dissolved in oil as opposed to a water-based solution

TABLE 8.2
Studies on the Effect of Capsiate on Thermogenesis and Appetite

References	Participants	Experimental Design/Intervention	Thermogenesis	Appetite
Galgani and Ravussin (2010)	78 ♂ in the United States (LA) Young adults overweight	Parallel-arm double blind Randomized to 1 of 3 supplements for 4 weeks: 1. 3 mg/day dihydrocapsiate (capsules) 2. 9 mg/day dihydrocapsiate (capsules) 3. 0 (placebo)	↑ RMR 54 kcal/day (3 mg and 9 mg groups combined) No effect on FAT oxidation, body wt, fat mass, or fat-free mass	n/a
Galgani et al. (2010)	13 ♂ in the United States (LA) Age 28.4 ± 1.4 years BMI 27.1 ± 1.0 kg/m² (mean ± SE)	Randomized crossover double blind 1. 1 mg capsinoids (capsules) 2. 3 mg capsinoids (capsules) 3. 6 mg capsinoids (capsules) 4. 12 mg capsinoids (capsules) 5. 0 (placebo) Capsinoids (capsiate, dihydrocapsiate, nordihydrocapsiate in a 70:23:7 ratio)	No effect on RMR, FAT oxidation, or axillary temperature	n/a
Josse et al. (2010)	12 ♂ in Canada (Ontario) Age 24.3 ± 3 years BMI 25.5 ± 1.7 kg/m² (mean ± SD)	Randomized crossover double-blind ingested capsules 30 min before 90-min cycling and 30-min recovery 1. 10 mg capsinoids (capsules) 2. 0 (placebo) Capsinoids (capsiate, dihydrocapsiate, nordihydrocapsiate in a 70:23:7 ratio)	↑ SNS activation, EE (VO₂), and FAT oxidation	n/a

(Continued)

TABLE 8.2 (CONTINUED)
Studies on the Effect of Capsiate on Thermogenesis and Appetite

References	Participants	Experimental Design/Intervention	Thermogenesis	Appetite
Lee et al. (2010)	26 ♂ and 20 postmenopausal ♀ in the United States (CA) BMI 26.9–38 kg/m²	Parallel-arm double blind Randomized to 1 of 3 supplements for 4 weeks (while following an 800 kcal/day, 120 g/day PRO diet): 1. 3 mg/day dihydrocapsiate (capsules) 2. 9 mg/day dihydrocapsiate (capsules) 3. 0 (placebo)	↑ PPEE (9 mg > 3 mg > placebo) ↑ FAT oxidation (3 and 9 mg > placebo) No effect on body wt, fat mass, or BMR	n/a
Snitker et al. (2009)	40 ♂ and 40 ♀ in the United States (NJ) Age 42.6 ± 8 y BMI 25–35 kg/m² (mean ± SD)	Parallel-arm double blind Randomized to 1 of 2 supplements for 12 weeks: 1. 6 mg/day capsinoids (capsules) 2. 0 (placebo) Capsinoids (capsiate, dihydrocapsiate, nordihydrocapsiate in a 70:23:7 ratio)	↓ Abdominal adiposity (correlated with change in body wt) Tended to ↑ FAT oxidation No effect on RMR	n/a
Inoue et al. (2007)	44 ♂ and postmenopausal ♀ in Japan Age 30–65 years BMI ≥ 23 kg/m² (BMI ≥ 25, n = 28)	Parallel-arm double blind Randomized to 1 of 3 supplements for 4 weeks: 1. 3 mg/day capsinoids (capsules) 2. 10 mg/day capsinoids (capsules) 3. 0 (placebo) Capsinoids (capsiate, dihydrocapsiate, nordihydrocapsiate)	↑ FAT oxidation positively correlated with BMI ↑ VO₂ (10 mg, BMI ≥ 25 kg/m² only) Tended to ↑ EE and FAT oxidation (3 and 10 mg, BMI ≥ 25 kg/m² only) Tended to ↓ body wt and BMI (3 mg and 10 mg)	Tended to ↑ PRO intake (10 mg only) No effect on energy, FAT, CHO, cholesterol, or fiber

Kawabata et al. (2006)	7 ♂ (capsiate group) and 5 ♂ (control) in Japan young adults BMI 17–30 kg/m²	Parallel arm 1. Capsinoids (0.4 g/kg/day for 2 weeks: divided between 3 meals, ingested uncooked, and frozen before meals) 2. Control (received no supplemental food)	↓ Body wt, BMI, fat mass, fat-free mass, total fat area, and RQ Tended to ↑ FAT oxidation and SNS activity Tended to ↓ visceral FAT area No effect on subcutaneous fat area, resting VO₂, CHO oxidation, RMR, or PSNS activity	n/a
Ohnuki et al. (2001)	7 ♂ and 4 ♀ in Japan Age 21–32 years	Crossover 1. CH-19 sweet: 0.1 g/kg (containing 0.3–1 mg/g capsiate ingested orally) 2. California-Wandar: 0.1 g/kg (containing neither capsiate or capsaicin ingested orally)	↑ Core body (tympanic membrane of ear) and body surface (forehead, wrist, and neck) temperature ↑ VO₂ No effect on substrate oxidation	n/a

Note: BMR: basal metabolic rate; CHO: carbohydrate; n/a: not applicable; PRO: protein; PSNS: parasympathetic nervous system; RMR: resting metabolic rate; RP: red pepper; VO₂: oxygen consumption.

TABLE 8.3

Studies on the Effect of Both Capsaicin and Capsiate on Thermogenesis and Appetite

References	Participants	Experimental Design/Intervention	Thermogenesis	Appetite
Reinbach et al. (2009)	10 ♂ and 17 ♀ in the Netherlands Age 26.9 ± 6.3 years BMI 22.2 ± 2.7 kg/m² Likers of hot spices (mean ± SD)	Randomized crossover (3 weeks positive and 3 weeks negative EB) 5 test days in which the following treatments were consumed in capsule form with 3 meals (standardized breakfast, standardized lunch, and ad libitum dinner): 1. Capsaicin (0.510 g RP; 40,000 SHU) 2. Green tea and capsaicin (0.510 g RP; 40,000 SHU) 3. Green tea (19.2 g) 4. CH-19 Sweet (2.3 mg capsiate) 5. Placebo	n/a	CH-19 Sweet ↓ EI (positive EB) No effect on EI (negative EB); desire to eat, fullness, hunger, and satiety (positive or negative EB) capsaicin ↑ Fullness and satiety (negative EB) ↓ Hunger (positive EB) No effect on hunger (negative EB); fullness or satiety (positive EB); EI and desire to eat (positive or negative EB) (results for CH-19 Sweet and capsaicin only)
Hachiya et al. (2007)	5 ♂ and 7 ♀ in Japan Age 22–25 years	Crossover 0.1 g/kg body wt (0.1 mg/kg dry weight capsiate and capsaicin) (ingested at 37°C with water, in 2 min, after 30 chews): 1. CH-19 Sweet (capsinoids) 2. Cayenne Long Slim (capsaicinoids) 3. California Wonder (control, containing neither capsinoids nor capsaicinoids)	↑ SNS activity ↑ Forehead and neck temperature (capsaicinoids > capsinoids > control) ↑ Tympanic (core) temperature (capsaicinoids = capsinoids > control) No effect on PSNS activity	n/a

Note: EB: energy balance; PSNS: parasympathetic nervous system; RP: red pepper; SHU: Scoville Heat Unit.

(Lawless et al 1985; Ludy and Mattes 2012). A practical challenge to the utility of use of capsaicin in clinical practice in weight loss management is that of compliance, since in thermogenic doses, its pungency exceeds tolerability of the typical Western diet (Diepvens et al. 2007).

A critical review of the sensory mechanisms involved in thermogenesis by Ludy et al. (2012), tables of which are reproduced here, is worthy of the readers' attention. They performed a meta-analysis of published studies and cautiously concluded that capsaicin has a dose-dependent effect in its thermogenic action. Ludy et al. (2012) also addressed the anorexigenic action of capsaicin. Their review suggested that capsaicin reduces the desire to consume a wide spectrum of food flavors including fatty, hot, sweet, and salty; capsaicin also causes a general reduction in desire to eat as manifested by the reduction in preoccupation with food and hunger and increase in satiety; although other studies found just the opposite, with no effect on appetite and consumption (see Tables 8.2 and 8.3).

Such discrepant conclusions are rationalized based on different experimental groups, i.e., cultural background and gender.

Clearly, further investigation into this fertile chemosensory arena and its impact on nutrition is warranted.

REFERENCES

Alimohammadi, H., and W.L. Silver. 2002. Chemesthesis: Hot and cold mechanisms. *ChemoSense* 4:2:1–6, 9.

Belza, A., and A.B. Jessen. 2005. Bioactive food stimulants of sympathetic activity: Effect on 24-h energy expenditure and fat oxidation. *European Journal of Clinical Nutrition* 59:733–741.

Carden, L.A., M.P. Penfield, and A.M. Saxton. 1999. Perception of heat in cheese sauces as affected by capsaicin concentration, fat level, fat mimetic and time. *Journal of Food Science* 64:175–179.

Chaiyata, P., S. Puttadechakum, and S. Komindr. 2003. Effect of chili pepper (*Capsicum frutescens*) ingestion on plasma glucose response and metabolic rate in Thai women. *Journal of the Medical Association of Thailand* 86:854–860.

Diepvens, K., K.R. Westerp, and M.S. Westerterp-Plantenga. 2007. Obesity and thermogenesis related to the consumption of caffeine, ephedrine, capsaicin, and green tea. *American Journal of Physiology. Regulatory, Integrative and Comparative Physiology* 292:R77–R85.

Galgani, J.E., and E. Ravussin. 2010. Effect of dihydrocapsiate on resting metabolic rate in humans. *American Journal of Clinical Nutrition* 92:5:1089–1093.

Hachiya, S., F. Kawabata, K. Ohnuki et al. 2007. Effects of CH-19 sweet, a non-pungent cultivar of red pepper, on sympathetic nervous activity, body temperature, heart rate, and blood pressure in humans. *Bioscience, Biotechnology, and Biochemistry* 71:3:671–676.

Henry, C.J.K., and B. Emery. 1986. Effect of spiced food on metabolic rate. *Human Nutrition; Clinical Nutrition* 40C:165–168.

Hill, J.O., M. DiGirolamo, and S.B. Heymsfield. 1985. Thermic effect of food after ingested versus tube-delivered meals. *American Journal of Physiology* 248:3:E370–E374.

Inoue, N., Y. Matsunaga, H. Satoh, and M. Takahashi. 2007. Enhanced energy expenditure and fat oxidation in humans with high BMI scores by the ingestion of novel and non-pungent capsaicin analogues (capsinoids). *Bioscience, Biotechnology, and Biochemistry* 71:2:380–389.

Josse, A.R., J.E. Tang, M.A. Tarnopolsky, and S.M. Phillips. 2010. Body composition and strength changes in women with milk and resistance exercise. *Medicine and Science in Sports and Exercise* 42:6:1122–1130.

Kawabata, F., N. Inoue, S. Yazawa, T. Kawada, K. Inoue, and T. Fushiki. 2006. Effects of CH-19 sweet, a non-pungent cultivar of red pepper, in decreasing the body weight and suppressing body fat accumulation by sympathetic nerve activation in humans. *Bioscience, Biotechnology, and Biochemistry* 70:12:2824–2835.

Ku, Y., and S. Choi. 1990. *The Scientific Technology of Kimchi.* Seoul: Korean Institute of Food Development, pp. 33–34, as quoted in Yoshioka, M., L. Kiwon, S. Kikuzato, A. Kiyonaga, H. Tanaka, M. Shindo, and M. Suzuki. 1995. Effects of red-pepper diet on the energy metabolism in men. *Journal of Nutritional Science and Vitaminology* 41:647–656.

Lawless, H.T., and D.A. Stevens. 1990. Differences between and interactions of oral irritants. In *Chemical Senses, Vol. 2. Irritation,* eds. B.G. Green, J.R. Mason, and M.R. Kare, Ch. 10, pp. 197–216. New York: Marcel Dekker.

Lawless, H., P. Rozin, and J. Shenker. 1985. Effects of oral capsaicin on gustatory, olfactory, and irritant sensations and flavor identification in humans who regularly or rarely consume chili pepper. *Chemical Senses* 10:579–589.

LeBlanc, J., and L. Brondel. 1985. Role of palatability on meal-induced thermogenesis in human subjects. *American Journal of Physiology* 248:3:E333–E336.

LeBlanc, J., D. Richard, and D. Lupien. 1981. Thermogenesis: An adaptive reaction controlled by food intake (Abstract). *Federation Proceedings* 40:94 as quoted in LeBlanc, J., M. Cabanac, and P. Samson. 1984. Reduced postprandial heat production with gavage as compared with meal feeding in human subjects. *American Journal of Physiology* 246:E95–E101.

LeBlanc, J., M. Cabanac, and P. Samson. 1984. Reduced postprandial heat production with gavage as compared with meal feeding in human subjects. *American Journal of Physiology* 246:E95–E101.

Lee, T.Y.A., Z. Li, A. Zerlin, and D. Herber. 2010. Effects of dihydrocapsiate on adaptive and diet-induced thermogenesis with a high-protein very low calorie diet: A randomized control trial. *Nutrition & Metabolism* 7:78.

Lejeune, M.P.G.M., E.M.R. Kovacs, and M.S. Westerterp-Plantenga. 2003. Effects of capsaicin on substrate oxidation and weight maintenance after modest body-weight loss in human subjects. *British Journal of Nutrition* 90:651–659 as referenced in Ludy, M.J., G.E. Moore, and R.D. Mattes. 2012. The effects of capsaicin and capsiate on energy balance: Critical review and meta-analysis of studies in humans. *Chemical Senses* 37:103–121.

Lim, K., M. Yoshioka, S. Kikuzato et al. 1997. Dietary red pepper ingestion increases carbohydrate oxidation at rest and during exercise in runners. *Medicine and Science in Sports and Exercise* 29:3:355–361.

Ludy, M.J., and R.D. Mattes. 2011. The effects of hedonically acceptable red pepper doses on thermogenesis and appetite. *Physiology & Behavior* 102:251–258.

Ludy, M.J., and R.D. Mattes. 2012. Comparison of sensory, physiological, personality, and cultural attributes in regular spicy food users and non-users. *Appetite* 58:19–27.

Ludy, M.J., G.E. Moore, and R.D. Mattes. 2012. The effects of capsaicin and capsiate on energy balance: Critical review and meta-analysis of studies in humans. *Chemical Senses* 37:103–121.

Malick, A., M. Jakubowski, J.K. Elmquist, C.B. Saper, and R. Burstein. 2001. A neurohistochemical blueprint for pain-induced loss of appetite. *Proceedings of the National Academy of Sciences* 98:17:9930–9935.

Manuela, P.G., M. Lejeune, E.M.R. Kovacs, and M.S. Westerterp-Plantenga. 2003. Effect of capsaicin on substrate oxidation and weight maintenance after modest body-weight loss in human subjects. *British Journal of Nutrition* 90:651–659.

Matsumoto, T., C. Miyawaki, H. Ue, T. Yuasa, A. Miyatsuji, and T. Moritani. 2000. Effects of capsaicin-containing yellow curry sauce on sympathetic nervous system activity and diet-induced thermogenesis in lean and obese young women. *Journal of Nutritional Science and Vitaminology* 46:309–315.

Mattes, R.D. 1997. Physiologic responses to sensory stimulation by food: Nutritional implications. *Journal of the American Dietary Association* 97:406–413.

Montell, C., and M.J. Caterina. 2007. Thermoregulation: Channels that are cool to the core. *Current Biology* 17:R885–R887.

Muraki, S. 1989. Physiological role of spices. In *Function of Components of Spice*, eds. K. Iwai, and N. Nakatani, pp. 1–18. Tokyo: Kousei-kan.

Ohnuki, K., S. Niwa, S. Maeda, N. Inque, S. Yazawa, and T. Fushiki. 2001. CH-19 sweet, a non-pungent cultivar of red pepper, increased body temperature and oxygen consumption in humans. *Bioscience, Biotechnology, and Biochemistry* 65:9:2033–2036.

Reinbach, H.C., A. Smeets, T. Martinussen, P. Moller, and M.S. Westerterp-Plantenga. 2009. Effects of capsaicin, green tea and CH-19 sweet pepper on appetite and energy intake in humans in negative and positive energy balance. *Clinical Nutrition* 28:260–265.

Reinbach, H.C., T. Martinussen, and P. Moller. 2010. Effects of hot spices on energy intake, appetite and sensory specific desires in humans. *Food Quality and Preference* 21:655–661.

Shin, K.O., and T. Moritani. 2007. Alterations of autonomic nervous activity and energy metabolism by capsaicin ingestion during aerobic exercise in healthy men. *Journal of Nutritional Science and Vitaminology* 53:124–132.

Smeets, A.J., and M.S. Westerterp-Plantenga. 2009. The acute effects of a lunch containing capsaicin on energy and substrate utilization, hormones, and satiety. *European Journal of Nutrition* 48:229–234.

Smutzer, G.S., J.C. Jacob, D.I. Shah, J.T. Tran, and J.C. Stull. 2014. Modulation of chemosensory properties of capsaicin in the human oral cavity. *Association for Chemoreception Sciences (AChemS) Abstract Book*, 36th Annual Meeting, Bonita Springs, FL, 179:98–99.

Snitker, S., Y. Fujishima, H. Shen et al. 2009. Effects of novel capsinoid treatment on fatness and energy metabolism in humans: Possible pharmacogenetic implications. *American Journal of Clinical Nutrition* 89:45–50.

Sochtig, M.A., M.A. Sochtig, and F. Muller. 2014. Olfactory trigeminal interaction. (Abstract). *Chemical Senses* 39:1:110–111.

Szolcsanyi, J. 1990. Capsaicin, irritation, and desensitization. In *Chemical Senses, Vol. 2. Irritation*, eds. B.G. Green, J.R. Mason, and M.R. Kare, Ch. 8, 141–169. New York: Marcel Dekker.

Westerterp-Plantenga, M.S., A. Smeets, and M.P.G. Lejeune. 2005. Sensory and gastrointestinal satiety effects of capsaicin on food intake. *International Journal of Obesity* 29:682–688.

Yoshioka, M., L. Kiwon, S. Kikuzato et al. 1995. Effects of red-pepper diet on the energy metabolism in men. *Journal of Nutritional Science and Vitaminology* 41:647–656.

Yoshioka, M., S. St. Pierre, M. Suzuki, and A. Tremblay. 1998. Effects of red pepper added to high-fat and high-carbohydrate meals on energy metabolism and substrate utilization in Japanese women. *British Journal of Nutrition* 80:503–510.

Yoshioka, M., S. St. Pierre, V. Drapeau et al. 1999. Effects of red pepper on appetite and energy intake. *British Journal of Nutrition* 82:115–123.

Yoshioka, M., M. Imanaga, H. Ueyama et al. 2004. Maximum tolerable dose of red pepper decreases fat intake independently of spicy sensation in the mouth. *British Journal of Nutrition* 91:991–995.

9 The Look and Feel of Food

Sanford S. Sherman, Mary Beth Gallant-Shean, and Alan R. Hirsch

CONTENTS

9.1 Introduction 193
9.2 Texture 194
9.3 Size 195
9.4 Viscosity 196
9.5 Astringency 197
9.6 Burn/Sting 197
References 198

9.1 INTRODUCTION

In addition to the smell and taste of foods, the look and feel of food also plays an important role in appeal and satiation. Texture, viscosity, crunch, and color are all sensory factors that affect the desirability and satiation effect of the substances that we ingest. Energy content has also been shown to play a role. There have been numerous studies that have looked at these factors, many of which are conducted in relation to industrial marketing.

The food industry spends a large amount of resources in an attempt to promote their products for marketing purposes. This begins with the packaging itself. Piqueras-Fiszman et al. studied the packaging of potato crisps in the United Kingdom. They have found a correlation between package colors and participants' perception of flavor (Piqueras-Fiszman and Spence 2011). When package coloring was incongruent with expectations, participants had difficulty guessing the flavor correctly. They postulated that choosing the appropriate packaging across flavor varieties, through such an expectation effect, should help achieve immediate product recognition and consumer satisfaction.

Once the consumer opens the package, then the texture, color, consistency, and size of the product, along with the smell and taste, become factors in food product desirability. Actually, even before opening the package, the sound of the crunchiness of the potato chips migrating within the moving bag, or the sound of the breaking of the seal as the bottle top of soda is opened, impacts upon perceived freshness, quality, and hedonics of the consumables within (see Chapter 10 of this book).

The somesthetic quality of food varies depending on the degree of mastication and madification. Crackiness, crispiness, and hardness are sensations perceived at the start of the chewing epoch. This is followed by brittleness and lightness in the middle, ending with perception of stickiness (Lenfant et al. 2009). Despite the shifting transitions in somatosensory sensation, in this chapter, we have attempted to categorize these based on texture, viscosity, astringency, and prickliness or burn.

The ultimate variation in texture could be viewed as solid versus liquid. This was assessed in 43 non-obese elderly (average age of 72 years old). On different test days, subjects consumed isocaloric meal replacement shakes or meal replacement bars. Greater satiety and lower ghrelin resulted from consumption of the solid than the liquid (Leidy et al. 2010). Such results are consistent with less sensory-specific satiety with consumption of liquids (see Chapter 11 of this book). This suggests that a solid rather than a liquid diet would demonstrate greater effect in weight control.

9.2 TEXTURE

Texture differences have been shown to have a significant effect on the satiation factors of solid and semisolid foods. For instance, thicker yogurt and custards had a greater enhancing effect on expected satiation than less thick versions (Hogenkamp et al. 2011). Texture is "the manifestation of the structural elements of food in terms of appearance, feel, and resistance to applied forces" (Szczesniak 1979, p. 1). Appearance can clearly affect the perceived textures, overriding somesthetic input (deWijk et al. 2004). The input of vision is described further in Chapters 6 and 7 of this book.

Perception of a texture is thus generated as food is manipulated and deformed in the oral cavity (Christensen 1984). Tongue movements enhance the intensity of not only flavor (through enhanced retronasal smell) but also mouthfeel, representing a variety of somesthetic perceptions including temperature, thickness, homogeneity, speed of melting, creaminess, hardness, smoothness, prickliness, and astringency (Baek et al. 1999; deWijk et al. 2003).

Mastication shears food by macerating and grinding. Such kinesthetic action generates not only proprioceptive information (for position) and stretch receptor discharge (for hardness and size). The extent of salivary modification also influences the perception of texture, although taste can impact this as well: while high concentrations of sodium chloride and sucrose are weak inducers of salivation, trigeminal stimulants such as alcohol and chili pepper are sialagogues (Martin and Pangborn 1971; Pangborn and Chung 1981; Rozin et al. 1981). The texture of liquids is manifested as thickness or thinness, which is characterized here as viscosity (Szczesniak 1979). Texture may also be derived from sounds generated from mandibulation (see Chapter 10 of this book; Drake 1963, 1965). Such manducation generates vibrations as well as sound, and the Pacinian corpuscle discharge associated with this may, independent of the sound produced, be the mediator of textural perception (Christensen and Vickers 1981). Zijlstra et al. (2010) studied hard and soft versions of specially developed luncheon meats. They found that eating rates varied between the two textures, with the rates being significantly slower for the hard versions. However, the mean total intake did not differ significantly between the two versions. Also noted was that the number of subjects who ate more of the soft version outnumbered those who ate more of the hard version. It was expected that the hard version may have taken more oral processing time, but the correlation with reduced overall food intake was not confirmed.

However, an orosensory time/intake reciprocal relationship was found with consumption of tomato soup (Bolhuis et al. 2011). Here, a shorter exposure in the oral cavity was associated with a 34% greater ad lib intake possibly due to minimization of sensory-specific satiety (see Chapter 11 of this book).

9.3   SIZE

Bite size may also play a role. Ruijschop et al. (2011) hypothesized that consuming foods either in multiple small bites or with a longer duration of oral processing may evoke higher cumulative nasal aroma stimulation, which may lead to increased feelings of satiation and decreased food intake. They studied 21 young, healthy normal-weight subjects consuming dark, chocolate-flavored custard. In a crossover design, the subjects were exposed to both free and fixed bite size and free and fixed duration of oral processing. Consumption of multiple small bites resulted in a significantly higher cumulative extent of retronasal aroma released per gram consumed, compared with a smaller amount of large bite sizes. They also found that a longer-duration oral processing tended to result in a higher cumulative extent of retronasal aroma release per gram consumed. They concluded that by adapting the bite size or duration of oral processing, meal termination can be accelerated by increasing the extent of retronasal aroma released, and subsequently satiation.

Sip size of beverages also has been shown to play a role in sensory-specific satiation. Weijzen et al. (2009) investigated the sip size of orangeade. In particular, they investigated the differences between large and small sip size in both high- and no-energy beverages of the same flavor. Part of the purpose of the study was to eliminate some of the variables present in other studies, such as chewing effort and the viscosity of the food, isolating the duration of the orosensory exposure as the principle study variable. Along with sip size, the energy level of the drink was also varied. What the investigators found was that with small sips, the mean intake of both low- and high-energy drinks was lower than with large sips. With small sips, the subjective desire was higher for the no-energy drink without a significant difference in the mean intake between the two energy levels. However, with large sips, the mean intake of the no-energy drink was lower than that of the high-energy drink. The large sip resulted in lower orosensory exposure per swallow, thus reducing any inhibiting effect of sensory-specific satiety, whereas the small sip maximized orosensory exposure and thus sensory-specific satiety (German et al. 2004; Zijlstra et al. 2008). They postulated that the intake of sweet drinks is stimulated but as a result of energy level and metabolic reward value, homeostatically balanced through inhibition by sensory-induced satiation. Weijzen et al. (2009) concluded that narrowing straws or bottle openings may decrease sip size, prolong the duration of drink exposure, promote satiation, and thus reduce energy intake, which ultimately would aid in management of obesity.

Beverages appear to promote increased intake because of their weak influence on satiety. Ingestion of soda containing high-fructose corn syrup leads to increased energy intake and weight gain compared to diet beverages. The energy from beverages adds to, rather than substitutes for, the energy intake from other sources. A number of studies have also compared the ingestion of solids or semisolids such as purees versus liquid juices with essentially the same caloric value (Haber et al. 1977; Bolton et al. 1981; Wadden et al. 1985). Solid foods that contain the same caloric intake led to significantly greater reduction in hunger as compared to liquids. Increasing the fiber content of beverages, especially soluble fiber, generally increases the satiety ratings.

9.4 VISCOSITY

Viscosity, or the ease of deformation of flow, is another sensory characteristic of food that affects appetite, satiety, food consumption, and nutrition (Stokes 2012). Thus, viscosity requires a liquefied or semisolid substance. The quality of viscosity applies to solid foods only once they have been modified to a partially liquefied state. Highly viscous foods, such as those with high fiber content, require more time to swallow, thus providing greater sensory stimulation, facilitating sensory-specific satiety and associated reduced appetite and consumption (Blundell and Halford 1994). Furthermore, viscous solutions have a specific mouthfeel, which may in and of itself induce satiety (Lyly et al. 2009).

The relative viscosity of beverages also plays a role in sensory satiety. Mattes and Rothaker (2001) found that viscosity is inversely related to postprandial hunger. They studied the ingestion of vanilla shakes that were matched on weight, volume, temperature, and energy but varied in viscosity. Appetite ratings were obtained over the next 4 h, and dietary intake was then recorded over the next 24 h. Significantly greater and more prolonged reductions in hunger were observed with the thicker shake. They concluded that viscosity exerts an independent inverse effect on hunger. They found that hunger ratings were significantly lower following ingestion of the more viscous version. Similarly, high-viscosity locust bean gum beverage was a greater satiety inducer than the low-viscosity equivalent (Marciani et al. 2001).

While such findings would support utilization of thick beverages as a potential treatment of obesity, this enthusiasm must be tempered—while hunger ratings were reduced for 4 h, no significant effects were found on the first meal or the 24-h energy intake (Mattes and Rothacker 2001).

Viscosity has an even greater influence on satiety than the protein content of a beverage. In a crossover study of alginate and whey protein drinks, greater inhibition of hunger occurred through ingestion of the high-viscosity/low-protein variant than the low-viscosity/high-protein variant (Solah et al. 2010).

Cross-modal sensory interaction, whereby one sense impacts the perception of another, in the form of taste, can also impact upon viscosity (Verhagen and Engelen 2006). Increasing sweetness results in enhanced perceived viscosity, whereas citric acid reduces viscosity perception (Christensen 1980). Odors also impact in a cross-modal fashion. Rose odor changes the perception of a surface to appear softer and smoother, whereas sandalwood has the opposite effect (Nishino et al. 2011).

Further, cross-modal interaction may exist in the arena of touch. Increasing viscosity decreases the astringency of grape seed tannin (Smith et al. 1996). Fat, by acting as a lubricant and reducing friction, also reduces astringency (deWijk and Prinz 2005).

In an opposite fashion, astringent rinses, as with grape seed extract, reduce oral lubrication sensation (fattiness and slipperiness). This possibly accounts for why astringent beverages, like tea or red wine accompanying a fatty meal, result in an oral sensation of *cleanliness* (Peyrot des Gachons and Breslin 2011).

Thus, high-viscosity foods or drinks could potentially be utilized as a nutritional aid to reduce consumption in obese or overweight subjects (Zijlstra et al. 2008). For instance, low-calorie, high-viscosity beverage can be served as a preload prior to a meal, leading to reduced hunger and thus reduced food intake (Kristensen and Jensen 2011).

9.5 ASTRINGENCY

Astringency is the perception of drying or puckering, as is prototypically seen in response to tannic acid in dry wine or the mouth somesthetic sensation in response to the introduction of strong lemon juice (Bates-Smith 1954). Such a sensation may reflect a combination of touch receptors, through Meissner's corpuscles, and mechano-receptors for deformation, with activation of Pacinian corpuscles. Such activation may come directly from the consumed thermal stimulus or indirectly, as a result of salivary production inhibition inducing physiological changes to the oral epithelium and thus greater sensitivity to chemical external stimuli (Joslyn and Goldstein 1964). Supporting such a theory, tannic acid-induced astringency (or dryness) was reduced by the addition of the sialagogue sucrose (Lyman and Green 1990). The astringency of a food is partially dependent on its ability to precipitate salivary proteins (Noble 1995). Such precipitants reinforce astringency (Green 1993). Cross-linking of proteins may enhance tension, thus stimulating mechanoreceptors.

The perception of texture, astringency, and, to an extent, viscosity is all influenced by the underlying oral sensory capacities of the individual. For instance, 6-n-propylthiouracil (PROP) supertasters have a greater capacity to detect small particles on the tongue (Tepper and Nurse 1997; Chopra et al. 2002). Supertasters are also more sensitive to tactile qualities of graininess and grittiness (Kirkmeyer and Tepper 2004). In response to red wine, PROP supertasters demonstrated a greater perception of astringency as reflected in a perceived particulate size, smoothness, and grip/adhesiveness (Pickering and Robert 2006).

9.6 BURN/STING

The feel of burn and sting is mediated through the trigeminal nerve and is discussed more specifically in Chapter 8 of this book. While at sufficiently high levels, nearly all olfactory stimuli induce trigeminal sensation, the areas of the brain involved are very different (Luebbert et al. 2011). Such trigeminal stimulation, demonstrated in fMRI studies of anosmic subjects, is processed primarily in the left supplementary motor area of the frontal lobe, the right superior middle gyri of the temporal lobe, the left parahippocampal gyrus of the limbic lobe, and the sublobar regions of the left putamen and right insula. Both olfactory and trigeminal stimuli activate the cerebellum and the right premotor frontal cortex (Iannilli et al. 2007). Different tastes can modulate the trigeminal response. Sucrose reduces burn from capsaicin and piperine (Sizer and Harris 1985; Stevens and Lawless 1986). On the other hand, capsaicin and piperine reduce sweet, bitter, and sour tastes (Lawless and Stevens 1984). Such gustatory and somatosensory input is integrated at the single-neuron level (Simon et al. 2008).

Trigeminal sensation also impacts upon olfaction. Irritants reduce olfactory ability and retronasal smell; some studies suggest that capsaicin reduces the intensity of vanilla and orange flavor (Prescott and Stevenson 1995). Alternatively, Cajun pepper, with associated trigeminal stimulation, enhances the retronasal perception of grape jelly (Stamps and Bartoshuk 2011). This implies that trigeminal stimuli may be utilized to enhance flavor perception in those with nutritional difficulties associated with impaired chemosensation. Contrarily, sweet taste reduces capsaicin-induced pain sensation (Schoebel et al. 2011).

Static pressure on the tongue increases irritation from alcohol (Green 1990). On the other hand, 60-Hz vibration reduces burn and pain on the lip, possibly due to its distraction effect (Green 1990) or through the gate control theory of pain with large fiber stimulation.

Heating increases trigeminal irritation as a result of enhancing small-fiber C-polymodal nociceptor firing (Green 1986). Contrarily, cooling decreases such discharge—and thus capsaicin-induced trigeminal sensation of irritation, pain, and burn (Szolcsanyi 1977).

In summary, multiple factors play a role in the perception of hunger and the satiety value of the foods and beverages that we ingest. Color, texture, crunch value, and beverage viscosity all play a role in their appeal. Accounting for these factors may allow for higher satiety and decreased caloric intake.

REFERENCES

Baek, I., R.S.T. Linforth, A. Blake, and A.J. Taylor. 1999. Sensory perception is related to the rate of change of volatile concentration in-nose during eating of model gels. *Chemical Senses* 24:155–160, as referenced in deWijk, R.A., L. Engelen, and J.F. Prinz. 2003. The role of intra-oral manipulation in the perception of sensory attributes. *Appetite* 40:1–7.

Bates-Smith, E.C. 1954. Astringency in foods. *Food Processing Industry* 23:124–127, as referenced in Lyman, B.J., and B.G. Green. 1990. Oral astringency: Effects of repeated exposure and interactions with sweeteners. *Chemical Senses* 15:2:151–164.

Blundell, J.E., and J.C. Halford. 1994. Regulation of nutrient supply. The brain and appetite control. *Proceedings of the Nutrition Society* 53:407–418, as referenced in Kristensen, J., and M.G. Jensen. 2011. Dietary fibres in the regulation of appetite and food intake. Importance of viscosity. *Appetite* 56:65–70.

Bolhuis, D.P., C.M.M. Lakemond, R.A. deWijk, P.A. Luning, and C. deGraaf. 2011. Both longer oral sensory exposure to and high intensity of saltiness decrease ad libitum food intake in healthy normal-weight men. *The Journal of Nutrition* 141:2242–2248.

Bolton, R.P., K.W. Heaton, and L.F. Burroughs. 1981. The role of dietary fiber in satiety, glucose, and insulin: Studies with fruit and fruit juice. *American Journal of Clinical Nutrition* 34:211–217.

Chopra, A., G. Essick, and F. McGlone. 2002. Are supertasters also superfeelers? *European Chemoreception Organization Satellite Symposium on Sensitivity to PROP: Measurement, Significance and Implications.* Erlangen, Germany, as referenced in Pickering, G.J. and G. Robert. 2006. Perception of mouthfeel sensations elicited by red wine are associated with sensitivity to 6-n-propylthiouracil. *Journal of Sensory Studies* 21:249–265.

Christensen, C.M. 1980. Effects of taste quality and intensity on oral perception of viscosity. *Perception & Psychophysiology* 28:4:315–320, as referenced in Verhagen, J.V., and L. Engelen. 2006. The neurocognitive basis of human multimodal food perception: Sensory integration. *Neuroscience and Biobehavioral Reviews* 30:613–650.

Christensen, C.M. 1984. Food texture perception. In *Advances in Food Research, Vol. 29*, pp. 159–199, eds. E.E.M. Mrak, C.O. Chichester, and B.S. Schweigert. Orlando, FL: Academic Press.

Christensen, C.M., and Z.M. Vickers. 1981. Relationships of chewing sounds to judgments of food crispness. *Journal of Food Science* 46:574–578, as referenced in Christensen, C.M. 1984. Food texture perception. In *Advances in Food Research, Vol. 29*, pp. 159–199, eds. E.E.M. Mrak, C.O. Chichester, and B.S. Schweigert. Orlando, FL: Academic Press.

deWijk, R.A., and J.F. Prinz. 2005. The role of friction in perceived oral texture. *Food Quality and Preference* 16:121–129.

deWijk, R.A., L. Engelen, and J.F. Prinz. 2003. The role of intra-oral manipulation in the perception of sensory attributes. *Appetite* 40:1–7.

deWijk, R.A., I.A. Polet, L. Engelen, R.M. vanDoorn, and J.F. Prinz. 2004. Amount of ingested custard dessert as affected by its color, odor, and texture. *Physiology & Behavior* 82:397–403.

Drake, B.K. 1963. Food crushing sounds. An introductory study. *Journal of Food Science* 28:233–241, as referenced in Christensen, C.M. 1984. Food texture perception. In *Advances in Food Research, Vol. 29*, pp. 159–199, eds. E.E.M. Mrak, C.O. Chichester, and B.S. Schweigert. Orlando, FL: Academic Press.

Drake, B.K. 1965. Food crushing sounds. Comparisons of objective and subjective data. *Journal of Food Science* 30:556–559, as referenced in Christensen, C.M. 1984. Food texture perception. In *Advances in Food Research, Vol. 29*, pp. 159–199, eds. E.E.M. Mrak, C.O. Chichester, and B.S. Schweigert. Orlando, FL: Academic Press.

German, R.Z., A.W. Crompton, T. Owerkowicz, and A.J. Thexton. 2004. Volume and rate of milk delivery as determinants of swallowing in an infant model animal (*Sus scrofia*). *Dysphagia* 19:3:147–154, as referenced in Pascalle, L., G. Weijzen, P.A.M. Smeets, and C. deGraff. 2009. Sip size of orangeade: Effects on intake and sensory-specific satiation. *British Journal of Nutrition* 102:1091–1097.

Green, B.G. 1986. Sensory interactions between capsaicin and temperature. *Chemical Senses* 11:371–382.

Green, B.G. 1990. Effects of thermal, mechanical, and chemical stimulation on the perception of oral irritation. In *Irritation*, pp. 171–192, eds. B.G. Green, J.R. Mason, and M.R. Kare. New York: Marcel Dekker, as referenced in Verhagen, J.V., and L. Engelen. 2006. The neurocognitive basis of human multimodal food perception: Sensory integration. *Neuroscience and Biobehavioral Reviews* 30:613–650.

Green, B.G. 1993. Oral astringency: A tactile component of flavor. *Acta Psychologica (Amst)* 84:1:119–125.

Haber, G.B., K.W. Heaton, D. Murphy, and L.F. Burroughs. 1977. Depletion and disruption of dietary fibre. Effects on satiety, plasma-glucose, and serum-insulin. *Lancet* 2:679–682.

Hogenkamp, P.S., A. Stafleu, M. Mars, J.M. Brunstrom, and C. deGraaf. 2011. Texture, not flavor, determines expected satiation of dairy products. *Appetite* 57:635–641.

Iannilli, E., J. Gerber, J. Frasnelli, and T. Hummel. 2007. Intranasal trigeminal function in subjects with and without an intact sense of smell. *Brain Research* 1139:235–244.

Joslyn, M.A., and J.L. Goldstein. 1964. Astringency of fruits and fruit products in relation to phenolic content. *Advances in Food Research* 13:179–217, as referenced in Lyman, B.J., and B.G. Green. 1990. Oral astringency: Effects of repeated exposure and interactions with sweeteners. *Chemical Senses* 15:2:151–164.

Kirkmeyer, S.V., and B.J. Tepper. 2004. A current perspective on creaminess perception and 6-n-propylthiouracil taster status. In *Genetic Variation in Taste Sensitivity*, pp. 117–135, eds. J. Prescott, and B.J. Tepper. New York: Marcel Dekker, as referenced in Pickering, G.J., and G. Robert. 2006. Perception of mouthfeel sensations elicited by red wine are associated with sensitivity to 6-n-propylthiouracil. *Journal of Sensory Studies* 21:249–265.

Kristensen, M., and M.G. Jensen. 2011. Dietary fibres in the regulation of appetite and food intake. Importance of viscosity. *Appetite* 56:65–70.

Lawless, H.T., and D.A. Stevens. 1984. Effects of oral chemical irritation on taste. *Physiology & Behavior* 32:995–998, as referenced in Verhagen, J.V., and L. Engelen. 2006. The neurocognitive basis of human multimodal food perception: Sensory integration. *Neuroscience and Biobehavioral Reviews* 30:613–650.

Leidy, H.J., J.W. Apolzan, R.D. Mattes, and W.W. Campbell. 2010. Food form and portion size affect postprandial appetite sensations and hormonal responses in healthy, nonobese older adults. *Obesity* 18:293–299.

Lenfant, F., C. Loret, N. Pineau, C. Hartmann, and N. Martin. 2009. Perception of oral food breakdown: The concept of sensory trajectory. *Appetite* 52:659–667.

Luebbert, M., J. Kyerene, M. Rothermel, K.P. Hoffmann, and H. Hatt. 2011. Activation of the trigeminal system by odorous substances. *AChemS Annual Meeting Abstract Book* P65:48.

Lyly, M., K.H. Liukkonen, M. Salmenkallio-Marttila, L. Karhunen, K. Poutanen, and L. Lahteenmaki. 2009. Fibre in beverages can enhance perceived satiety. *European Journal of Nutrition* 48:251–258, as referenced in Kristensen, M., and M.G. Jensen. 2011. Dietary fibres in the regulation of appetite and food intake. Importance of viscosity. *Appetite* 56:65–70.

Lyman, B.J., and B.G. Green. 1990. Oral astringency: Effects of repeated exposure and interactions with sweeteners. *Chemical Senses* 15:2:151–164.

Marciani, L., P.A. Gowland, R.C. Spiller, P. Manoj, R.J. Moore, P. Young, and A.J. Fillery-Travis. 2001. Effect of meal viscosity and nutrients on satiety, intragastric dilution, and emptying assessed by MRI. *American Journal of Physiology—Gastrointestinal and Liver Physiology* 280:G1227–G1233, as referenced in Kristensen, M., and M.G. Jensen. 2011. Dietary fibres in the regulation of appetite and food intake. Importance of viscosity. *Appetite* 56:65–70.

Martin, S., and R.M. Pangborn. 1971. Human parotid secretion in response to ethyl alcohol. *Journal of Dental Research* 50:485–490, as referenced in Christensen, C.M. 1984. Food texture perception. In *Advances in Food Research, Vol. 29*, pp. 159–199, eds. E.E.M. Mrak, C.O. Chichester, and B.S. Schweigert. Orlando, FL: Academic Press.

Mattes, R., and D. Rothacker. 2001. Beverage viscosity is inversely related to postprandial hunger in humans. *Physiology and Behavior* 74:551–557.

Nishino, Y., D.W. Kim, J. Liu, and H. Ando. 2011. Interaction between olfactory and somatosensory perception: Do odors influence stiffness and roughness perception? *Chemical Senses* 36:J17.

Noble, A.C. 1995. Applications of time-intensity procedures for the evaluation of taste and mouthfeel. *American Journal of Enology and Viticulture* 45:128–133, as referenced in Verhagen, J.V., and L. Engelen. 2006. The neurocognitive basis of human multimodal food perception: Sensory integration. *Neuroscience and Biobehavioral Reviews* 30:613–650.

Pangborn, R.M., and C.M. Chung. 1981. Parotid salivation in response to sodium chloride and monosodium glutamate in water and broths. *Appetite* 2:380–385, as referenced in Christensen, C.M. 1984. Food texture perception. In *Advances in Food Research, Vol. 29*, pp. 159–199, eds. E.E.M. Mrak, C.O. Chichester, and B.S. Schweigert. Orlando, FL: Academic Press.

Peyrot des Gachons, C., and P.A.S. Breslin. 2011. Effects of astringency sensations on oral fat perception. *AChemS Annual Meeting Abstract Book* P188:90.

Pickering, G.J., and G. Robert. 2006. Perception of mouthfeel sensations elicited by red wine are associated with sensitivity to 6-n-propylthiouracil. *Journal of Sensory Studies* 21:249–265.

Piqueras-Fiszman, B., and C. Spence. 2011. Crossmodal correspondences in product packaging. Assessing color–flavor correspondences for potato chips (crisps). *Appetite* 57:753–757.

Prescott, J., and R.J. Stevenson. 1995. Effects of oral chemical irritation on tastes and flavors in frequent and infrequent users of chili. *Physiology & Behavior* 58:6:1117–1127.

Rozin, P., M. Mark, and D. Schiller. 1981. The role of desensitization in capsaicin in chili pepper ingestion and preferences. *Chemical Senses* 6:23–30, as referenced in Christensen, C.M. 1984. Food texture perception. In *Advances in Food Research, Vol. 29*, pp. 159–199, eds. E.E.M. Mrak, C.O. Chichester, and B.S. Schweigert. Orlando, FL: Academic Press.

Ruijschop, R.M., N. Zijlstra, A.E. Boelrijk, A. Dijkstra, M.J. Burgering, C. deGraff, and M.S. Westerterp-Plantenga. 2011. Effects of bite size and duration of oral processing on retro-nasal aroma release—Features contributing to meal termination. *British Journal of Nutrition* 105:307–315.

Schoebel, N., A. Minovi, and H. Hatt. 2011. Sweet taste and taste nerve lesion modify trigeminal capsaicin perception in adult human subjects. *AChemS Annual Meeting Abstract Book* 70:50.

Simon, S.A., I.E. deAraujo, J.R. Stapleton, and M.A.L. Nicoletis. 2008. Multisensory processing of gustatory stimuli. *Chemosensory Perception* 1:95–102.

Sizer, F., and N. Harris. 1985. The influence of common food additives and temperature on threshold perception of capsaicin. *Chemical Senses* 10:279–286, as referenced in Verhagen, J.V., and L. Engelen. 2006. The neurocognitive basis of human multimodal food perception: Sensory integration. *Neuroscience and Biobehavioral Reviews* 30:613–650.

Smith, A.K., H. June, and A.C. Noble. 1996. Effects of viscosity on the bitterness and astringency of grape seed tannin. *Food Quality and Preference* 7:3:161–166, as referenced in Verhagen, J.V., and L. Engelen. 2006. The neurocognitive basis of human multimodal food perception: Sensory integration. *Neuroscience and Biobehavioral Reviews* 30:613–650.

Solah, V.A., D.A. Kerr, C.D. Adikara, X. Meng, C.W. Binns, K. Zhu, A. Devine, and R.L. Prince. 2010. Differences in satiety effects of alginate- and whey protein-based foods. *Appetite* 54:485–491, as referenced in Kristensen, M., and M.G. Jensen. 2011. Dietary fibres in the regulation of appetite and food intake. Importance of viscosity. *Appetite* 56:65–70.

Stamps, J.L., and L.M. Bartoshuk. 2011. Rescuing flavor perception in the elderly. *Chemical Senses* 31:A32–A33.

Stevens, D.A., and H.T. Lawless. 1986. Putting out the fire: Effects of tastants on oral chemical irritation. *Perception & Psychophysics* 39:5:346–350, as referenced in Verhagen, J.V., and L. Engelen. 2006. The neurocognitive basis of human multimodal food perception: Sensory integration. *Neuroscience and Biobehavioral Reviews* 30:613–650.

Stokes, J.R. 2012. "Oral" rheology. In *Food Oral Processing*, Ch. 11, pp. 227–263, eds. J. Chen, and L. Engelen. Oxford: Blackwell Publishing.

Szczesniak, A.S. 1979. Classification of mouthfeel characteristics of beverages. In *Food Texture and Rheology*, p. 1, ed. P. Sherman. New York: Academic Press.

Szolcsanyi, J. 1977. A pharmacological approach to elucidation of the role of different nerve fibres and receptor endings in mediation of pain. *Journal of Physiology (Paris)* 73:251–259, as referenced in Verhagen, J.V., and L. Engelen. 2006. The neurocognitive basis of human multimodal food perception: Sensory integration. *Neuroscience and Biobehavioral Reviews* 30:613–650.

Tepper, B., and R. Nurse. 1997. Fat perception is related to PROP taster status. *Physiology & Behavior* 61:949–954, as referenced in Pickering, G.J., and G. Robert. 2006. Perception of mouthfeel sensations elicited by red wine are associated with sensitivity to 6-n-propylthiouracil. *Journal of Sensory Studies* 21:249–265.

Verhagen, J.V., and L. Engelen. 2006. The neurocognitive basis of human multimodal food perception: Sensory integration. *Neuroscience and Biobehavioral Reviews* 30:613–650.

Wadden, T.A., A.J. Stunkard, K.D. Brownell, and S.C. Day. 1985. A comparison of two very low calorie diets: Protein-sparing modified fast versus protein–formula–liquid diet. *American Journal of Clinical Nutrition* 41:533–539.

Weijzen, P.L., P.A. Smeets, and C. deGraff. 2009. Sip size of orangeade: Effects on intake and sensory-specific satiation. *British Journal of Nutrition* 102:7:1091–1097.

Zijlstra, N., M. Mars, R.A. DeWijk, M.S. Westerterp-Plantenga, and C. deGraaf. 2008. The effect of viscosity on ad libitum food intake. *International Journal of Obesity (London)* 32:4:676–683, as referenced in Pascalle, L., G. Weijzen, P.A.M. Smeets, and C. deGraff. 2009. Sip size of orangeade: Effects on intake and sensory-specific satiation. *British Journal of Nutrition* 102:1091–1097.

Zijlstra, N., M. Mars, A. Stafleu, and C. deGraff. 2010. The effect of texture differences on satiation in 3 pairs of solid foods. *Appetite* 55:3:490–497.

10 Auditory System and Nutrition

Alan R. Hirsch

When queried, the ubiquitous penultimate sensation is hearing. It may seem trivial, but the music of manduction, the trope of mastication, and the symphony of mandibulation affect consumption. Who has not reveled in the crisp crunch of fresh lettuce, the snap, crackle, and pop of the modification of Rice Krispies®, or the burst of a bubble gum? Such acoustic accompaniments augment the hedonics of the gustatory experience and serve to confirm the expectations about the axiopisty of foods (Vickers 1983). Alternatively, lack of expected sounds may lead to negative hedonics toward the consumable and the rejection of ingestion.

The sounds of manduction, or munching music, will vary in volume, pitch, and tempo depending on the food consumed (Drake 1963). The hedonics toward a food is thus influenced by the noise generated in the process of mandibulation (Vickers 1991). The value of a food (such as celery, turnip, and crackers) in terms of its freshness is in part defined by its crispiness, crunchiness, and hardness (Zampini and Spence 2010). These traits are delineated through auditory and oromandibular tactile, proprioceptive, and mechanoreceptor cues—and it is the auditory that may be the most important (Vickers 1981). The auditory indicators of crispiness include the loudness of the crunch and a predominance of high-frequency sounds (Vickers and Christensen 1980). Mastication of crispy foods produces louder high-pitched sounds of frequency greater than 5 kHz (Dacremont 1995). Changing just one component of sound—increasing the high-amplitude frequencies—is sufficient to enhance the hedonics of Pringles® potato chips as to be fresher and to the maderization, or flatness, of sparkling water (Zampini and Spence 2004, 2005). The perceived madification, or extent of moisturization of crackers, is also influenced by the music of maceration: when white noise is played over headphones, the ability to identify a degree of pretzel moisturization is impaired (Masuda et al. 2008). These results are not uniformly accepted. Assessment of crispiness (almost the opposite of moist or softened by moisture) as determined by sensations during mandibulation was unaffected by headphone background noise (Christensen and Vickers 1981).

External sounds outside of the body, extrasomatic acoustics if you will, also can influence eating behavior. A long-recognized phenomenon by restaurateurs and bartenders is that of enhancement of imbibing in the spirits among patrons when background music is present. Since the social environment has been demonstrated to modify food intake, it is unclear how much direct influence sounds have on this behavior (Edelman et al. 1986). Increased consumption in response to increase in music tempo has been found. The reason for such is unclear but may partly be due to tempo-entrained mandibulation and deglutition, since the increase in the number of bites correlates with music speed (Roballey et al. 1985).

Others have found the opposite: slower-tempo background music actually enhanced consumption. To address this, 1392 diners were monitored in a Texas restaurant for how much they ate and spent (Milliman 1986). Compared to nights when fast ambient music was broadcast, in the presence of slow music, the diners remained 11 min longer and spent an average of $8.38 more on drinks (although no change in money spent for food was observed). Slow music increased the time spent dining and restaurant bills, even when controlling for music volume, temperature, and lighting conditions (Caldwell and Hibbert 2002). Furthermore, college students drank faster with slow-tempo music in the background (McElrea and Standing 1992).

Not only tempo but also volume impact upon consumption. Auditory stimulation increased the consumption of soda, and the louder the music, the more soft drinks the patrons drank (McCarron and Tierney 1989). When loud (88–91 dB) top 40 music is broadcast, bar customers drank more than when the same music of lower volume was played (Gueguen et al. 2008). In another study, 10 men were exposed to low-volume noise (70 dB), high-volume noise (90 dB), loud noise of their individual choice (90 dB), and a silent control period while tasting sweet and salty solutions (Fantino and Goillot 1986). The volume of noise was selected because it simulated the levels at a public cafeteria. While no effect on hedonics was seen for salt solution, at a 90-dB sound, sucrose was rated more pleasant. The mechanism of such action was postulated to be due not to the direct effect of noise or music but rather to the loud sounds causing a stress response, with increase in endorphins, which then increase hedonics toward sucrose.

While hyperphagia had been demonstrated in response to such noise-induced stress, the direct effect of noise on sensory perception had not been explored until the last half of this century (Ferber and Cabanac 1987). In an attempt to eliminate auditory input, subjects occluded their external auditory canal with their digits. In this condition, the perception of sweetness of sugar, the saltiness of salt, and the odor of asafetida changed but not in a consistent direction (Srinivasan 1955).

The exact genre of music with the greatest efficiency in promoting consumption remains controversial. Studies support classical, jazz, pop, or no music at all (North and Hargreaves 1996; North et al. 2003). Pop music enhances hedonics toward soap odor compared to listening to white noise and theoretically may enhance food odor hedonics as well (Miyazaki and Sakai 2008). Background rock music increased patrons' imbibing in alcohol (Lindman et al. 1986). Background classical music enhanced the amount spent on wine as compared to that of background popular music (Areni and Kim 1993). One can only speculate what the music of Justin Bieber would do to alcohol consumption.

To further elucidate the mechanism of music-induced enhanced consumption, the eating habits of 78 college students, with an average age of 20, over a seven-day period were assessed (Stroebele and deCastro 2006). When music was placed in the background of a meal, 447 kJ more was eaten, 93 g more liquid was drank, and 222 kJ more fat was consumed than without music. This was true in normal-weight and overweight subjects. Meal duration was also longer with musical background by 11.26 min. However, unlike other studies, no effect of volume, tempo, or type of music was seen on meal size or duration.

Possible mechanisms for enhanced consumption include music-induced change in affect or distraction-induced inhibition of sensory-specific satiety and associated disinhibition of appetite, culminating in greater consumption (see Chapter 11 of this book).

Viewing this from another perspective, if music increases consumption, does absence of music (or sound) reduce consumption and thus reduce weight? Studies suggest that this is not the situation—if anything, the opposite is the case. Recurrent otitis media is associated with taste loss (with damage of the chorda tympani nerves), hearing loss, and childhood and adult obesity (Bartoshuk et al. 2012). Furthermore, age-related hearing impairment is associated with increased waist circumference and increase in body mass index (Fransen et al. 2008; Hwang et al. 2009). While association does not prove causation, it could indicate the same pathology affecting both hearing and mechanisms of weight regulation. Such coincidence invites speculation and further exploration.

The mechanism whereby music impacts nutrition and consumption is unclear but may reflect a direct effect of sound on chemosensation (Srinivasan 1955; Fantino and Goillot 1986). Or music may act on arousal, or on mood, which then secondarily affects appetite or chemosensation (Zampini and Spence 2010). Alternatively, like odors, music may impact on time perception, and thus assessment of time duration consuming a meal, leading to more time eating (perceived as less) and ultimately leading to overconsumption (Eghil et al. 2010; Zampini and Spence 2010).

Contextual congruence also plays a role in the impact of music on consumption. Background French music increased French and decreased German wine purchases, whereas German music increased the purchase of German wines and reduced that of French wines (North et al. 1999). The nature of the specific sound that would have the greatest effects on hedonics is unclear, but it is possible that congruency is the most relevant aspect (Seo et al. 2014). In normal subjects, specific tastes are paired with distinct sounds. Sour tastes as in lemons, vinegar, and pickle are associated with low-pitched sounds, whereas both sweet, such as candy, and bitter tastes, such as beer, coffee, and tonic water, are paired with high-pitched sounds (Crisinel and Spence 2009, 2010). In pathological synesthetes, a tone at 50 cps and 10 dB induces the perception of taste of sweet and sour borscht, whereas 200 cps and 113 dB caused a taste of briny pickle (Luria 1968). Piano, strings, woodwinds, and brass increase hedonics toward the aroma of crème brûlée and a variety of other aromas (Crisinel et al. 2013). Theoretically, *La Cucaracha* may enhance the hedonics toward salsa and nachos but may have little or opposite effects on bananas foster.

Incongruent stimuli, but endowed with the same affective tone, can enhance positive hedonics toward olfactory stimuli. For instance, the sound of a baby laughing enhanced the positive hedonics to both pleasant and unpleasant odors (Seo and Hummel 2011). Seo et al. (2014, p. 225) posited that "congruent sounds increase odor familiarity and facilitate odor identification, thereby enhancing odor pleasantness." Thus, "Jingle Bells" enhances the hedonics of cinnamon odor more than "YMCA." Hedonic pairing of sound to consumables is most likely through a learned process (Seo et al. 2014). Years of hearing snap, crackle, and pop set up expectations for these sounds when milk modifies Rice Krispies, whereas such sounds emanating from a hotdog upon appliance of condiments would be, to say the least, disturbing (the halo and Horn effect of sensory stimulation) (Seo and Hummel 2011). Congruent sensory stimuli enhance not only odor hedonics but also detection, identification, duration, and intensity (Zellner et al. 1991; Gottfried and Dolan 2003; Sakai et al. 2005; Dematte et al. 2009; Seo and Hummel 2011).

Hence, the auditory system impacts appetite and nutrition. As more research in this relatively unexplored realm is conducted, new uses of sound for clinical application (for instance, to enhance weight gain in tabescent oncology patients) will, without a doubt, be forthcoming. For more details in this arena, an outstanding comprehensive review of the impact of sound on consumers by Zampini and Spence (2010) is highly recommended.

REFERENCES

Areni, C.S., and D. Kim. 1993. The influence of background music on shopping behavior: Classical versus top-forty music in a wine store. *Advances in Consumer Research* 20:236–340.

Bartoshuk, L.M., H. Hoffman, H. Logan, and D.J. Snyder. 2012. Taste damage (otitis media, tonsillectomy and head and neck cancer), oral sensations and BMI. *Physiology & Behavior* 107:4:516–526.

Caldwell, C., and S.A. Hibbert. 2002. The influence of music tempo and musical preference on restaurant patron's behavior. *Psychology and Marketing* 19:895–917.

Christensen, C.M., and Z.M. Vickers. 1981. Relationships of chewing sounds to judgments of food crispness. *Journal of Food Science* 46:574–578.

Crisinel, A.S., and C. Spence. 2009. Implicit association between basic tastes and pitch. *Neuroscience Letter* 464:39–42.

Crisinel, A.S., and C. Spence. 2010. A sweet sound? Exploring implicit association between basic tastes and pitch. *Perception* 39:3:417–425.

Crisinel, A.S., C. Jacquier, O. Deroy, and C. Spence. 2013. Composing with cross-modal correspondences: Music and odors in concert. *Chemical Perception* 6:45–52.

Dacremont, C. 1995. Spectral composition of eating sounds generated by crispy, crunchy and crackly foods. *Journal of Texture Studies* 26:27–43.

Dematte, M.L., D. Sanabria, and C. Spence. 2009. Olfactory discrimination: When vision matters? *Chemical Senses* 34:103–109.

Drake, B.K. 1963. Food crunching sounds. An introductory study. *Journal of Food Science* 28:233–241.

Edelman, B., D. Engel, P. Bronstein, and E. Hirsch. 1986. Environmental effects on the intake of overweight and normal-weight men. *Appetite* 7:71–83.

Eghil, M.M.M., S. Yakov, A.R. Hirsch, A. Kaur, S. Freels, and M.F.A. Gamra. 2010. Effects of odor on time perception. *Chemical Senses* 32:A49.

Fantino, M., and E. Goillot. 1986. Hyperphagic induite par le stress chez l'homme. *Cahiers de Nutrition et de Dietetique* 21:51 as referenced in Ferber, C., and M. Cabanac. 1987. Influence of noise on gustatory affective ratings and preference for sweet or salt. *Appetite* 8:229–235.

Ferber, C., and M. Cabanac. 1987. Influence of noise on gustatory affective ratings and preference for sweet or salt. *Appetite* 8:229–235.

Fransen, E., V. Topsakal, J.J. Hendrickx et al. 2008. Occupational noise, smoking, and a high body mass index are risk factors for age-related hearing impairment and moderate alcohol consumption is protective: A European population-based multicenter study. *Journal of the Association for Research in Otolaryngology* 9:264–276.

Gottfried, J.A., and R.J. Dolan. 2003. The nose smells what the eye sees: Crossmodal visual facilitation of human olfactory perception. *Neuron* 39:375–386.

Gueguen, N., C. Jacob, H. LeGuellec, T. Morineau, and M. Lourel. 2008. Sound level of environmental music and drinking behavior: A field experiment with beer drinkers. *Alcoholism: Clinical and Experimental Research* 32:10:1795–1798.

Hwang, J.H., C.C. Wu, C.J. Hsu, T.C. Liu, and W.S. Yang. 2009. Association of central obesity with the severity and audiometric configurations of age-related hearing impairment. *Obesity* 17:1796–1801.

Lindman, R., B. Lindfors, E. Dahla, and H. Toivola. 1986. Alcohol and ambience: Social and environmental determinants of intake and mood. In *Proceedings of the 3rd Congress of International Society for Biomedical Research on Alcoholism*, eds. K.O. Lindros, R. Ylikahri, and K. Kiianmaa, pp. 385–388. Oxford: Pergamon.

Luria, A.R. 1968. *The Mind of a Mnemonist*. Cambridge, MA: Harvard University Press.

Masuda, M., Y. Yamaguchi, K. Arai, and K. Okajima. 2008. Effects of auditory information on food recognition. *IEICE Technical Report* 108:36:123–126.

McCarron, A., and K.J. Tierney. 1989. The effect of auditory stimulation in the consumption of soft drinks. *Appetite* 13:155–159.

McElrea, H., and L. Standing. 1992. Fast music causes fast drinking. *Perceptual and Motor Skills* 75:362.

Milliman, R.E. 1986. The influence of background music on behavior of restaurant patrons. *Journal of Consumer Research* 13:286–289.

Miyazaki, A., and N. Sakai. 2008. Attention for listening to music effects on perception of soap odor. *ChemoSense* 11:1:17.

North, A.C., and D.J. Hargreaves. 1996. The effect of music responses to a dining area. *Journal of Environmental Psychology* 16:55–64.

North, A., D. Hargreaves, and J. McKendrick. 1999. The influence of in-store music on wine selections. *Journal of Applied Psychology* 84:271–276.

North, A.C., A. Shilcock, and D.J. Hargreaves. 2003. The effect of musical style on restaurant consumers' spending. *Environment and Behavior* 35:712–718.

Roballey, T.C., C. McGreevy, R.R. Rongo et al. 1985. The effect of music on eating behavior. *Bulletin of the Psychonomic Society* 23:221–222.

Sakai, N., S. Imada, S. Saito, T. Kobayakawa, and Y. Deguchi. 2005. The effect of visual images on perception of odors. *Chemical Senses* 30:1:i244–i245.

Seo, H.S., and T. Hummel. 2011. Auditory–olfactory integration: Congruent or pleasant sounds amplify odor pleasantness. *Chemical Senses* 36:301–309.

Seo, H.S., F. Lohse, and C.R. Luckett. 2014. What makes the congruent sound-enhanced odor pleasantness? *The Association of Chemoreception Sciences 36th Annual Meeting Abstract Book* 298:141–142.

Seo, H.S., F. Lohse, C.R. Luckett, and T. Hummel. 2014. Congruent sound can modulate odor pleasantness. *Chemical Senses* 39:215–228.

Srinivasan, M. 1955. Has the ear a role in registering flavour? *Bulletin of the Central Food Technology Research Institute Mysore (India)* 4:136.

Stroebele, N., and J.M. deCastro. 2006. Listening to music while eating is related to increases in people's food intake and meal duration. *Appetite* 47:285–289.

Vickers, Z.M. 1981. Relationships of chewing sounds to judgments of crispness, crunchiness and hardness. *Journal of Food Science* 47:121–124.

Vickers, Z.M. 1983. Pleasantness of food sounds. *Journal of Food Science* 48:783–786.

Vickers, Z. 1991. Sound perception and food quality. *Journal of Food Quality* 14:87–96.

Vickers, Z.M., and C.M. Christensen. 1980. Relationship between sensory crispness and other sensory and instrumental parameters. *Journal of Texture Studies* 11:291–307.

Zampini, M., and C. Spence. 2004. The role of auditory cues in modulating the perceived crispness and staleness of potato chips. *Journal of Sensory Studies* 19:347–363.

Zampini, M., and C. Spence. 2005. Modifying the multisensory perception of carbonated beverage using auditory cues. *Food Quality and Preference* 16:632–641.

Zampini, M., and C. Spence. 2010. Assessing the role of sound in the perception of food and drink. *Chemosensory Perception* 3:57–67.

Zellner, D.A., A.M. Bartoli, and R. Eckard. 1991. Influence of color on odor identification and liking ratings. *American Journal of Psychology* 104:547–561.

11 Sensory-Specific Satiety and Nutrition

Alan R. Hirsch

Satiety, or the perception of fullness, is the result of myriad sensory inputs ranging from allesthesia due to firing of interoceptive muscle stretch receptors on the stomach wall to cerebral glucostat receptors. Also contributing to satiety are visual and chemosensory influences. Chapter 6 of this book elucidated the visual aspects, and this chapter will review many of the chemosensory influences on satiety.

The search for the mechanism of satiety, not unlike Indiana Jones's search for the Holy Grail, has been punctuated with twists and turns into the minutiae of sensory system physiology and behavior. To understand this fully, let us review this from a historical perspective.

Anecdotally and through personal experience, it has been a dogma that hunger originated from signals from the stomach. Institutively, this is logical since food deprivation induces hunger and *hunger pangs*, which are a vague sense of abdominal emptiness as contrasted to the postholiday gorging and abdominal and stomach distension and fullness experienced with overeating.

But do stomach and abdominal distension truly induce a state of fullness? Such stretch receptor-induced allesthesia (or change in pleasantness of sensory input produced by internal signals—in this instance, satiety resulting from physiological effects of ingestion) has been the prevailing precept in the field, promoted by the legendary physiologist, Walter B. Cannon, who is associated with the promulgation of the concept of homeostasis, first proposed by Claude Bernard (Bernard 1878; Rolls 2004).

This principle was called into question when it was demonstrated that even after total gastrectomy, hunger persisted (Wangensteen and Carlson 1931). Half a century later, Novin (1983, p. 242) continued to try to chip away at the *stomach as satiety organ* concept, "The optimal utilization and storage of nutrients occurs when nutrient intake engages the entire alimentary tract and viscera. Our leading principle is that hunger and satiety mechanisms are ultimately controlled by the need to regulate a balance between energy input and output, and also needs for specific substances. This makes it unreasonable to expect that hunger and satiety arise out of a single depletion or that control resides in a single organ."

Conceptual inertia is ubiquitous in medicine. How else can one explain why the *stomach is full* concept of satiety had even persisted that long? In what should have been the final-nail-in-the-coffin study of this concept, more than 40 years ago, Jordan (1969) assessed the effect on fullness on four male volunteers who ingested 558 meals, of which 344 were provided through nasogastric intubation. Food was introduced orally, intragastrically, or both simultaneously. He found that intragastric presentation of food had less of a satiating effect than that of oral ingestion (Jordan 1969).

The final nail in the coffin of stomach stretch receptor-induced satiety occurred when it was demonstrated that orally ingested food diverted prior to reaching the stomach induced satiety, whereas food placed directly in the stomach, bypassing the mouth and nose, had minimal effect on hunger (Cecil et al. 1998a,b). Thus, the concept evolved that orosensory stimuli were integral to induction of satiety.

Thus, the satiety center migrated from the stomach rostrally to land in the skull—in particular, the ventromedial nucleus of the hypothalamus. This theory was supported by animal studies: lesion of the ventroposterior medial nucleus of the hypothalamus in guinea pigs produced hyperphagia, weight gain, and an apparent elimination of satiety. Labeled the ventromedial hypothalamic (VMH) syndrome, it suggests that the VMH directly inhibits the feeding area in the lateral hypothalamus: lesion of the VMH thus leads to lateral hypothalamic disinhibition (Miller et al. 1950). It has been postulated that VMH lesions cause a decrease in short-term satiety, which induces a reduction in meal termination and thus an increase in ingestion (Brooks et al. 1946; Teitelbaum and Campbell 1958). Expanding the role of sensory systems in satiety, Powley (1977) concluded that olfactory, gustatory, visual, and visceral sensations modify the lateral hypothalamic discharge and thus feeding.

The basic concept of sensory-specific satiety was elucidated by Scott. Scott (2010) observed, "Hungry people describe a glucose solution as sweet, strong, and pleasant. After they have consumed a filling meal, they describe the same solution as sweet, strong, but no longer pleasant (Thompson et al. 1976, p. 12). The hedonic reaction changes; the perceptual analysis does not."

In a plethora of studies, Cabanac (1979) demonstrated that ingestion of a meal can convert the hedonic ratings of food odors and tastes from pleasant to unpleasant. He further demonstrated that the hedonic change was intersensory-specific (food consumption did not modify thermal pleasure) and intrasensory-specific (eating led to a reduction of hedonics toward food-related odors but not nonfood odors). As a precursor to sensory-specific satiety, he refined the concept even further to a sensory-specific hedonic transformation. For instance, he observed that ingestion of peanut oil reduced hedonics to peanut oil but not to other food smells or tastes. Such *post-ingestive negative alliesthesia* contributed to satiety and corresponded with the contemporary definition of sensory-specific satiety.

However, the couple who put sensory-specific satiety on the chemosensory stage, the Marie and Pierre Curie of appetite, was Barbara and Edmund Rolls. For the last 35 years, their comprehensive investigations into the mechanisms and limitations of sensory-specific satiety essentially defined the concept as it is known today. They literally named their findings *sensory-specific satiety*.

They found, for instance, in response to a preload of the same food, that subjects ate less and had lower pleasantness ratings as opposed to a preload of different foods (Rolls et al. 1980). Thus, they posited, by providing a varied sensory eating experience, that one could limit sensory-specific satiety and induce obesity (similar to what may be seen in an all-you-can-eat buffet). Not only did they carve out the realm of sensory-specific satiety regarding specificity, but they also extended the concept both intersensorily and intrasensorily. For instance, preloading with sausage, cheese, and water caused a decrease in pleasantness to the sight of these items (intersensory generalization) (Thompson et al. 1977; Rolls et al. 1983). Intrasensorial effects (or sensory-generalized satiety) were seen after preloading with sausage, whereby the hedonics of the sight and taste of sausage as well as cheese and Smarties was also seen (albeit to a lesser degree than to that of sausage).

Not only did sensory-specific satiety affect hedonics, but it also actually leads to a reduction in ingestion. Rolls et al. (1982) found that after preloading, relatively little of that food is eaten in a second course, but the intake of novel foods remains relatively high.

Sensory-specific satiety effects were observed with changes in visual sensation as well. Rolls et al. found that in children presented with colored Smarties, the decrease in pleasantness of the color eaten was greater than for the colors not eaten—even though they had the same taste. The same sensory-specific satiety effects of preloading with a specific shape of pasta were found. When second courses provided multiple shapes of the same pasta, the preload shape was liked less and eaten less (Rolls et al. 1982).

So, in what manner do sensory-specific satiety and hedonic factors influence nutrition and food intake? Part of their influence is in food selection, and the other end is on meal termination. A cornucopia of factors integrate together to regulate food intake. These range from underlying metabolic and pathological states to social pressure and aversions (Castonguay et al. 1983). Hedonic assessment is of particular importance for nutritional intake. It is apparent that if the taste of a food is disliked, it will not be selected for consumption and it will not be eaten. But the hedonics toward a food change acutely with sensory-specific satiety and chronically with the monotony effect. Rolls (1986, p. 93) observed that "...when more than one food is available there is a natural tendency to switch between foods rather than just consume the most preferred food."

With unrelenting exposure to the same food, the hedonics and desire for the food show a steep and long-lasting decline. This is intuitive and corresponds with personal experience. Even if nutritionally balanced, who could stand having the same food everyday for each meal?

Newly weaned infants demonstrate this in that when given a choice of their preferred food or a varied diet, they would consistently choose a varied diet (Davis 1928, 1939).

This monotony effect (possibly a chronic variant of sensory-specific satiety) has been well documented. Restaurants and meal providers routinely rotate their menus to help provide for such diversity and novelty. Seen with chocolate but not with other desserts or French fries, this monotony effect has been demonstrated in those who are forced to eat the same main course each day: army rations—baked beans and canned ham (Schutz and Pilgrim 1958; Hetherington et al. 2000)—and among those in an Ethiopian refugee camp (Rolls and de Waal 1985).

Time preference curves have even been described whereby foods not consumed for 3 months are highly desired as opposed to foods eaten the day before (Moskowitz 1980). Such an effect is less in those foods with high fat or protein, explaining why bread, salad, and potatoes may be a daily staple of meals. Such long-term impairment of food acceptance, chronic sensory-specific satiety, monotony effect, or, as Rolls delineated, *wear out* may be viewed as a cognitive satiety and may explain why diets of only a few of the same foods (grapefruit diet, for instance, or monotonous liquid diet) may work by reducing the desire to eat (Hashim and Van Itallie 1965; Cabanac and Rabe 1976). Furthermore, in a blow to mothers mandating their children to *eat your vegetables*, forcing people to eat foods that they have not chosen for themselves decreases the preference for these foods (Birch et al. 1961; Kamen and Peryam 1961). On the other hand, Rolls (1986, p. 99) concluded, "It seems likely that, in affluent societies where there is continual appetite stimulation by both successive and simultaneous variety within and between meals, there will be little opportunity to compensate for overeating due to variety without conscious limitation of intake."

The possibility that sensory-specific satiety may act to help terminate eating is an appealing approach for the treatment of obesity but with certain limitations. Particularly important, given the current demographic and the *graying of America*, is the question of the efficacy of sensory-specific satiety in the elderly population, a group with impaired olfactory ability (Doty et al. 1984). Rolls's experiments demonstrated impaired sensory-specific satiety to taste or odor in the elderly, independent of olfactory function, depression, or dietary restraint (Rolls and McDermott 1991). Why the elderly have a reduced sensory-specific satiety response is unknown— maybe it is based on a central cognitive dysfunction. It would be enlightening to see if sensory-specific satiety is less impaired in cognitively normal normosmic elderly as opposed to mild cognitively impaired normosmic elderly. Such determination may help elucidate the origin for the reduced sensory-specific satiety in the older population.

Sensory-specific satiety has also been labeled orosensory habituation (Swithers and Hall 1994). Its effect has been demonstrated not just on hedonics but also on reduced eating and earlier meal termination (Hetherington 1996), as well as physiological responses. After preloading with cheeseburgers and pizza, both consumption and salivatory responses were reduced upon representation of these same foods (Wisniewski et al. 1992). The onset of sensory-specific satiety occurs immediately after consumption with change in food pleasantness (Rolls et al. 1988a). How long does sensory-specific satiety persist? In animals and humans, it appears to be long-lasting, anywhere from tens of minutes to a few hours, although its maximum effect is seen after 2 min (Harris 1943; Thompson and Spencer 1966; Dethier 1976; Booth 1977; Rolls et al. 1988b; Hetherington et al. 1989; Epstein et al. 1992; Johnson and Vickers 1993; Rolls and Rolls 1997). While not seen with pears in light syrup, there is even evidence that sensory-specific satiety can persist as long as 7 days after eating cheese biscuits to satiety (Weenen et al. 2005).

Not only can consumption induce sensory-specific satiety, but chewing and expectorating without swallowing, or smelling the food for as long a duration as is required to eat the same food also induces sensory-specific satiety (Rolls and Rolls 1997). This implies that one may reduce food intake by presenting the olfactory equivalent of the food to be consumed for several minutes prior to eating (see Chapter 13 of this book). Inexplicably, such findings are at odds with a study of 34 anosmics who would be anticipated to have a dysfunction of sensory-specific satiety. No positive or negative influence was found (Havermans et al. 2010). Furthermore, slow eating may reduce consumption by providing a cumulation of olfactory and gustatory sensations, thus inducing sensory-specific satiety (Rolls and Rolls 1997).

These studies also localize sensory-specific satiety to the brain as opposed to the gastrointestinal system and its inhibition to a cerebral consumption feedback system (Rolls and Rolls 1997; Rolls 2005, 2006a). Further narrowing down the site of control of sensory-specific satiety, a positron emission tomography (PET) study demonstrated that odor activates the pyriform cortex and the right orbitofrontal cortex (Zatorre et al. 1992). The orbitofrontal cortex is where pleasantness of flavors and palatability of food are located (Rolls 2007). Functional magnetic resonance imaging (MRI) demonstrated that activation of the orbitofrontal cortex occurs in odor-induced sensory-specific satiety (O'Doherty et al. 2000; Rolls 2006b).

Event-related functional MRI has shown a satiation-induced reduction of activity in the orbitofrontal cortex, amygdala, and hypothalamus (Haase et al. 2005).

Practically applying the concept of sensory-specific satiety, Holt et al. (1995) delineated the degree of satiety (satiety index) of 38 foods believed primarily to be due to chemosensory stimulation. Thus, a diet could be designed based on the satiety value of food as opposed to the amount of fats or carbohydrates that a food contains (Zeolla 2003). Foods of high satiety index would theoretically induce earlier and longer satiety, resulting in reduced consumption with weight loss. Wedderburn (1999, p. 4) suggests, "...meals that take into consideration the satiety quotient of a given food within a particular calorie allotment can aid the person trying to eat below maintenance in alleviating hunger pangs." Such sentiment was echoed by Sorensen et al. (2003), who observed, "...knowledge about what flavor combinations improve satiety most is very useful in order to be able to produce low energy foods that both taste good and increase satiety. This may be relevant because it will make it easier for people to maintain energy balance in the long term and to prevent the development of overweight and obesity." Indeed, Vander Wal et al. (2005, p. 1162) found that both in obese and normal weight women, two scrambled eggs, two slices of toast, and one tablespoon of reduced-calorie fruit spread produced greater satiety with an average reduction over one-and-a-half days of 1104-kJ energy intake compared to an isocaloric breakfast of bagel and cream cheese and 3 oz of nonfat yogurt.

Expanding on the concept of sensory-specific satiety has been the idea of the generalization of sensory-specific satiety. While clearly, sensory-specific satiety has the greatest effect when presented with the identical type of food that had been given as a preload, there also is an impact on other foods as well. The greater the degree of similarity to the preload, the greater the sensory-specific satiety effect with reduced hedonics and ingestion. Thus, a sweet preload has the greatest effect on other sweet foods and savory on other savory foods (Rolls et al. 1981, 1983, 1984; De Graaf et al. 1993; Guinard and Brun 1998)—but not hedonic inhibition of savory on sweet or a sweet on a savory (De Graaf et al. 1993). Such sensory-generalized satiety could theoretically be utilized to facilitate weight loss by dichotomizing foods into savory and sweet and providing corresponding sensory stimuli to maximize the orosensory experience and thus any satiating effect (see Chapter 13 of this book).

The mechanism underlying sensory-specific satiety remains unclear. At first glance, it would appear to be due to olfactory or gustatory adaptation. In this model, the time spent eating or retronasally smelling the food would rapidly lead to olfactory or gustatory adaptation. Such adaptation would reduce the sensory experience of continuing to eat the food, thus reducing hedonics and consumption. However, this explanation is unlikely since the changed hedonics toward a recently consumed food is independent of the perceived intensity of the foods (Rolls et al. 1983; Rolls and Rolls 1997). Such findings are consistent with the essential role of a cerebral satiety center.

A natural extension of the concept of sensory-specific satiety would be into its role in disease states. In conditions of anorexia, is sensory-specific satiety intensity escalated to a pathological degree? Alternatively, in obesity, is impaired sensory-specific satiety the essential pathophysiological feature? In two experiments, one with sandwiches and one with snacks, Smoek et al. (2004) set out to answer the latter. No difference in sensory-specific satiety between 21 obese and 23 normal-weight women was found, suggesting that impaired sensory-specific satiety is not the mechanism of obesity. However, while sensory-specific satiety and hedonics or *liking* for the foods was normal, obese subjects had a higher appetite rating or *wanting* for more food after ad lib consumption. The difference between obese and normal-weight subjects is thus not in how much they liked the food but in wanting to eat more of the food (Berridge 1996). An intrinsic difference is that the obese want to eat more food, even if they do not enjoy or like it as much, whereas the normal-weight ones will not eat the food if they do not like it (Havermans et al. 2009). Brondel et al. (2007) extended these findings to obese men as well as women, determining that sensory-specific satiety developed equally to the normal-weight ones and the obese, and thus, dysfunction of sensory-specific satiety is not the primary mediator of obesity.

Beverages, like black tea, a liquid carbohydrate, tend to have very low effects on sensory-specific satiety compared to their solid equivalents (Chung and Vickers 2007; Pan and Hu 2011). Possibly, this is due to the quick intraoral transit time and therefore with relatively little retronasal olfactory stimulation. Prolonging oropharyngeal transit time may thus enhance the sensory-specific satiety of a beverage. This was shown with small versus large sips of orangeade (Weijzen et al. 2009). The small sip size caused a prolonged orosensory exposure and greater sensory-specific satiety with reduced desire to drink. Thus, substances with prolonged orosensory stimulation should have a greater effect on sensory-specific satiety. An example of such would be a noningested orosensory stimulator—like gum. Lavin et al. (2002) had shown that chewing sucrose-containing pastilles for 10 min reduced intake by 10% and thus was a small leap to progress to the question of the effect of chewing gum on sensory-specific satiety. Hetherington and Boyland (2007) examined this exact model; they found that chewing aspartame or sugar-sweetened gum reduced energy intake by 36 cal, and there was a reduced desire to eat sweet snacks, posited to be due to sensory-specific satiety. Such effect of gum as a mediator of sensory-specific satiety was broadened to include a wide variety of sugar-free and specialty gums in children (Hirsch et al. 2012, 2013a,b), suggesting that such a mediator could have efficacy as a tool in weight management.

It is apparent that sensory-specific satiety, or sensory-generalized satiety, has an impact upon both the hedonics and consumption of food. It has potential practical application in the management of obesity. Why does sensory-specific satiety exist in humans? Sensory-specific satiety is a logical evolutionary adaptation. If the type of food corresponds with nutrients, then sensory-specific satiety is a physiological way to prevent nutrient excess and switch consumption to other foods with other needed nutrients. While cafeteria-style food would act to reduce the effect of sensory-specific satiety and increase weight, flavoring all food eaten in a similar manner should act to decrease consumption. The problem with such monotonous diet is a matter of compliance. Possibly, a diet based on satiety index or using other modalities to enhance sensory-specific satiety (see Chapter 13 of this book). would be one mechanism of overcoming such monotony effect while still maximizing this homeostatic and physiologic mechanism of sensory-specific satiety.

REFERENCES

Bernard, C. 1878. *Leçons sur les Phénomènes de la Vie Communs aux Animaux et aux Végétaux Vol 2.* Paris: Ballière, p. 121, as quoted in Weingarten, H.P. 1985. Stimulus control of eating: Implications for a two-factory theory of hunger. *Appetite* 6:387–401.

Berridge, K. 1996. Food reward: Brain substrates of wanting and liking. *Neuroscience & Biobehavioral Review* 20:1–25, as quoted in Smoek, H.M., L. Huntjens, L.J. vanGemert, C. de Graaf, and H. Weenen. 2004. Sensory-specific satiety in obese and normal-weight women. *American Journal of Clinical Nutrition* 80:823–831.

Birch, L.L., D. Birch, D.W. Marlin, and L. Kraemer. 1961. Effects of instrumental consumption on children's food preference. *Appetite* 3:125–134.

Booth, D.A. 1977. Satiety and appetite are conditioned responses. *Psychosomatic Medicine* 39:79–81, as quoted in Swithers, S.E., and W.G. Hall. 1994. Does oral experience terminate ingestion? *Appetite* 23:113–138.

Brondel, L., M. Romer, V. Van Wymelbeke et al. 2007. Sensory-specific satiety with simple foods in humans: no influence of BMI? *International Journal of Obesity* 31:987–995.

Brooks, C.M., R.A. Lockwood, and M.L. Wiggins. 1946. A study of the effect of hypothalamic lesions on the eating habits of the albino rat. *American Journal of Physiology* 147:735–741.

Cabanac, M. 1979. Sensory pleasure. *The Quarterly Review of Biology* 54:1:1–29.

Cabanac, M., and E.F. Rabe. 1976. Influence of a monotonous food on body weight regulation in humans. *Physiologic Behavior* 17:675–678.

Castonguay, T.W., E.A. Applegate, D.E. Upton, and J.S. Stern. 1983. Hunger and appetite: Old concepts/new distinctions. *Nutrition Reviews* 41:101–110.

Cecil, J.E., K. Castiglione, S. French, J. Francis, and N.W. Read. 1998a. Effects of intragastric infusions of fat and carbohydrate on appetite ratings and food intake from a test meal. *Appetite* 30:1:65–77.

Cecil, J.E., J. Francis, and N.W. Read. 1998b. Relative contributions of intestinal, gastric, oro-sensory influences and information to changes in appetite induced by the same liquid meal. *Appetite* 31:3:377–390.

Chung, S.J., and Z. Vickers. 2007. Influence of sweetness on the sensory-specific satiety and long-term acceptability of tea. *Food Quality and Preference* 18:256–264.

Davis, C.M. 1928. Studies in the self-selection of diet by young children. *American Journal of Diseases of Children* 36:651–679.

Davis, C.M. 1939. Results of the self-selection of diets by young children. *Canadian Medical Association Journal* 41:257–261.

De Graaf, C., A. Shreurs, and Y.H. Blauw. 1993. Short-term effects of different amounts of sweet and nonsweet carbohydrates on satiety and energy intake. *Physiology & Behavior* 54:833–843, as quoted in Sorensen, L.B., P. Moller, A. Flint, M. Martens, and A. Raben. 2003. Effect of sensory perception of foods on appetite and food intake: A review of studies on humans. *International Journal of Obesity* 27:1152–1166.

Dethier, V.G. 1976. *The Hungry Fly*. Cambridge, MA: Harvard University Press, as quoted in Swithers, S.E., and W.G. Hall. 1994. Does oral experience terminate ingestion? *Appetite* 23:113–138.

Doty, R.L., P. Shaman, S.L. Applebaum, R. Giberson, L. Siksorski, and L. Rosenberg. 1984. Smell identification ability: Changes with age. *Science* 226:1441–1443.

Epstein, L.H., J.S. Roderfer, L. Wisniewski, and A.R. Caggiula. 1992. Habituation and dishabituation of human salivatory responses. *Physiology and Behavior* 51:945–950, as quoted in Swithers, S.E., and W.G. Hall. 1994. Does oral experience terminate ingestion? *Appetite* 23:113–138.

Guinard, J., and P. Brun. 1998. Sensory-specific satiety: Comparison of taste and texture effects. *Appetite* 31:141–157, as quoted in Sorensen, L.B., P. Moller, A. Flint, M. Martens, and A. Raben. 2003. Effect of sensory perception of foods on appetite and food intake: A review of studies on humans. *International Journal of Obesity* 27:1152–1166.

Haase, L.B., B. Cerf-Ducastel, A. Fowler et al. 2005. The effect of a nutritional preload on gustatory activation: An ER-FMRI study. *AChemS XXVIIth Annual Meeting Abstract Book* 122:31.

Harris, J.D. 1943. Habituatory response decrement in the intact organism. *Psychological Bulletin* 40:385–422, as quoted in Swithers, S.E., and W.G. Hall. 1994. Does oral experience terminate ingestion? *Appetite* 23:113–138.

Hashim, S.A., and T.B. Van Itallie. 1965. Studies in normal and obese subjects with a monitored food-dispensing device. *Annals of the New York Academy of Sciences* 131:654–661.

Havermans, R.C., T. Janssen, J.C.A.H. Giesen, A. Roefs, and A. Jansen. 2009. Food liking, food wanting, and sensory-specific satiety. *Appetite* 52:222–225.

Havermans, R.C., J. Hermanns, and A. Jansen. 2010. Eating without a nose: Olfactory dysfunction and sensory-specific satiety. *Chemical Senses* 35:735–741.

Hetherington, M.M. 1996. Sensory-specific satiety and its importance in meal termination. *Neuroscience Behavior Review* 20:113–117, as quoted in Sorensen, L.B., P. Moller, A. Flint, M. Martens, and A. Raben. 2003. Effect of sensory perception of foods on appetite and food intake: A review of studies on humans. *International Journal of Obesity* 27:1152–1166.

Hetherington, M.M., and E. Boyland. 2007. Short-term effects of chewing gum on snack intake and appetite. *Appetite* 48:397–401.

Hetherington, M.M., B.J. Rolls, and V.J. Burley. 1989. The time course of sensory-specific satiety. *Appetite* 12:57–68, as quoted in Sorensen, L.B., P. Moller, A. Flint, M. Martens, and A. Raben. 2003. Effect of sensory perception of foods on appetite and food intake: A review of studies on humans. *International Journal of Obesity* 27:1152–1166.

Hetherington, M.M., A. Bell, and B.J. Rolls. 2000. Effects of repeat consumption on pleasantness, preference and intake. *British Food Journal* 102:7:507–521.

Hirsch, J.W., S.R. Aiello, and A.R. Hirsch. 2012. Relative satiety value of candy and gum: Potential therapies for childhood obesity. *Journal of Obesity and Weight Loss Therapy* 2:1–8.

Hirsch, J.W., M.O. Soto, and A.R. Hirsch. 2013a. As American as apple pie gum: A study of satiety. *Chemical Senses* 38:7:A646.

Hirsch, J.W., M.O. Soto, and A.R. Hirsch. 2013b. The satiety value of sugar-free Orbit Bubblemint chewing gum. *AChemS XXXIVth Annual Meeting Abstract Book* 38:3:262.

Holt, S.H, J.C. Miller, P. Petocz, and E. Farmakalidis. 1995. A satiety index of common foods. *European Journal of Clinical Nutrition* 49:9:675–690, as quoted in Wedderburn, R. 1999. Practical application of the satiety index. *Journal of Performance Enhancement* 1:2:1–7.

Johnson, J., and Z. Vickers. 1993. Effects of flavor and macronutrient composition of food servings on liking, hunger and subsequent intake. *Appetite* 21:25–39, as quoted in Sorensen, L.B., P. Moller, A. Flint, M. Martens, and A. Raben. 2003. Effect of sensory perception of foods on appetite and food intake: A review of studies on humans. *International Journal of Obesity* 27:1152–1166.

Jordan, H.A. 1969. Voluntary intragastric feeding: Oral and gastric contributions to food intake and hunger in man. *Journal of Comparative and Physiological Psychology* 68:4: 498–506.

Kamen, J.M., and D.R. Peryam. 1961. Acceptability of repetitive diets. *Food Technology* 15:173–177.

Lavin, J.H., S.J. French, C.H. Ruxton, and N.W. Read. 2002. An investigation of the role of oro-sensory stimulation in sugar satiety? *International Journal of Eating Disorders* 39:341–345, as quoted in Hetherington, M.M., and E. Boyland. 2007. Short-term effects of chewing gum on snack intake and appetite. *Appetite* 48:397–401.

Miller, N.E., C.J. Bailey, and J.A.F. Stevenson. 1950. Decreased "hunger" but increased food intake resulting from hypothalamic lesions. *Science* 112:256–259.

Moskowitz, H.R. 1980. Psychometric evaluation of food preferences. *Journal of Foodservice Systems* 1:149–167.

Novin, D. 1983. The integration of visceral information in the control of feeding. *Journal of the Autonomic Nervous System* 9:233–246.

O'Doherty, J., E.T. Rolls, S. Francis et al. 2000. Sensory-specific satiety-related olfactory activation of the human orbitofrontal cortex. *NeuroReport* 11:893–897.

Pan, A., and F.B. Hu. 2011. Effects of carbohydrates on satiety: Differences between liquid and solid food. *Current Opinion in Clinical Nutrition and Metabolic Care* 14:4:385–390.

Powley, T.L. 1977. The ventromedial hypothalamic syndrome, satiety, and a cephalic phase hypothesis. *Psychological Review* 84:1:89–126.

Rolls, B.J. 1986. Sensory-specific satiety. *Nutrition Reviews* 44:3:93–101.

Rolls, B.J., and T.M. McDermott. 1991. Effects of age on sensory-specific satiety. *American Journal of Clinical Nutrition* 54:988–996.

Rolls, B.J., E.T. Rolls, E.A. Rowe, and K. Sweeney. 1980. Sensory-specific satiety in man. *Physiology & Behavior* 27:137–142.

Rolls, B.J., E.A. Rowe, E.T. Rolls, B. Kingston, A. Megson, and R. Gunary. 1981. Variety in meal enhances food intake in man. *Physiology & Behavior* 26:215–221, as quoted in Sorensen, L.B., P. Moller, A. Flint, M. Martens, and A. Raben. 2003. Effect of sensory perception of foods on appetite and food intake: A review of studies on humans. *International Journal of Obesity* 27:1152–1166.

Rolls, B.J., E.A. Rowe, and E.T. Rolls. 1982. How flavour and appearance affect human feeding. *Proceedings of the Nutrition Society* 41:109–117.

Rolls, B.J., P.M. Van Duijvenvoorde, and E.T. Rolls. 1984. Pleasantness changes and food intake in a varied four-course meal. *Appetite* 5:337–348, as quoted in Sorensen, L.B., P. Moller, A. Flint, M. Martens, and A. Raben. 2003. Effect of sensory perception of foods on appetite and food intake: A review of studies on humans. *International Journal of Obesity* 27:1152–1166.

Rolls, B.J., M. Hetherington, and V.J. Burley. 1988a. The specificity of satiety: The influence of foods of different macronutrient content on the development of satiety. *Physiology & Behavior* 43:145–153, as quoted in Sorensen, L.B., P. Moller, A. Flint, M. Martens, and A. Raben. 2003. Effect of sensory perception of foods on appetite and food intake: A review of studies on humans. *International Journal of Obesity* 27:1152–1166.

Rolls, B.J., M. Hetherington, and V.J. Burley. 1988b. Sensory stimulation and energy density in the development of satiety. *Physiology & Behavior* 44:727–733, as quoted in Sorensen, L.B., P. Moller, A. Flint, M. Martens and, A. Raben. 2003. Effect of sensory perception of foods on appetite and food intake: A review of studies on humans. *International Journal of Obesity* 27:1152–1166.

Rolls, E.T. 2004. Smell, taste, texture, and temperature multimodal representations in the brain, and their relevance to the control of appetite. *Nutrition Reviews* 62:1:S193–S204.

Rolls, E.T. 2005. Taste, olfactory, and food texture processing in the brain, and the control of food intake. *Physiology & Behavior* 85:45–56.

Rolls, E.T. 2006a. Brain mechanisms underlying flavour and appetite. *Philosophical Transactions of the Royal Society B* 361:1123–1136.

Rolls, E.T. 2006b. Olfaction and food intake: Electrophysiological and neuroimaging data in human and primate. *Chemical Senses* 31:E68.

Rolls, E.T. 2007. Understanding the mechanisms of food intake and obesity. *Obesity Reviews* 8:1:67–72.

Rolls, E.T., and A.W.L. de Waal. 1985. Long-term specific satiety: Evidence from an Ethiopian refugee camp. *Physiological Behavior* 34:1017–1020, as quoted in Weenen, H., A. Stafleu, and C. de Graaf. 2005. Dynamic aspects of liking: Post-prandial persistence of sensory-specific satiety. *Food Quality and Preference* 16:528–535.

Rolls, E.T., and J.H. Rolls. 1997. Olfactory sensory-specific satiety in humans. *Physiology & Behavior* 61:3:461–473.

Rolls, E.T., B.J. Rolls, and E.A. Rowe. 1983. Sensory-specific and motivation-specific satiety for the sight and taste of food and water in man. *Physiology & Behavior* 30:185–192.

Schutz, H.E., and F.J. Pilgrim. 1958. A field study of monotony. *Psychological Reports* 4:559–565.

Scott, T.R. 2010. Taste, reward, and physiology. *Chemosensory Perception* 3:3–15.

Smoek, H.M., L. Huntjens, L.J. van Gemert, C. de Graaf, and H. Weenen. 2004. Sensory-specific satiety in obese and normal-weight women. *American Journal of Clinical Nutrition* 80:823–831.

Sorensen, L.B., P. Moller, A. Flint, M. Martens, and A. Raben. 2003. Effect of sensory perception of foods on appetite and food intake: A review of studies on humans. *International Journal of Obesity* 27:1162.

Swithers, S.E., and W.G. Hall. 1994. Does oral experience terminate ingestion? *Appetite* 23:113–138.

Teitelbaum, P., and H.A. Campbell. 1958. Ingestion patterns in hyperphagic and normal rats. *Journal of Comparative and Physiological Psychology* 51:135–141.

Thompson, D.A., H.R. Moskowitz, and R.G. Campbell. 1976. Effects of body weight and food intake on pleasantness for a sweet stimulus. *Journal of Applied Physiology* 41:77–83, as quoted in Scott, T.R. 2010. Taste, reward, and physiology. *Chemosensory Perception* 3:3–15.

Thompson, D.A., H.R. Moskowitz, and R.G. Campbell. 1977. Taste and olfaction in human obesity. *Physiology & Behavior* 19:335–337.

Thompson, R.F. and W.A. Spencer. 1966. Habituation: A model phenomenon for the study of neuronal substrates of behavior. *Psychological Review* 73:16–43, as quoted in Swithers, S.E., and W.G. Hall. 1994. Does oral experience terminate ingestion? *Appetite* 23:113–138.

Vander Wal, J.S., J.M. Marth, P. Khosta, K-L.C. Jen, and N.V. Dhurandhar. 2005. Short-term effect of eggs on satiety in overweight and obese subjects. *Journal of the American College of Nutrition* 24:6:510–515.

Wangensteen, O.H. and H.A. Carlson. 1931. Hunger sensations in a patient after total gastrectomy. *Proceedings of the Society of Experimental Biology* 28:545–547, quoted in Novin, D. 1983. The integration of visceral information in the control of feeding. *Journal of the Autonomic Nervous System* 9:233–246.

Wedderburn, R. 1999. Practical application of the satiety index. *Journal of Performance Enhancement* 1:2:1–7. Available at http://members.tripod.com?JPE_Sportsscience/Saiety%20Index%20html.html (accessed June 22, 2012).

Weenen, H., A. Stafleu, and C. de Graaf. 2005. Dynamic aspects of liking: Post-prandial persistence of sensory-specific satiety. *Food Quality and Preference* 16:528–535.

Weijzen, P.L.G., P.A.M. Smeets, and C. de Graaf. 2009. Sip size of orangeade: Effects on intake and sensory-specific satiation. *British Journal of Nutrition* 102:1091–1097.

Wisniewski, L., L. Epstein, and A.R. Caggiula. 1992. Effect of food change on consumption hedonics and salivation. *Physiology and Behavior* 52:21–26, as quoted in Swithers, S.E., and W.G. Hall. 1994. Does oral experience terminate ingestion? *Appetite* 23:113–138.

Zatorre, R.J., M. Jones-Gotman, A.C. Evans, and E. Meyer. 1992. Functional localization and lateralization of human olfactory cortex. *Nature* 360:399–340, as quoted in O'Doherty, J., E.T. Rolls, S. Francis et al. 2000. Sensory-specific satiety-related olfactory activation of the human orbitofrontal cortex. *NeuroReport* 11:893–897.

Zeolla, G.F. 2003. Lifestyle changes for maintained body fat loss. Available at http://www .fitnessforoneandall.com/general/article/lifestyle.htm. (accessed June 22, 2012).

12 Chemosensory Influences on Eating and Drinking, and Their Cognitive Mediation

David A. Booth

CONTENTS

12.1   Introduction 223
12.2   Basic Theory of Ingestive Behavior 223
12.3   Excitation and Inhibition of Ingestion by Level of Sweetness 224
      12.3.1   Saccharin Preference as the Model of Appetite 224
      12.3.2   Ingestive Responses to Sweet Solutions 225
      12.3.3   Reflex-Ingestive Movements to Sweet Taste 227
      12.3.4   Sensory Motivation without Pleasure or Reward 227
      12.3.5   Learnt Preferences for Levels of Sweetness 227
      12.3.6   Conditioned Taste Aversion 229
      12.3.7   Conditioned Taste Preference 229
12.4   Learnt Peak of Preference for Level of Sweetener 230
      12.4.1   Preferred Strengths of Sweet Taste 230
      12.4.2   Most Preferred Strength 230
      12.4.3   Somatic Contexts of Sweet Preference 231
      12.4.4   Evidence That Human Sensory Preferences Are Learnt 234
      12.4.5   Peak of Learnt Facilitation by Any Sensory Factor 234
      12.4.6   Learnt Likings for Levels of Bitterness 235
      12.4.7   Conditioned Appetite for Caffeine 236
      12.4.8   Ideal Point for Bitterness of Caffeine in Own Coffee 236
      12.4.9   Development of Preference for Bitter Foods and Drinks 236
      12.4.10 6-*n*-Propylthiouracil and Food Preferences 238
      12.4.11 Human Preference for the Taste of Salt 239
      12.4.12 Tastes, Smells, Colors, and Textures 240
12.5   Missing the [Ideal] Point 240
      12.5.1   Group-Averaged Scores for Preference 240
      12.5.2   Food Preferences and PROP Genetics 241
      12.5.3   Food Preferences and Obesity 241

              12.5.3.1 Sweet Taste 242
              12.5.3.2 Fat *Taste* 244
       12.5.4 Family Paradox..245
       12.5.5 Ingestive Appetite and Food Preference Responses 246
       12.5.6 Sensations or Sensed Characteristics?..246
       12.5.7 Preference or Appetite? 246
       12.5.8 Hunger Is Appetite for Food..247
       12.5.9 Words for Energy Intakes and Appetite Ratings............................248
12.6   Words for Gustatory and Olfactory Intensities and Preferences.................250
       12.6.1 Intensities...250
       12.6.2 Preferences 250
       12.6.3 Pleasant versus Pleasurable 250
       12.6.4 Motivating Stimulus or Associative Reward?.............................252
       12.6.5 Strength of an Influence..252
       12.6.6 Each Food Has a Different Taste 253
       12.6.7 Amount of Taste, Not Just the Sort of Taste 254
       12.6.8 Which Level?..254
12.7   Cognitive Mechanisms That Convert Sensing into Ingesting....................255
       12.7.1 Causal Processes from Chemical Stimulation to Ingestive
              Movement..255
       12.7.2 Mixing It..256
       12.7.3 Configured Ideal Points 257
              12.7.3.1 Mixture Statistics..257
              12.7.3.2 Scientific Measurement of Context....................258
              12.7.3.3 Identical or Configured Influences 260
12.8   Gustatory Configurations in Ingestion..261
       12.8.1 Balance of Sweet and Sour in Oranges 261
       12.8.2 Direct Stimulation of Preference 262
       12.8.3 Sensations versus Thoughts Controlling Preference 263
       12.8.4 Monosodium Glutamate: The Complex Savory Taste..................265
       12.8.5 Amino Acid Detectors in the Mouth and Brain.....................267
       12.8.6 Savory Complex or a Fifth Simple Taste?.............................268
       12.8.7 All Sensory Vocabularies Are Learnt Social Names....................268
       12.8.8 Quantity of MSG and Quality of a Food 269
       12.8.9 Direct Route to Food Quality..269
12.9   Olfactory Configurations in Ingestion 270
       12.9.1 Good Balance among Components 270
       12.9.2 Aroma of Fresh Strawberries..271
       12.9.3 Cognitive Analysis of Concentrations and Ratings 272
       12.9.4 Analytical and Configured Norms....................................275
       12.9.5 Flavor..276
       12.9.6 Flavors of Cuisines, Not Nutrients 278
12.10 Long-Term Effects of Taste on Nutrition 281
       12.10.1 Salt and Strokes 281
       12.10.2 Sugar and Teeth 283

12.11 Conclusions 283
 12.11.1 Mechanisms versus Tests 283
 12.11.2 Chemosensory Influences on Nutrition 284
References...284

12.1 INTRODUCTION

The only way that chemical senses can affect nutrition is by influencing selection among the amounts of foods and drinks to ingest. Fundamental to the science of nutrition, therefore, is a correct theoretical understanding of the mechanisms by which tasted and smelled molecules affect the choice of each mouthful and hence also the number of mouthfuls consumed of each material available on a particular occasion.

Nutritional state and other states of the body can also influence choices of what to put in the mouth and swallow. So can the external environment, both physical and socioeconomic. In the human case, social influences can dominate established habits, for example, through verbal and numerical signals of information such as the source of the flavoring in a manufactured food, a serving's nutrient content, and how much of the product people usually eat at one time (Booth 2008). Nevertheless, all the physiological and social factors in selective eating and drinking have to operate through taste, smell, touch, sight, and other senses, because some sensory information is essential to identifying a food or a drink at the point of choice.

In addition, generalist feeders such as humans, dogs, and rats have to learn this sensory recognition of a food and any contextual factor that influences that food's selection (Booth 1972a, 1985, 2013; Booth and Freeman 1993). Therefore, a scientific understanding of ingestive behavior cannot be built merely on measurements of the intake of a food or the verbally expressed strength of disposition to eat it, such as scores for preference or ratings of appetite. It is equally necessary to measure the major influences on each act of ingesting a food or on the rated liking for that item in those circumstances. Only then it is possible to work out how those influences interact to produce that physical or symbolic response to an item—that is, how the chemosensory factors in behavior are cognitively mediated.

12.2 BASIC THEORY OF INGESTIVE BEHAVIOR

Neglect of the above considerations has allowed the continuation of a traditional conception of the controls of intake, which is erroneous in each of its basic tenets. The size of a meal is not determined by competition between a fixed palatability of each ingested material and a sequence of invariant postingestional satiety signals. After a material has been consumed for the very first time or two, the innate gustatory reflexes to stimulation by sugars, acids, sodium salts, alkaloids, etc., cease to play any role in that material's acceptance or rejection or the rate of licking the fluid or of biting and chewing the solid. The reflexes are superseded by direct controls of mouthful selection by learnt reactions to many combined attributes, such as salty and sour tastes, a yellow–brown color, crisp texture, and peer approval. Once a dietary pattern has become familiar, chemical sensing of digestion products in the small intestine and of circulating hormones and metabolites in the brain no longer simply

excites or inhibits further ingestion of food. The postingestional signals become integrated in the mind with each item's sensed characteristics and social roles into the
state of appetite of the moment, including the depth of its sating by previous ingestion (Booth 1972a, 2013).

For example, a food that was accepted enthusiastically at its first mouthful in a
meal becomes uninteresting or even slightly aversive a number of mouthfuls later
(Duclaux et al. 1973; Rolls et al. 1981a). This particular satiety effect within a meal
is specific to the food that has just been eaten and not to a particular sensed characteristic in itself. Rather, the senses are needed to recognize the food that is now
less attractive. This mechanism of appetite suppression arises from still unidentified
factors such as the specific food's role in the meal, the eater's habitual portion size,
a growing boredom with that food, and/or habituation of the sensorimotor pathways
of its ingestion (Booth 1976; Meillon et al. 2013).

Hence, as illustrated by the first set of data in Section 12.3.5, there is no such
thing as persisting preference for sweetness as such in human children or adults or
nonhuman primates, pet dogs, or laboratory rats. Rather, each individual member of
an omnivorous species most prefers a particular level of sweetness that is different
for each food or drink and each context of signals from the internal and external
environments (Booth 1985, 2013). This chapter reviews the long-standing and recent
evidence that ingestion is controlled by those particular learnt combinations of levels
of chemosensory and other signals. The decision on an item in context is read out
from a standard in memory built during previous occasions, through readily measured but sometimes unconscious mental processes, into acceptance of an option for
the next mouthful.

12.3 EXCITATION AND INHIBITION OF INGESTION BY LEVEL OF SWEETNESS

12.3.1 SACCHARIN PREFERENCE AS THE MODEL OF APPETITE

Eating a meal accompanied by a drink is a pleasant activity. Nevertheless, the ingestion itself is often a routine and subsumed under other thoughts and/or interactions
with other people. When attention is paid to a mouthful, its flavors and textures
may be recognized and enjoyed. The expected sensory characteristics may help to
motivate the selection of an item from the shelf or menu, the choice from a buffet,
or the next forkful from the plate. Unless someone has become very disturbed, for
example, about the shape of the body, ingestion in itself is not emotional, although
the meaning of the occasion or the involvement with a companion may be intensely
affecting. Seldom if ever does the sensing of a food or drink generate a physical
thrill.

Despite this highly differentiated character of human motivation to eat and drink,
animal laboratory research was dominated at one time by the idea that the ingestion
of food was completely unselective—merely a general excitement in anticipation
of the scheduled return of food after it had been withheld for a day (Campbell and
Sheffield 1953; Sheffield and Campbell 1954). Ingestion as a side effect of nonspecific arousal was such a deep conviction that it was suggested that learning to avoid

dangerous materials was sufficient to explain the appetite for nutritious food (Garcia et al. 1974).

There are indeed very few materials that laboratory rats can be reliably induced to ingest without food deprivation. Even the single complete food on which they are brought up and maintained is eaten in very variable small amounts, unless it has been withheld for several hours (Le Magnen and Tallon 1966). Rats will drink strong solutions of salt when they are in sodium deficit but not otherwise. Only a very sweet solution of saccharin is consumed reliably on first access by an unfasted rat. Hence, the volume consumed of a novel saccharin solution was and still is used to measure the conditioning of aversion by association with poisoning or unfamiliar drug effects (Garcia et al. 1955; Massei and Cowan 2002; Verendeev and Riley 2012). Saccharin has been mixed with sour or bitter agents in order to suppress its intake sufficiently for nutrient-conditioned preferences to be seen (Pain and Booth 1968; Booth and Davis 1973).

The distinctive taste shared by saccharin, sucrose, and glucose was once regarded as the key to scientific theory of food and water intake, its neuroscience, and its societal roles (Pfaffmann 1960, 1964; Pfaffmann et al. 1977). The blow-fly's consumption of sugar provided an impressively simple model (Dethier 1962). When its crop is empty, the fly extends its proboscis to secrete fluid onto a lump of sugar and sucks up the solution until the crop is sufficiently distended; then the meal stops.

A solution of saccharin or sugar was treated as the model food and drink for generalist feeders as well. This was despite the fact that major foods (for wild or laboratory rats or for people) do not taste sweet at all. The model of responses to a single taste cannot address the fact that all foods and drinks have other sensed characteristics such as shape, color, opacity, odor, other tastes, and a great variety of textures to touch by the fingers, the eating utensil, and the mouth. Yet, when laboratory research began on the effects of physiological manipulations on sensory factors in human appetite for food, the test material was purely saccharin or glucose dissolved in water (e.g., Cabanac et al. 1968; Cabanac and Duclaux 1970a,b; Thompson et al. 1976; Thompson and Campbell 1977; Blundell and Hill 1986). Unflavored sugar water is not liked even by children unless they were given it as a baby (Beauchamp and Moran 1982). In order for there to be ingestive appetite, a learnt sensory context for sweetness is needed.

12.3.2 Ingestive Responses to Sweet Solutions

What then does a sweet taste do to ingestion? We and other omnivores are indeed born with a reflexive reaction, "the sweeter, the better" (Tatzer et al. 1985). Sweetness in itself speeds and shapes suckling in babies (Crook and Lipsitt 1976). Sweetness gets young children to consume new foods and drinks. Plainly, though, nobody could ever have lived on sugar alone or on ripe fruit or honey.

The story becomes more complex if the tested sweet taste comes from glucose (the sugar in mammalian blood) or other sugars (monosaccharides or disaccharides). When solutions are presented one at a time, cumulative intake increases with concentration only to a point: considerably less is ingested of a strong solution of sugar than of a weak solution. This effect is readily explained by an appetite-suppressing effect that develops shortly after ingestion of stronger solutions of sugar has started (McCleary 1953). This postingestional effect has often been assumed to be metabolic or caloric (e.g., Jacobs 1958, 1962; Jacobs and Sharma 1969; Cabanac and Duclaux 1970a). Nevertheless, there is clear evidence that the inhibition from concentrated sugars is osmotic (Smith and Duffy 1957; Shuford 1959; Smith 1966).

Hence, to understand the effect of sweet taste on ingestion, we need to use a molecule that has no other effect than sweet taste or at least to present a sweet sugar for such a short time that the ingestive behavior is not influenced by after-effects. Brief tests of rates of licking of glucose solution in rats showed a clear increase in rate with concentration (Davis 1973). A laboratory rat is provided with water all its life through a spout from an inverted bottle. Hence, it drinks by wipes of the tongue across the opening of the spout that draws water out into the mouth. These licks become as rapid as possible with rests every second or so. The greater rate of licking averaged over a minute or so induced by a stronger sweet taste comes from a reduction of the time between the bursts of licking at a fast fixed rate (Davis 1973).

This facilitatory effect of sweet taste on ingestion increases through all the tested levels if they are presented briefly one after the other in sequences randomized across rats: the sweeter the stimulus, the stronger the response. That is, the graph of response vigor on stimulus intensity is monotonic (unpeaked). The function is unlikely to be linear, however. It might follow a curve similar to that constructed by Beidler (1954) for responses to tastes in general. This allows for proportionately weaker responses to undetectably low levels and to high levels approaching saturation of the taste receptor. (A similar receptor-binding function fits data for odor as well; see Chastrette et al. 1998.)

Such monotonicity is the defining characteristic of an unlearned reflex mechanism. The stronger the stimulus, the more vigorous the response (Figure 12.1).

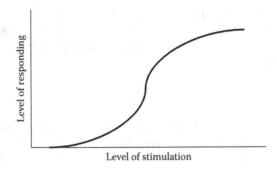

FIGURE 12.1 Dependence of the vigor of responding on the intensity of stimulation in a reflex mechanism. The monotonic shape of this output/input function is not mathematically determinate, but the vigor of the response rises continuously with the strength of stimulation, from detection of the stimulus at a low level to the approach to saturation of the receptors at high levels.

12.3.3 Reflex-Ingestive Movements to Sweet Taste

The newborn infants of omnivorous and frugivorous mammalian species show a fixed action pattern in response to the taste of sugar (Steiner 1977; Steiner et al. 2001). These movements center on configurations of the tongue that facilitate the transfer of milk from the breast to the throat. The tongue moves forward as far as necessary to squeeze the nipple against the upper gum, expressing milk as the tongue is drawn back into the mouth. In the absence of a nipple, this movement can be visible as a central protrusion of the tongue. The tongue also rolls into a U shape that helps to confine the milk to a flow directly into the pharynx (Iwayama and Eishima 1997). This curling of the tongue may also be visible if the lips are parted.

These ingestive movements can be observed when a sweet fluid is infused into the mouth of a rat (Grill and Norgren 1978). Furthermore, if the subcortical regions of the brain critical to ingestion are disrupted pharmacologically, the infusate is not swallowed but dribbles out of the mouth (Berridge et al. 1989). This is consistent with other evidence that the elicitation of these movements by a sweet taste can be mediated by the brainstem alone. Nevertheless, the sweet taste also acts on a part of the diencephalic region activated by ordinary food (Pecina and Berridge 2005). Hence, the sweet taste elicits innate ingestive movements via a subset of the general mechanisms of eating and drinking.

12.3.4 Sensory Motivation without Pleasure or Reward

These reflexive movements of rats and human neonates in response to sweet fluid have been interpreted as a sign of pleasure (Berridge and Grill 1983; Steiner et al. 2001) and not just as sensory facilitation of suckling. That separation of hedonic experience from the propensity to ingest was then extended to human adults on the basis of their scores for *liking* or *pleasantness*. Yet, sensual pleasure cannot be separated from pleasant eating or drinking merely by differently worded ratings (Booth et al. 1982; Booth 1990, 1991, 2009a; see Section 12.6 on the vocabulary of preferences). Distinguishing a pleasurable emotion from the usual pleasant motivation in adults would depend on the unlearnt ingestive movement reflex to sweetness breaking through a lifetime built norm for a food's particular levels of sweetness and other sensed characteristics (Booth 1991).

That dissociation between the reflex and normal learnt performance has recently been achieved by testing verbal responses to the appropriate combinations of stimuli involving different levels of sweet taste (Booth et al. 2010). Signs of the subjective experience of sensual pleasure were indeed seen at a level of sweetness far in excess of that tolerated in the familiar juice in which it was incorporated. Whether a newborn baby or an adult rat is capable of generating such an elaborate private world may be doubted. Adults are built to treat infants sympathetically regardless of what is actually going on in the latter's very young minds.

12.3.5 Learnt Preferences for Levels of Sweetness

Evidence against all preferences for sweetness being reflexively monotonic was first clearly seen in rats given a continuous choice between solutions of 10 and 35 g of glucose in 100 mL: the rats started by drinking more each day from the sweeter solution but soon switched to the less sweet solution and stuck with it (Jacobs 1958). That remarkable observation was readily replicated (Experiment 1 in Booth et al. 1972; see Figure 12.2, leftmost group). The unlearnt reflexive increase in preference with concentration of saccharin or sucrose (Figure 12.1) was also seen in initial choices in all subsequent experiments on other pairs of solutions: each group of rats started by drinking more of the sweeter of the two solutions (Figure 12.2, upper row of panels).

The replication of the switch from 35% to 10% glucose was followed up by a long series of experiments testing various explanations in terms of a fixed mechanism, such as suppression of sweet palatability by sugar satiety, and a more specific proposal that the acceptance of sweet taste is an innate appetite for calories that is progressively sated by consumption of glucose (Cabanac and Duclaux 1970a). None of those theories gained support from this reversal of "the sweeter, the better" (Figure 12.1).

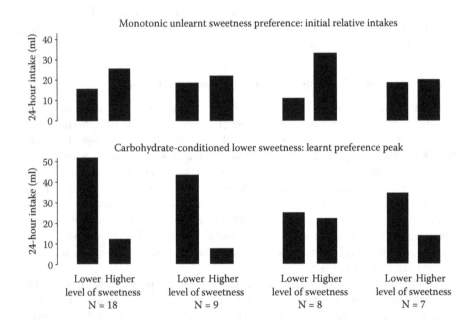

FIGURE 12.2 Dependence of the vigor of responding on the intensity of stimulation in a learnt acceptance response to a sensory stimulus, contrasted with the initially unlearnt reflex. The response was group mean 24-h intake volume of each of two simultaneously presented solutions having different levels of sweetness from saccharin and monosaccharides, disaccharides, and oligosaccharides. Greater intake (preference) was reinforced by the postingestional action of carbohydrate content (even at low concentrations). Less intake (aversion) was reinforced by osmotic effects at high concentrations of the monosaccharides glucose and fructose and the disaccharides sucrose and maltose. The initial gradient of preference for stronger glucose was already somewhat reduced by some learning within the first 24 h to prefer the lower concentration. (Data from Booth, D.A. et al., *Journal of Comparative and Physiological Psychology,* 78:485–512, 1972 in Figures 1, 12, 13 and 14.)

Finally, the two solutions were redesigned to test for explanations in terms of learning from associations between taste and postingestional consequences. Evidence was found for two new examples of classical conditioning, both starting to occur in the first hours of continuous access to the choice between 10% and 35% glucose (Booth et al. 1972).

12.3.6 CONDITIONED TASTE AVERSION

One mechanism is the conditioning of sensory aversion by osmotic effects. A 35% solution of glucose is extremely hypertonic. (A mere 5% of glucose generates the same osmotic pressure as body fluids.) Hence, even if the solution is somewhat diluted by saliva and digestive juices, it is still strong enough to draw water out of any cell that it touches. This creates rasping at innervated tissues of the throat, retention of ingested and digestive fluids in the stretch-sensitive stomach, and osmotic expansion of the volume in the duodenal lumen. Disaccharides such as sucrose and maltose are digested to the monosaccharides glucose and fructose inside the wall of the duodenum, doubling the osmotic pressure there from the sugars in the lumen. These postgastric osmotic signals are detected by sensory endings of the vagus nerve in the walls of the duodenum and the portal vein (Hunt and Pathak 1960; Hunt and Stubbs 1975; Kelly 1980; Mei and Garnier 1986).

The adverse effects of free sugars (Booth 1979; Booth et al. 2011b) classically condition an aversion to their sweet taste in the mouth, and/or they may reinforce avoidance of the solution that provides that sweet stimulus, which is discriminative of the upcoming osmotic punishment. This learnt sensory rejection may be independent of context such as food deprivation or recent feeding, as the suppressant effect of poisoning on saccharin intake can be (Garcia and Koelling 1966).

12.3.7 CONDITIONED TASTE PREFERENCE

The other mechanism involved in the switch from 35% to 10% glucose is postingestional conditioning of sensory preference. The wall of the duodenum has other receptors on the nerve endings of the afferent vagus that are chemically specific to glucose (Mei 1985). The same structures as gustatory receptors in the mouth have recently been found in the intestinal wall, although these receptors function in local regulation of glucose absorption (Mace et al. 2009). Glucose also stimulates chemospecific and metabolomic sensitivities in the brain and in other tissues that it reaches after absorption from the small intestine into the circulation (Levin et al. 1999). Stimulation from glucose infused directly into the stomach strongly reinforces preference for any flavor that accompanies or shortly precedes it through the mouth (Sclafani and Nissenbaum 1988; Sclafani 1995). Hence, the tastes of both 10% and 35% glucose become even more preferred than before learning. However, the punishment by the osmotic effects of 35% glucose is stronger than the reinforcement by its glucose-specific effects, and so a net aversion or avoidance of the stronger solution is seen in the relative intakes (Figure 12.2, bottom left-hand choice).

Glucose-conditioned preferences were revealed in a design that avoided immediate osmotic effects by use of isotonic or hypotonic solutions, e.g., no

more than 5% glucose or 10% sucrose or maltose, or of the soluble starch product, maltodextrin, in which the glucose molecules are bound to each other in
short chains. A 10%, 35%, or even 50% solution of maltodextrin is hypotonic (in
a version of that food product which contained only approximately 3% free glucose and 5% maltose). A stronger conditioned preference was seen for whichever
strength of sweet taste was associated with the high concentration of maltodextrin (Experiments 12–14 in Booth et al. 1972; the key data are redrawn here in
Figure 12.2).

When the stronger sweet taste was given to the more concentrated carbohydrate, the learnt slope was steeper than the slope of the initial innate preference
for the sweeter solution (data not shown here; see Figure 12.1). A qualitatively
stronger piece of evidence for glucose-conditioned sweet taste preference was provided by greater intake of the solution with the less sweet taste after pairing with the
effects of more concentrated maltodextrin, reversing the initial innate slope (Figure
12.2, right-hand three choices, lower panel). The same reversal was produced even
by the mildly hypertonic 10% glucose alongside 3% glucose made to taste sweeter
with saccharin (Experiment 12 in Booth et al. 1972).

12.4   LEARNT PEAK OF PREFERENCE FOR LEVEL OF SWEETENER

12.4.1   PREFERRED STRENGTHS OF SWEET TASTE

The most important aspect of those findings for the whole field of the chemical
senses and nutrition is that the learnt preferences (and aversions) are not for a taste as
such. The acquired acceptance is not for a sweet compound regardless of its concentration. The learnt sensory motivation of ingestion is from the particular level of the
sweet taste that has been reinforced by some biologically or socially significant event
or that has become familiar within a context of ingestion. Every detail of the rest of
this chapter follows from that single general fact.

Both the conditioned stimuli in these experiments were sweet (Figure 12.2). The
learnt difference in preference, whether in the innate or reverse direction, is between
two levels of sweet taste presented side by side. Therefore, the learning in each case
must be for a particular range or level of sweet taste and not for the sweet taste in
general.

12.4.2   MOST PREFERRED STRENGTH

The level of sweet taste that is ingested in greater amount after learning (lower panel
in Figure 12.2) is likely to be the most preferred level if different levels were tested
in short-term tests of relative acceptance. That is, the intake would go down at higher
levels than the conditioned level as well as go down at lower levels, as in the innate
reflex. A decrease in preference with a less sweet taste occurs with the unlearnt
reflex, but this decrease on the higher side as well as on the lower side of the learnt
level is a characteristic of learnt stimuli of all sorts, usually lacking a reflex.

The above implies another difference between unlearnt and learnt preferences.
The unlearnt reflex has smaller responses at lower levels, at all levels from the

highest to the lowest. In contrast, a learnt decline in responses with weaker stimuli starts below whatever level has been conditioned.

This principle of maximum response at the learnt level of a stimulus was established in the early years of research into learning processes. The learnt response became weaker as the strengths of test stimulus were made greater or smaller (Hovland 1937; Hull 1947). The learning was not general to all levels of the stimulus. Indeed, the generalization became weaker and weaker the further the tested level was from the trained level, either up or down. Another way of describing this gradient of decreased generalization is the detection of increasing dissimilarity between trained and tested stimulus levels (Shepard 1958).

Hence, measuring only the strength of a preference tells us nothing about what is going on. The variation of degree of preference with the amount of stimulation needs to be measured. Then, we know something about what the preference is for. Indeed, if we collect adequate data, we can estimate the most preferred level of the stimulus, i.e., which amount was trained (without ever observing the learning process), and even how sensitive the preference response is to the differences in the level of the stimulus.

Such characteristics of learnt acceptance of stimuli in foods and drinks are a foundation for a complete science of the sensory, somatic, and social controls of ingestive behavior. The rest of this chapter provides examples across the major chemosensory influences on the selection of mouthfuls.

12.4.3 SOMATIC CONTEXTS OF SWEET PREFERENCE

When a single sweet solution is presented to a rat that is strong enough in saccharin (0.2%) to elicit reflexive ingestion, the inclusion of a little glucose (3%—so little that it can barely be tasted on its own) conditions the preference for the sweet taste so powerfully that the rat rapidly comes to drink half its body weight of the solution each day (Valenstein et al. 1967). This extreme fluid intake does not occur with higher concentrations of glucose because of the immediate appetite-suppressant effects of their osmotic strength (Shuford 1959; Smith 1966), ahead of its associative conditioning of aversion to the taste. However, when the free glucose is replaced by its bound form in a soluble breakdown product of starch (maltodextrin), there are no longer immediate osmotic effects in the mouth and throat; osmotic effects can only arise after digestion frees the glucose. Then, the conditioned preference for the specific taste given to the solution induces increasingly large intake during a limited period of access to the single solution (Booth and Davis 1973; see Figure 12.3).

The specificity to the preference-conditioned taste was shown by providing a brief choice at the start of the daily test period between tastes previously paired with different concentrations of carbohydrate. In the 5-min choice period, more was drunk of the taste that had previously been paired with a high concentration of maltodextrin than of the taste paired with a low concentration of sugar and starch (Figure 12.3, lower panel). This showed that the larger amount of carbohydrate associatively conditioned the greater sensory preference.

Nevertheless, maltodextrin is eventually digested to glucose. First, maltose is released by amylases in the lumen of the duodenum. That disaccharide is then

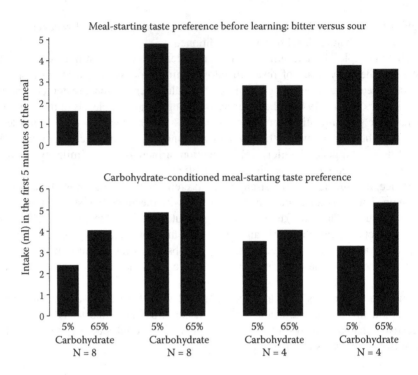

FIGURE 12.3 Meal-starting taste-specific intakes (mL in the first 5 min of 30-min access) at the start and end of pairing one taste with 65% carbohydrate (low-glucose maltodextrin, with no immediate osmotic effect) in 12 30-min test sessions (meals) and the other taste with 5% carbohydrate (3% starch gel, 2% glucose) in another 12 sessions (although the final difference began to emerge by the second to fourth sessions). The two solutions had similarly sweet tastes from glucose supplemented by maltose or saccharin and were differentiated by either citric acid at 200 mg/100 mL or quinine sulfate at 0.5 mg/100 mL, balanced across rats. Rats generally drank very little of each taste in the first 5 min of the initial sessions, and so the starting intakes (upper panel) are taken from the average of the first pair of sessions with substantial intake. Intakes in the final sessions (lower panel) showed that 65% maltodextrin conditioned a stronger preference to the initially aversive taste mixture than did the 5% carbohydrate. (From Booth, D.A., and J.D. Davis. *Physiology and Behavior*, 11:23–29, 1973.)

broken down to glucose on the inner side of the wall of the duodenum. Hence, the 65% maltodextrin could produce a high concentration of glucose at osmoreceptors as well as glucoreceptors in the wall of the duodenum and in the portal vein from the small intestine to the liver. If that occurred while a flavor was being consumed, the result could be a conditioned aversion.

In these experiments, however, the same flavor is being presented throughout the meal. The net effect of glucose-conditioned preference and osmotically conditioned aversion remains a preference at least at the start of the meal (Figure 12.4). Therefore, some other stimulus is needed to predict the transient osmotic signals from digestion of maltodextrin. The most reliable contrast with the start of the meal could be the amount in the stomach during the release of maltose in the lumen and glucose in the wall of the duo-denum. Hence, the relatively mild punishing effect of transient high osmotic strength of

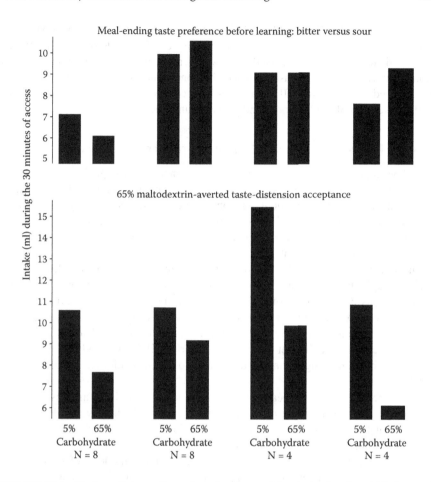

FIGURE 12.4 Taste–satiety configured meal volumes (30-min intakes in mL) before and after learning, showing a switch from larger meals on the thick and perhaps sweeter 65% maltodextrin to smaller meals (with taste the only difference, both tested in 35% carbohydrate), while the preference for 65% paired taste persist in choice tests between two bottles simultaneously. The switch is explicable only by the taste being configured with satiety signals, such as a substantial volume in the stomach or a decline in ghrelin secretion and that taste–satiety combination becoming averted by the delayed osmotic signal after duodenal digestion of maltodextrin (the conditioned satiety of Booth 1972b, 1985, 2009a, 2013). These meal sizes come from the same experiments as the meal-start data in Figure 12.3 (comparable with the design in Booth 1972a). (From Booth, D.A., and J.D. Davis. *Physiology and Behavior*, 11:23–29, 1973; see Figures 1 and 3.)

glucose from concentrated maltodextrin could counter much of the preference conditioned by glucose if it were tied to the combination of that level of sweet taste and a stimulus specific to the later part of a meal, such as a neural or hormonal signal from a relatively full stomach (Booth 1972a; Booth and Davis 1973; Booth et al. 1976).

In other words, this osmotically reduced facilitation (or actual inhibition) of acceptance is a learnt response to a level of gastric distension as well as to a level of sweetness (Booth 1985, 2009b, 2013). Therefore, for this interoceptive stimulus also, there should be a decline in learnt response on either side of the conditioned level of distension. Ingestion itself may well remain inhibited, nevertheless, even though distension has increased beyond the conditioned level, and so its satiating effect is reduced. The overall satiation is then coming from postgastric signals as well (Kissileff et al. 2008; Booth and Kissileff under review).

12.4.4   EVIDENCE THAT HUMAN SENSORY PREFERENCES ARE LEARNT

The above analysis implies its inverse. If a preference response peaks at a particular level of a stimulus, this is evidence that the preference has somehow been learned. That conclusion follows without any observation of the learning process. Such research into the human acquisition of preferences for novel materials is needed to elucidate factors that support or disrupt the learning process but not to establish that the preference has been learnt.

Indeed, demonstrating the learning of food preferences is a thankless task in adults brought up on a varied diet and flexible eating practices. The experimenter's manipulations have to build on a lifetime of learning. A successful experiment is likely to have exploited a higher-order mechanism for readily changing preferences rather than demonstrating the existence of a basic mechanism, such as habituation or reinforcement (see Kerkhof et al. 2009). Similarly, failures to condition preference can be attributed to designs that are unrealistic to routine choices (see Durlach et al. 2002).

Nevertheless, adequate measurement of the sensory basis of an existing preference can reveal something of the original learning whether by familiarization, conditioning, reward, or attitude transfer. The level of the stimulus at maximum preference points to the material and situation that the child or adult has learnt about. Widely available versions of a food or drink may differ in the level of sweetness or some other sensory factor, or in timing within the meal or other somatic or social factors. The most preferred sweetness and the appropriate stage in the meal are both liable to be the result of the use of the variant of the food that has that sweetness in that position within meals (Conner et al. 1988b).

12.4.5   PEAK OF LEARNT FACILITATION BY ANY SENSORY FACTOR

In the above experiments in rats (Booth and Davis 1973; see Figures 12.3 and 12.4), the two conditioned tastes at the start and end of ingestion had a similar level of sweet taste, and so, that was the location of the peak of the learnt sweet preference. However, citric acid was added to one sweet solution and quinine dissolved in the other in order to enable the rats to predict the distinction between their consequences. (The higher carbohydrate concentration was paired with the sweet-and-sour taste or the bitter-sweet taste in equal numbers of rats.) The implication is that both the sweet taste and the sour or bitter taste had each acquired its own peak preference level as we can see from later human data (Figure 12.5).

Mixtures of sweet and sour taste compounds commonly occur in fruits and in drinks prepared from them. When the levels of sweet taste and sour taste are varied

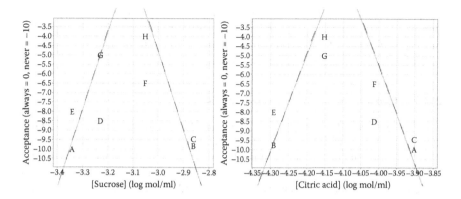

FIGURE 12.5 One assessor's degrees of preference for mixtures of sucrose and citric acid in a familiar orange-flavored still drink, plotted separately for the independently varied levels of sugar and acid. Sequence of presentation was from mixture A first to mixture H last. Ratios of tastant concentration are fitted to a symmetrical peak of preference rated from *always choose* (scored as zero) to *never choose* (–10). Linear fits account for much less of the variance. (Replotting of raw, unfolded data in Booth, D.A., *Psychology of Nutrition*. Bristol, PA: Taylor & Francis, 1994, Figure 5.3.)

independently of each other in a familiar orange-flavored drink, it becomes obvious that the learnt personal ideal for sour taste has a peak just as the learnt sweet taste preference does (Figure 12.5). The same presumably happens for the aroma and color of a breakfast drink, since an ideal point (IP) appears for the strength of a breakfast drink composed of flavoring and coloring as well as sugar and acid (McBride and Booth 1986).

Therefore, the default position has to be that any sensory facilitation of ingestion, including by tastes and smells, must have been acquired by personal experience. Indeed, preferences are likely to be so well learnt that changes in preference will be hard to induce in the laboratory or in life. The idea of acquiring a completely new preference is probably a misconception. In theoretical principle, even just trying a novel food or drink requires a preparatory context or some sampling incidental to existing habits. Once the shift in sensory stimulation has been experienced, its learning might be fast if there is a background to extend; otherwise, the learnt preference might be weak and its acquisition slow. Early laboratory evidence of learnt appetitive food stimuli in animals emerged only after prolonged training (Booth and Miller 1969) unless a single exposure was very intense (Booth and Simson 1971).

12.4.6 LEARNT LIKINGS FOR LEVELS OF BITTERNESS

The unlearnt reflex movements to a bitter taste are expulsive, such as gaping in rats and human neonates and spitting in older children. The expulsive reflex movements are suppressed, however, when the bitter substance is in an already familiar material that has become acceptable. Adults acquire ingestive preferences and appetites for intensely bitter materials, when the level of bitter taste is appropriate to the context of other sensed features such as aroma, color, and temperature. Strong coffee is a prime example. In some people, the learnt reaction may be a purely sensory preference, extending to the decaffeinated version of the usual brand of coffee. Nevertheless, drinking coffee can be the expression of a whole appetite for caffeine, involving expected pharmacological effect and current social context.

12.4.7 CONDITIONED APPETITE FOR CAFFEINE

An individual's adenosine neurotransmitter receptors can become adapted to high circulating levels of caffeine. The heavy user of caffeinated drinks may be sensitive to a decline in concentration in the blood when no caffeine has been ingested for several hours. Restoration of caffeine levels by consumption of a distinctively flavored caffeine-containing material can then condition a preference for that material. This caffeine-conditioned sensory preference is greater when blood levels of caffeine have declined again (Yeomans et al. 2000). That is, that material's consumption has become an appetite specific to the combination of the sensory characteristic of the material and a circulating concentration of caffeine below the adapted level.

12.4.8 IDEAL POINT FOR BITTERNESS OF CAFFEINE IN OWN COFFEE

As with sweet-tasting compounds, the learnt preference or appetite for the bitter taste of coffee (whether or not reinforced by the pharmacological effects of caffeine) proves to be an acceptance that peaks at a particular level of the coffee's bitter taste and not for the bitter taste at any intensity, either higher or lower. This ideal point (IP) for bitterness in the personally familiar drink of coffee was demonstrated in an experiment looking for variation with age in taste sensitivity to the differences in the concentration of caffeine (Booth et al. 1989, 2011c).

The roasting of coffee beans generates many bitter compounds that add to the taste of the caffeine already in the beans. Thus, the level of bitterness can be varied by adding different amounts of caffeine to a decaffeinated product. When the test session is spent on mouthfuls of the drinker's usual coffee with widely varying caffeine contents, the gustatory effects of caffeine are disconfounded from its pharmacological effects during or after the session, as well as from any expectation of later effects of ingested caffeine if the assessor believes that different strengths of roast are being compared rather than different levels of caffeine.

Acceptance of samples of the assessor's usual coffee varied only in caffeine content always peaked somewhere between the lowest and highest levels tested (Figure 12.6). Hence, the preference or appetite for the bitter-tasting drink had been acquired. It was not, for example, a reversal in direction of a monotonic reflex mechanism from expulsive to ingestive.

12.4.9 DEVELOPMENT OF PREFERENCE FOR BITTER FOODS AND DRINKS

Individuals' IPs and differential sensitivities for the taste of caffeine varied widely with no clear relation to age group or gender (Booth et al. 1989). It is important to note that those who had the lowest IPs or greatest sensitivities were still habitually

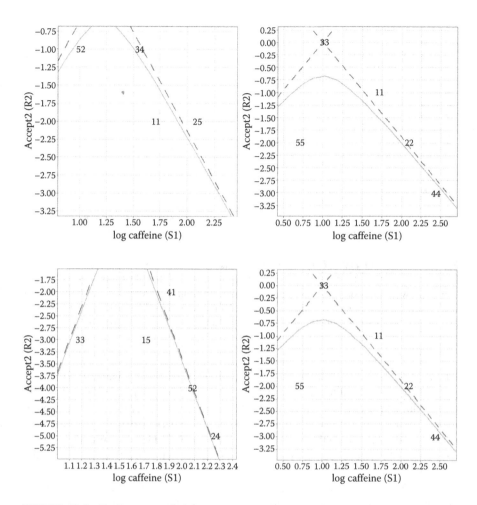

FIGURE 12.6 Preference peak (*always accept* = 0) for caffeine in the individual's usual coffee for two assessors at each quartile of that ideal level of coffee (total *N* = 52). Upper panels: lower quartile. Middle panels: median. Lower panels (on the next page): upper quartile. Caffeine concentrations in the $\log_{10}$ mg/cup (150 mL). Calculated by CoPro tool from data collected by Mark Conner for Booth et al. (1989). The group distribution of the personal ranges of IP was reported by Booth et al. (2011c).

(*Continued*)

drinking caffeinated coffee. Furthermore, IPs were not substantially correlated with sensitivities.

There is indeed no reason to expect adults' likings for coffee to be related to sensitivity in discriminating or detecting bitter-tasting compounds or indeed coffee's strongly sour constituents. There are many ways of preparing a drink of coffee and therefore at least as many routes to growing to like one or more of those versions. Young people may start drinking coffee with sugar or milk, or as a weak infusion,

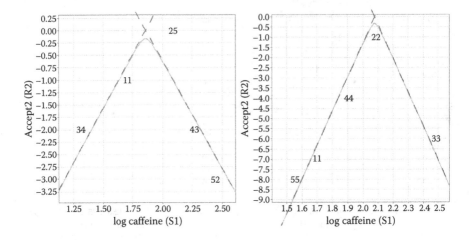

FIGURE 12.6 (CONTINUED) Preference peak (*always accept* = 0) for caffeine in the individual's usual coffee for two assessors at each quartile of that ideal level of coffee (total N = 52). Two panels on this page: upper quartile. Caffeine concentrations in the $\log_{10}$ mg/cup (150 mL). Calculated by CoPro tool from data collected by Mark Conner for Booth et al. (1989). The group distribution of the personal ranges of IP was reported by Booth et al. (2011c).

but in some societies, there is no standard adult version. Personal exploration or peers' habits may lead to strong infusions with or without sugar and/or milk, mild roasts with a little or a lot of milk, or other variants. Availability may shape a habit of using ground coffee or instant coffee. Good or bad experiences with pharmacological effects of caffeine on the brain or the kidneys and bladder may affect the choice of strength of coffee, and hence the preferred taste, as well as the frequency of coffee drinking.

The same diversity of options applies to the bitter tastes of chocolate, grapefruit, and cheese. The intensity of taste (and aroma) of a mature Cheddar or a blue cheese, which tastes very bitter to an individual, may lead to great enjoyment of a small piece with butter on a cracker, with a mild cheese being quite unacceptable. The main disruption to the normal acquisition of liking for a bitter-tasting food may be that the initially sampled taste is too strong and does not have any of the incentives that others have to try that food again, such as participation with peers or carers.

In short, even though bitter agents are innately rejected more vigorously at higher concentrations, familiarity and reinforcement of some bitter taste in a particular food or drink will create the most preferred level for bitter taste in that item when consumed in its usual context. *A fortiori*, the individual difference in inborn reflexes to a taste need bear no general relationships to preferences for foods having that taste.

12.4.10 6-*N*-PROPYLTHIOURACIL AND FOOD PREFERENCES

The principle of diversity of developmental pathways applies to any source of stimulation to the taste receptor family for plant poisons. A minority of people inherit a strong sensitivity to the bitterness of the compound, 6-*n*-propylthiouracil, commonly known as PROP (Bartoshuk et al. 1994).

It has been widely assumed that such people must dislike foods that stimulate the same part of the large family of bitter receptors. In fact, the evidence is far from conclusive that PROP sensitivity always puts people off bitter foods for life. An undergraduate project screened for high sensitivity to PROP by the standard filter paper test and found that such people tended to like medium-strength Cheddar cheese better than those who did not taste the PROP on the paper (Stroud and Booth 1999). Indeed, a simple cross-sectional relation of PROP sensitivity to aversion to bitter foods is far from clear in the literature. The chances that sensitivity to PROP relates systematically to nutritional health through dietary habits are therefore quite remote.

There are undoubtedly genetic influences on human behavior, as well as environmental factors. Nevertheless, genetic expression interacts strongly with environmental exposure continuously throughout life. Hence, a search for simple associations is highly questionable. Rather than the simplistic model of genetic determinism, it could be more productive to search for genetic vulnerabilities and environmental stressors with a view to specifying the variety of more prevalent interactions among them (see Rutter 2008).

12.4.11 Human Preference for the Taste of Salt

Many nonhuman omnivores have an innate appetite for sodium chloride (NaCl) (Denton 1982). That is, when the animal in the wild goes into sodium deficit, it seeks out materials tasting of salt and consumes them. Laboratory rats can learn ways to get salt before ever becoming sodium-deficient (Krieckhaus and Wolf 1968).

At birth, human infants are relatively insensitive to the taste of salt. Yet, within a few months, they are capable of discriminating between the levels of salt in human milk and in a supplementary or weaning food such as cereal or mashed potato, and preferring the level of salt they have been exposed to, with both abilities measured by how much they eat in a test session (Harris and Booth 1987; Harris et al. 1991). These findings have been replicated in a larger group of 6-month-olds using a contrast with exposure to fruit, which is much lower in salt content (Stein et al. 2012).

By young adulthood at the latest, preferences have developed for the particular levels of the taste of salt in each familiar food, including bread, mashed potatoes, and soups of chicken or tomato (Booth et al. 1983; Shepherd et al. 1984; Conner et al. 1988a). (These are all prepared foods with diverse conventional levels of salt; hence there is no possibility that each of these most preferred levels is innate.) Furthermore, there is a very sharp peak of personal preference when plotted against salt concentration in a test food close in other characteristics to the individual's usual version, as for the taste of sugar in a familiar food or drink (Figure 12.4). Adequately refined designs to identify increased preference for salt during sodium deficit, whether innate or learnt, should measure each individual's salt preference function and look for within-subject rises in IPs and/or increases in tolerance slope (Conner et al. 1988a). Individuals' preference scores by themselves cannot show what is going on, especially in tests on salt solutions out of the context of a familiar food (Cowart and Beauchamp 1986).

There is some evidence in human adults of temporarily increased intake of familiar higher-sodium foods after depletion of sodium ions by prolonged sweating (Leshem et al. 2008). That also could have been based on earlier learning from eating salty foods while body fluids were depleted. Any permanent enhancement of human salt intake by sodium depletion appears to be limited to the period around birth (Leshem 2009).

12.4.12 Tastes, Smells, Colors, and Textures

The evidence from rats and people therefore supports a generalization to any sensory factor in an individual preference for a particular item. The mechanisms for acquiring a maximum preference for a specific level of sweetness in each food and drink in the usual context of consumption are activated for any sensed characteristic of the familiar option. Indeed, also any somatic or social signal that is familiar or has been reinforced has an IP for each context in which that signal occurs.

The chemical senses extend beyond taste and smell. Irritation (mild pain) is also chemospecific (Dessirier et al. 2000). Irritative agents in foods and drinks that are liked at particular levels range from carbonation to ginger, pepper, and chili. The theory is that each substance has a peak-preferred level for each person in each familiar fizzy drink or spicy food. Color is a key part of flavor as ordinarily experienced and can be regarded as the photochemical sense: the retinal pigments differ in amino acid sequence at their photon-sensitive sites. Consumers' choices cluster around the intensity of hue given to a manufactured product (Conner et al. 1994).

The physical texture (mouthfeel) of a food or drink is also often included in everyday impressions of flavor. For example, the astringent *taste* of tea is in fact the texture of salivary proteins denatured by the polyphenols in the brew (Breslin et al. 1993; Horne et al. 2002).

Many other textures depend to a considerable extent on chemical composition, although purely physical factors are sometimes crucial, e.g., the distribution of fat globule sizes in dairy cream (Richardson and Booth 1993; Richardson et al. 1993; see Booth 2005). Nevertheless, the same principle applies. For example, each regular user of light cream has an ideal level of viscosity and does not act as though "the thicker, the better" (unless they really prefer superheavy cream in their coffee or butter in their tea in the Tibetan tradition). Users of cream in whole milk yogurt are also liable to have the most preferred range for the diameters of the fat globules. Similarly, the crispness of lettuce or the crunchiness of a type of cookie has an ideal level of each physical component of the heard or felt characteristic for each user, depending on the experience of the particular food (Vickers 1984; Booth et al. 2003a,b,c).

12.5 MISSING THE [IDEAL] POINT

12.5.1 Group-Averaged Scores for Preference

Failure to attend to the relationship of degree of preference to the amounts of chemical stimulation has repeatedly disrupted progress in research into the role of taste or smell in nutrition. The reality needs to be faced that each individual has the most preferred level of a sensory factor in a context of food choice and a particular sensitivity to deviations from that IP. Those are the characteristics of ingestive behavior that should be profiled across people and foods, as illustrated throughout the remainder of this chapter. Instead, the raw scores for quantities of pleasantness or ranks of liking have been averaged across groups. Worse, aversion has been confounded with preference by putting unpleasantness or dislike into those scores or rankings of preference using the term *pleasant* or *like*.

Yet, this poor measurement of degree of preference is not the most serious problem with these research areas. Whatever measure of degree of preference is used, it is the influences on preference that are relevant and not just how much a food is preferred.

12.5.2 FOOD PREFERENCES AND PROP GENETICS

Most of the research into genetic variation in the bitter taste of PROP (mentioned in Section 12.4.10) has been based on average scores for the degree of preference for each named food. Such scores convey no information about the contribution of bitter taste or any other factor to the individual's present acceptance of that food (by whatever pathways it developed). A simple illustration of the scientific use of preference scores was given above for the taste of caffeine. The IPs estimated in that experiment were distributed in a pattern reminiscent of that observed in much more complicated measures using the unscientific concept of an absolute threshold. That pattern of most preferred levels is as expected for a division of the population into tasters and nontasters of PROP, with a subcategory of generic supertasters (Booth et al. 2011c).

A realistic approach would start with specifying each individual's current frequency of use of foods having a substantial bitter taste, with a view to identifying foods eaten by a sufficiently high proportion of the sample to be useful for genetic analysis. Then, the influence of a constituent stimulating a broad profile of bitter taste receptors on the liking of each widely eaten food would be measured using samples that differed only in concentration of that constituent. This sensory contribution to preference for each of several common foods in each person is measured as the mathematically independent values of differential sensitivity (not detection sensitivity) and IP (not preference score). These are the two phenotypic characteristics for each food (or a multivariate if highly correlated) that should be used for genetic screening and differentiations between PROP tasters and nontasters (compare studies such as Ditschun and Guinard 2004; Chang et al. 2006; Tepper et al. 2008).

12.5.3 FOOD PREFERENCES AND OBESITY

The increasing prevalence of obesity has often been blamed on the attractiveness of sugars and fats. However, the leanest people eat attractive foods. So this attack on the commercial suppliers requires evidence that fatter people have stronger likings for the sensed characteristics of sugary and fatty foods.

12.5.3.1 Sweet Taste

Way before claiming that sugar is addictive, we first have to see if widely consumed foods or drinks are more preferred when given the sensed characteristics of extra sugar. As should be clear by now, this is an ill-formulated question, since there is not a one-to-one relation between combinations of sugar with other constituents and degrees of preference.

Whenever one sensory feature, but nothing else, is varied in a familiar food, each person is found to have acquired the most preferred level. This was established first for salt in soup and bread (Booth et al. 1983; Shepherd et al. 1984; Conner et al. 1988b). Then, it was shown many times for the sugar content of a variety of foods and drinks (Conner et al. 1986, 1988b; Conner and Booth 1988). Consistent with the IP being a product of learning, these personally most preferred levels cluster around the levels in the most popular brands of that food. This applies to sweet taste as much as to any other sensed characteristic (Figure 12.7).

Each participant's preference for the food or drink peaked at a particular level of sucrose rather than increasing indefinitely. Many people preferred even the relatively sour drink and a soup to contain less than 10% sucrose (1 $\log_{10}$ g/100 mL in Figure 12.7), a rule-of-thumb that has been suggested. Also, the mode for IP varied among the three tested materials. In each case, the mode was in the range of the levels available in the market and therefore expected by users of the product. The ranges of sucrose concentration and the widths of the five to six bins in Figure 12.7 may also reflect variability among participants in the most familiar version of the products. Indeed, the pattern of IPs differed between participants who used manufactured sweet foods and drinks, such as chocolate and fruit drinks, and users of fruits and sweet vegetables such as carrots (Conner and Booth 1988).

Plots of concentration of sweetener (or intensity of sweetness) against the individual's degree of preference (e.g., rated pleasantness) are seldom constructed correctly. The individual's peak preference for sweet taste in the test food is often not measured nor even allowed for in the presentation of the data. Indeed, for a long time, research into the role of sweet taste in obesity used plain solutions of sugar or saccharin, not universally familiar sweet drinks or foods, and did not anchor the ratings on the usual or most preferred version of each material in a particular use.

An early comparison of obese and lean people that plotted individuals' pleasantness ratings against sugar levels had the essential merit of testing a real food material, namely, fruit cordial (Witherley and Pangborn 1980). Likers of sweetness were expected to show a positive slope (as in Figure 12.1), whereas sweet haters were thought to give a negative slope, as to a purely aversive taste. The authors despaired at the variability of slopes in both the fatter and leaner groups, from a wobbly flat line to a steep slope that was sometimes positive and sometimes negative in each group. Yet, either slope can be created in the same individual by testing the levels of sweet taste in a familiar food that are all on one side of that person's ideal sweet intensity for that food. A positive slope shows that the levels in the samples are all below ideal or close to it. Samples solely or mostly above ideal should give a negative slope (e.g., top left panel in Figure 12.6). Furthermore, if the individual had never consumed the cordial on its own, an ideal sweet taste could not have been acquired,

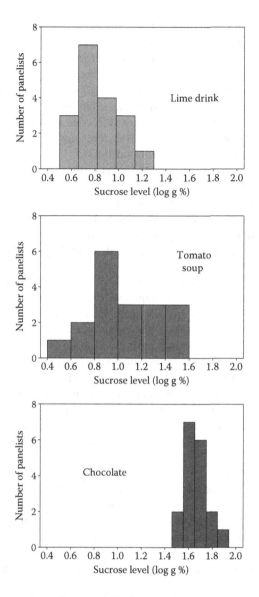

FIGURE 12.7 Distributions of personal IPs for sugar in an uncarbonated limeade, canned tomato soup, and chocolate in a panel of 18 assessors. (From Conner, M.T. et al., *Journal of Applied Psychology*, 73:275–280, 1988b.)

and the pleasantness/sucrose function might be flat. If the ratings of pleasantness had been anchored on the most preferred sweetness, it would have been simple to estimate each participant's IP and compare the distributions of this most relevant personal characteristic between the two groups.

Even more seriously, the usual practice then, and still to this date, has been to average the preference score for each tested material and plot those mean values against concentrations or intensities of the sensory factor. In statistically more elaborate analyses of grouped data, the profile of preference scores is smoothed by fitting the data to a polynomial regression or by nonmetric, multidimensional scaling. The result is a conflation of the raw data that have no theoretical basis in the mechanisms of sensory preference. Such neglect of individuals' precise achievements is unnecessary. The group's data are as clearly summarized in histograms of the prevalence of IPs in each range of sweet taste (see Figure 12.7; contrast the usual umbrella graphs and contour maps drawn from grouped raw scores, for example, in Drewnowski et al. 1982, 1985; Drewnowski and Greenwood 1983).

If fatter people do have higher IPs for sweet taste, or sweet taste makes stronger contributions to their preferences, that finding by itself does not show that a liking for sweetness causes obesity. Both obesity and IPs for sweetness come from eating habits. Whether or not a particular habit is fattening is a further question that has yet to be adequately addressed for any common pattern of eating or drinking, including one majoring on sweet materials (Booth et al. 2004; Laguna-Camacho and Booth under review).

In the United Kingdom, there appeared to be two forms of sugar preference (*sweet tooth*). One had lower maximum sweet preferences, coming from frequent use of fruit. The other had higher IPs attributable to frequent use of sweet packet foods (Conner and Booth 1988). A somewhat similar differentiation was evident more recently in the United States (Wansink et al. 2006). However, obesity cannot be caused by the mere existence of greater amounts of sugar in cookies and candy than in apples and carrots: the foods have to be ingested. The question is whether a switch in consumption from sugary foods and drinks to fruit and vegetables reduces daily energy intake after the amounts consumed of other sources of calories have adapted to the change. The experimental design needed to answer that question within and across localities has yet to be run several decades after it was formulated.

12.5.3.2 Fat *Taste*

Preferences for fats in foods have been attributed to the *taste* of fat. However, triglycerides do not stimulate gustatory receptors. Fats have aromas derived from their sources: a major factor in the attractiveness of butter and cream is their dairy aroma (a low level of the smell of the cow). Hydrolysis and oxidation of fats during cooking produce short-chain fatty acids, ketones, aldehydes, etc. Some of these compounds have sour and/or bitter tastes but again mostly an obvious and behaviorally influential aroma.

Liquid or solid fat by itself is not attractive. Even for those who like it as a dressing, it needs the taste and smell inherent in olive oil or added as vinegar. A lot of the attraction to fats in foods arises rather from tactile textures. Dairy cream is an emulsion with a thick and smooth texture. Such sensed physical characteristics such as high viscosity, low stickiness, and precise globule size distribution are critical to the authentic creaminess of yogurts (Richardson et al. 1993; Booth 2005; van Aken 2010). The fat in baked goods such as cookies forms planes along which rock-hard starch–protein matrix and sugar crystals can be pressed apart by the teeth (Vickers 1984; Booth et al. 2003a). The vegetable or animal fat in baked products such as cookies and cakes and fried foods such as potato slices and sticks creates microregions of softness within a matrix of hardened gels of starch and protein, generating various types of crispness, crunchiness, and crackling texture.

The fat in ice cream is crucial to retaining dairy, vanilla, and fruit aromas and to breaking up the hard texture of ice crystals. Nevertheless, fruit ices without fat are also popular. Hence, people might vary in their IPs for each element in the complex of sensory contributions from the amount of fat in ice cream. There are lots of sugar in both types of ice. Unfortunately, however, the data on personally ideal levels of fat and sugar in ice cream have been buried in polynomial regressions through raw preference scores. These profiles (or *umbrellas* fitted to preference scores for fat and sugar) provide very coarse measures, making group differences hard to replicate and limiting the breakdowns by age group and gender that are important in relating eating habits to obesity. It would be more productive to look for differences in frequencies of the use of foods that have divergent fat contents.

In fact, the usual approach of relating food preferences to obesity is ill-founded because of lack of evidence that patterns of consuming foods containing sugar and/ or fat do indeed fatten the individuals who have those habits. Hence, warning labels "Fattening. Keep off!" cannot be justified, unlike the message that smoking causes death on cigarette packs. Indeed, there remains no firm evidence that sugars are any more fattening than other sources of energy, although the timing of sugar sodas between meals may be a problem (Booth 1988; Booth et al. 2004). Fats are liable to be more fattening than carbohydrates or proteins, calorie for calorie, but there is still no measure how much weight is lost from reduction in frequency of eating any particular higher-fat option (French et al. 1999; Laguna-Camacho and Booth under review).

12.5.4 FAMILY PARADOX

Generations within a family share substantial backgrounds of both genes and environment. Hence, there is reason to think that they might share preferences among foods. Yet, very low correlations have been found between preference scores for common foods from students who have only recently left home and their parents (Rozin 1991).

A major flaw in these studies is that the hypothesis has not been tested scientifically. A score for preference, liking, or pleasantness of a named food, or a choice among food samples, does not measure what is preferred about the food. Each food is preferred for the levels of its attributes. That is, each family member has an IP and a differential sensitivity for each sensed and conceptualized characteristic of each food. At the very least, a familiar branded product or a sampled variant of a food will have an overall distance from the ideal of that food for each person in a particular context of use, involving social and somatic influences as well as sensory factors. It is these measures of the performance of preferring one material over another that should be tested for family associations and not the raw preference scores (see Pliner 1994; Guidetti et al. 2012).

Again too, it may be more productive to measure each person's current frequency of each eating and drinking habit. That is where the preferences come from during lifelong development through successive interactions between genomics and

upbringing. Furthermore, differences between parents and offspring in habit frequency might be a rather specific indicator of which environments they have not
shared.

12.5.5 INGESTIVE APPETITE AND FOOD PREFERENCE RESPONSES

A scientific theory cannot be tested effectively until the terms in which it is formulated are empirically realistic. The investigation of chemosensory and other
influences on ingestion has been greatly weakened by the assumption that differently worded ratings or differently named intake tests refer to distinct influences on
ingestion. When that presupposition is tested on the different measures, the evidence
shows that the various phrasings refer to one and the same phenomenon—the current
tendency to take a mouthful of the food on offer.

Hence, outputs by themselves cannot differentiate among different inputs or
mediating processes. Each proposed influence on preference or appetite has to be
measured as well as an integrative output such as disposition to accept the item in a
specified context.

12.5.6 SENSATIONS OR SENSED CHARACTERISTICS?

A rating by itself does not measure experienced sensations, contrary to the claims
for magnitude estimation (Stevens 1957) and indeed by the founder of psychophysics (Fechner 1860/1996). Ratings do not achieve perception either: the evidence of
perceiving comes from the relationship of the ratings to sources of stimulation to
the senses (e.g., Shankar et al. 2009). Measurements of chemical concentrations are
needed as well as all-or-none or graded responses in order to have the data on which
to justify a claim that either chemosensory perception has been achieved or a taste or
aroma sensation has been experienced.

Moreover, instead of being either an objective response to sweet constituents or
a subjective expression of the experience of a sensation of sweetness, the rating of
how sweet a sample is can reflect the use solely of the verbal concept of being *sweet*.
The tested sample may merely be put implicitly in a place along a graded series of
named foods, such as from honey to chocolate, and then banana and apple to bread.
Other processes that might generate a rating are describing (e.g., as being as sweet as
a ripe banana) and unconsciously sensing (e.g., an effect of sugar on preference without activating the concept *sweet*). The distinctions among these various cognitive
processes can be made by exact calculations from the raw data when an individual
makes one or more analytically relevant ratings as well as rating overall preference
(Booth and Freeman 1993; Booth et al. 2011d).

12.5.7 PREFERENCE OR APPETITE?

Acceptance is an act of the moment, whether the response is the physical movement of
a piece of material or the symbolic expression of the disposition to do so (rated preference). The mouthful or the rating is subject to present influences. The observation can
be assumed to generalize only to circumstances where the influences are identical.

Hence, no intake test or rated acceptance can measure the palatability of a food because that means that the food has a constant relative acceptability at all times and in any context, which has long been known to be untrue (Cabanac and Duclaux 1970b; Booth 1972b; Booth and Davis 1973; Duclaux et al. 1973; Rolls et al. 1981b; Booth 1990). Understandably, therefore, many participants get confused when asked repeatedly to rate how *palatable* a food is rather than how pleasant it is at each moment (Yeomans and Symes 1999). Pleasant, liked, preferred, or attractive can all mean the disposition just at that moment in those circumstances. The numbers do not become a measure of a context-free palatability because an investigator assumes that they are. Simply not wanting more of a food right now does not make it any less possible to enjoy the food on other occasions.

Indeed, literal palatability clearly does not exist. Acceptance of a food is highly contingent on circumstances that vary by the minute within a meal and after an hour or two later. Those people who love steak cannot tolerate it as a second dessert even if they have had no steak for days or weeks. Pieces of candy become quite boring if they are all the same taste, smell, and color (Rolls et al. 1981b). At the most, a subset of people in a community may have a fairly stable hierarchy of preferences among foods for each particular use, e.g., one rank order at breakfast, another when snacking on the move, and yet another in a main evening meal. Such survey numbers should not be expected to contribute to quantitative accounts of chemosensory influences on ingestion. Rather, if such data are needed, they should be aggregated from representative samples of what individuals prefer in commonly occurring situations.

It follows that daily intakes of foods or the sizes of test meals that constitute nearly all of the published data on food consumption tell us almost nothing about measurable influences on eating. Meal size is a mere physical epiphenomenon accumulated from a large number of cognitively discrete actions, with changing sensory, social, and somatic determinants across the minutes spent eating. Cultural appropriateness and physiological state do not have fixed influences either. Their effects depend on how they have interacted with each other and all the other influences on similar past occasions in the individual's life.

It also follows that important information about physiological influences on eating can be obtained from intakes of an unattractive food, so long as presented when the hypothesized signal is operating (e.g., Booth et al. 1970a,b). Indeed, intake from a buffet of diverse and tempting foods could well be insensitive to a physiological signal of appetite or satiety. Even more importantly, such tests make it impossible to analyze interactions among social and sensory factors that vary among those foods. It is far better to measure intake, portion by portion, of one food presented at a time that is regarded by the eater as appropriate to the occasion (e.g., Booth et al. 1976, 1982; Dibsdall and Booth 1996, 2014; Dibsdall et al. 1996).

12.5.8 Hunger Is Appetite for Food

There has been a tendency to assign the terms *hunger* and *thirst* to a bodily need for energy or water, respectively, or to require the presence of a physiologically signaled deficit in energy or water, while reserving the word *appetite* for ingestion attributed solely to external factors such as the aroma of cooking or the sight of a beer or a soda.

However, a half-full stomach and an incompletely covered plate can either inhibit or facilitate ingestion depending on the context of gastrointestinal hormones, eating or drinking companions, or other items to consume. There may be some force in the joke that optimists see a glass as half full, whereas pessimists regard it as half empty. Yet, the basic fact remains that they both tend to take more mouthfuls from the glass when the beverage is halfway to the top. What influences such mundane actions?

Hunger is not a purely bodily state that compels the ingestion of food. Appetite is not a mental state driven solely by sight or other sensing of food, drink, or other objects of desire. Rather, ingestive appetite is the cognitive-behavioral tendency to take a mouthful or more of a food and/or a drink whatever the causes of that disposition are on a particular occasion. Appetite for food (usually in solid form) simply is hunger motivation. Similarly, thirst motivation is the appetite for a watery fluid.

Some people sometimes have rumblings or pangs in the upper abdomen when they want to eat or a dry mouth or rough throat when they would like a drink. However, these sensations typical of hunger or thirst for some are not the same as the tendencies to ingest selectively. Rather, the individual's privately experienced epigastric pang has become associated by that person with the publicly observable desire for food.

The word *sensation* should not be used to refer to a physiological signal either, especially in the metaphysically dualistic phrase *central sensation* or the self-contradictory concept of an *unconscious sensation*. Neural activation that stimulates appetite for foods or fluids is just that, whether central or peripheral, or conscious or unconscious. Metabolic or hormonal induction of food intake is not having a hunger sensation; there may be no awareness of the operation of the signal but only an increase in the motivation to eat. Osmotic or hypovolemic stimulation of water intake is not a sensation of thirst. The osmoreceptors and baroreceptors generate central signals of water deficit of which we may not be aware. Tactile receptors sensitive to the drying of oral mucosa generate peripheral signals from reduced salivation. These signals are dispensable to the appetite for water, but the dryness is likely to come to consciousness.

12.5.9 WORDS FOR ENERGY INTAKES AND APPETITE RATINGS

A great variety of words have been presented to human participants to assess the current level of appetite for food. People can be asked how hungry or full they are, whether they would eat a great amount, how strongly they want to eat or desire food, how pleasant it would be to eat a food, and so on. The answers have been claimed to measure distinct sensations, motivations, bodily states, or social signals.

Many words have also been used in reports by investigators to label the weight of foods and volumes of drinks that have been swallowed (intakes) and the numbers assigned to positions between phrases about eating and drinking (ratings). Usually, each label has been assumed to refer to the measure of a different process influencing that intake or rating, such as an unconscious physiological signal, the subjective experiencing of a sensation, or unwittingly or deliberately following a social convention. Yet, no evidence is provided that the assumed process does indeed influence the numbers postulated to measure it, let alone more so than other numbers from other physical or verbal tests of hunger/satiety, i.e., the present strength or weakness of the appetite for food.

Contrary to all that, the first scientific step required for any multiple measures is to test for correlations between them in order to check if they measure a single underlying variable. When that has been done for responses to a mouthful of a particular food, by itself or at one stage in a meal, the weights consumed and the words rated are found to be highly correlated (e.g., Booth et al. 1982, 2011b; Hill et al. 1984). Indeed, recently, it was found that the amounts of foods that a person wanted to eat at a particular moment correlated highly with the expected pleasantness of eating those named items (Booth et al. 2011b). That is, all the differently worded or labeled numbers measure the preference for that food in that context. If the dependency on the context is also characterized, such as a difference between the start and end of a meal, then the measure is of present appetite for that food. There is one single phenomenon, the acceptance of a tasted, seen, or named food (or drink), in an implicit or explicit context of bodily and social signals.

The sign of a correlation is secondary: a negative correlation merely means that one of the two numbers reflects reduced acceptance. If that reduction of appetite comes from an effect of recent eating, whether sensory, social, or somatic, then the rating or mouthful intake is a measure of the degree of sating of appetite for that food or perhaps for many foods. The word *fullness* or *satiety* does not have to be mentioned in order to measure the present depth to which appetite has been sated during or after a meal. The degree of specificity of the partly satiated state depends on further evidence and not mere assumption that the inhibition of appetite is specific to sensory modality, nutritional state, or culinary category. Indeed, an increase or decrease in the rate of intake or appetite score may have nothing to do with appetite itself; it could come from a general excitement or lassitude or even some malaise (Booth et al. 2011b).

For example, the ratings of how *full* someone is at the time are negatively correlated with how *hungry* that person is then or how much she or he *likes* a familiar food at that moment. That merely means that the rater is less predisposed to take a mouthful of that food. Saying "I'm full" is not evidence of a sensation of stretching in the upper abdomen nor of how much food is in the stomach. Often, it merely means that the eater has had enough (of that food or of all food), i.e., has less of an appetite (Booth 1976, 1990, 2009a; Booth et al. 1982).

Hence, it is a disastrously bad research practice to plot a separate time series of each differently worded rating. A single latent variable for the strength of hunger and its sating should first be extracted from each of several representative points in time and that one number analyzed and reported (Booth et al. 2011b). The only role for presenting data on differently presented tests of intake or variously wording ratings of appetite is to find out if one of the measures is consistently most sensitive to an influence that has been manipulated (Booth et al. 1982, 2010). This strategy is illustrated in this chapter for the cognitive machinery through which the chemical senses influence food choice and intake.

12.6 WORDS FOR GUSTATORY AND OLFACTORY INTENSITIES AND PREFERENCES

The same scientific mistake about alternative words for the same phenomenon has plagued research into sensory intensities and food preferences.

12.6.1 INTENSITIES

Elaborate sets of vocabulary are presented to sensory panels without routine statistical checking of which words achieve distinctions among sensed factors. Each word is presented on a separate point of a star diagram of rated intensities. Yet, typically two or more of these words appear on effectively the same vector in graphs constructed from factor analysis or multidimensional scaling. This information should be used to weed out redundant terms for theoretical coherence and practical convenience. The reduced vocabulary then needs to be validated on measured variations among food samples of the sort to be assessed and not by training on an artificial model of the technically intended meaning of each term.

Statistical reduction of experts' vocabulary also uncovers the stabilities in their expression of the subtler distinctions that they have incorporated into their memory. Native speakers who eat the foods in life have already learnt the accurate uses of the words in their culture's language (Wittgenstein 1953). The word most heavily loaded on a principal component in factor analysis is therefore likely to be the most precise name for the actual sensed influence on perception.

12.6.2 PREFERENCES

Preference is the scientifically most useful term for a set of influences on acts of eating or drinking. Influences can be cultural, via symbolic communications such as labels on foods, or interpersonal such as sight or knowledge of what someone else is eating. Hence, influences from the sensed physicochemical characteristics of foods and drinks are more clearly identified by the term *sensory preferences.*

Strictly speaking, what is meant is by *preference* a greater degree of acceptance of the *preferred* item over alternatives. Nevertheless, the term *relative acceptance* is too pernickety for general use. *Acceptance* by itself is better used for the act of accepting a single item as distinct from a factor influencing that physical or symbolic action.

Many other terms are used in ordinary English for preferring something, such as liking it, finding the item pleasant, having an appetite for it, desiring the item, wanting it, and so on. Sometimes, these terms are assumed to refer specifically to the sensory component of preference, but the evidence is that they all refer to the same phenomenon of responding to the cognitive integration of current social and somatic signals as well as of sensed information.

12.6.3 PLEASANT VERSUS PLEASURABLE

A major disadvantage of words other than preference and acceptance is that they are taken by many people, including some scientists, to mean that something extra must be going on besides the observable preferring or accepting of an item. Preference is evident in the performance of selecting one food over others, more vigorous ingestive movements than in response to other foods, or rating a sample as more attractive than other samples. Perhaps the scientifically most important and longest-standing example of misnaming of this greater acceptance is the term *hedonic* (Booth 1991).

This misconception of preference entered the research literature on behavioral nutrition in the applied area of designing military rations (Peryam and Haynes 1957). The mistake now pervades the neuroscience of motivation, emotion, and learning, and the social science of well-being, care of the needy, and treatment of disease. The degree of preference for a food was assessed by checking one of a rank-ordered set of nine phrases from *like extremely* to *dislike extremely* (Peryam and Pilgrim 1957). It is a still widespread mistake to use more than two anchor phrases (specifying a straight line against the determinants of preference; see Booth 2009a) because, inevitably, three or more anchors are unequally spaced (Jones et al. 1955). Among early research users, these categories of food preference (and aversion) were called a *hedonic scale* (Peryam and Girardot 1952). That adjective comes from the classical Greek word for pleasure, *hedonē*. The presumption is that liking a food is the subjective experiencing of a pleasurable thrill while eating it. Unfortunately, for ambitious suppliers of food, but perhaps conveniently for those who eat every few hours, sensual thrills from attractive foods are rather more unusual than those from erotic activity and other activities providing intense excitement such as a ride on a roller coaster.

The universal assumption that liking is a subjective experience rather than a public performance was exposed by the proposal of a food action scale (Schutz 1965). The anchor words referred explicitly to observable activities with foods that indicated higher or lower rates of acceptance. Unfortunately, the use of nine anchor phrases was continued instead of just the two needed to keep responses in a straight line against levels of stimulation (Booth et al. 1982, 1983; Booth 2009a).

The error of equating preference with pleasure has been compounded by the verbal similarity between the word *pleasure* and the word used in a common measure of preference or appetite (and satiety) for an item—its rated pleasantness (Rolls et al. 1981b; Booth et al. 1982). A whole theory of the biological roles of pleasure has been built on ratings of the pleasantness of gustatory and thermal stimuli (Cabanac 1971, 1979). Any desired activity is a pleasant prospect. Yet, even when bodily sensations such as taste (or texture) are involved in the activity, as with eating and drinking, those conscious experiences need not be sensually pleasurable (Booth 1991). Recently, at last, the preference for a food and pleasure from the food have been dissociated experimentally (Booth et al. 2010). It seems that revoltingly strong sweetness can activate some of the innate reflex to sweetness, so that the taster feels the characteristic movements in the mouth. Furthermore, in an adult, such feelings can be pleasurable, raising mood and even creating a sense of smiling (Booth et al. 2010). Further, careful cognitive and electromyographic investigation is needed to determine if some of the muscles that can be recruited by intense sweetness are the same as some of the muscles involved in a smile, and whether the pleasure comes from actual or incipient contractions or directly from the taste of sweetness.

12.6.4   Motivating Stimulus or Associative Reward?

The immediately observed motivating effect of a food stimulus is often called *food reward*, without any evidence from later observations that the presentation of that stimulus had any associative effects, i.e., did any rewarding. The fact that a pattern of sensory input is preferred implies nothing about its contribution to learning through the reinforcement of either instrumental responses (reward) or reactive movements to stimuli in classical conditioning (Berridge and Robinson 2003; Epstein and Leddy 2006; Booth et al. 2012).

The need for terminological clarity is further emphasized by the demonstration that sweet taste by itself can serve as a reward in human subjects, creating an incentive stimulus out of a previously neutral odor (Yeomans and Mobini 2006; Yeomans et al. 2006; see Stevenson et al. 1998). Furthermore, such reinforcing associations of cues with consequences have to be distinguished from associations between cues, which does not require reinforcement but can occur with habituation or familiarization. We now turn to this learning of combined stimuli, starting with mixtures of taste compounds.

12.6.5   Strength of an Influence

These problems with experimenters' assumptions about words are sidestepped in this chapter by starting and remaining with the phenomena to which the wordings put onto ratings or used to name intake tests are meant to refer. Whichever the wording chosen for a response, the stimuli that influence that rating are sought before proceeding any further toward even just summarizing the data, let alone interpreting any response or claiming to observe any effect, quantitative (graded) or categorical (yes/no).

What matters is the strength of influence of a stimulus on a response and not a merely statistical prediction. These response–stimulus functions are familiar in biomedical science as dose–response relationships. If the amounts of the stimulus can be transformed into units that give a linear relationship to amounts of the response, the scientifically relevant measurement is the slope of the regression from stimulus levels to response levels (b) and not the regression coefficient (β). The reliability of the numerical value for the slope needs to be assessed of course, but confidence limits are the best indicator of the precision of an estimate. P values depend on the number of data, whereas the only facts of scientific interest are the numerical values derived from the response–stimulus data pairs, however few or many there are.

Best of all would be a single measure of the strength of an influence on a response that takes into account both the value of the slope of response levels on stimulus levels and the variability in the level of response to each particular level of stimulus. Psychology has been sitting on just such a measure of causal strength for 170 years. The strength of influence of levels of a stimulus on a response is identical to the sensitivity of the response to the stimulus levels. E.H. Weber (1843/1996) measured the minimum change in touch on the skin that would change the response. For medium levels of stimulation, the fractional change was constant across a wide range of medium levels (for four tastants, see McBride 1983; for concentrations of a familiar mixture, see McBride and Booth 1986). Weber and many others repeated the measurement of differential acuity in other sensory modalities and found that the fraction was constant across medium ranges of a particular stimulus. Weber's fraction divides the error in the responses by the slope of the response/stimulus function, generating a single number instead of three numbers, the slope and its two confidence limits.

The Weber fraction (or, strictly speaking, the ratio of levels that the fraction represents) is better known as the *just noticeable difference*. However, distinguishing between the levels of a stimulus has nothing to do with subjectively noticing a difference in strengths of a particular sensation. Preference or familiarity ratings can discriminate between stimulus levels without ever mentioning sensory vocabulary. Weber's fraction is an objectively observed difference in the level of response to a disparity between levels of measured stimulus, halfway between perfect discrimination when the two levels are far enough apart and the random responding that necessarily occurs when the two stimulus levels are identical. Hence, it can be called the half-discriminated fraction (HDF).

For chemical and physical stimuli, the disparities are linear against response stimulation when the stimulus levels are plotted in ratios of the physical level, such as concentration. Concentrations of taste or smell compounds should therefore always be converted in logarithms. Otherwise, a bowed curve is inevitable. Without the levels in logs, the distribution of slopes across individuals will be skewed as well.

12.6.6 EACH FOOD HAS A DIFFERENT TASTE

It is readily acknowledged that each species of food plant has a different aroma. Each fruit and vegetable emits a wide variety of volatile compounds and so could have a unique olfactory signature. It seems to be less widely appreciated that the taste of each food is also distinctive. How could that work when there are only a few distinct tastes to share among hundreds of foodstuffs? A key to the answer is that each taste presented by itself has at least about 10 distinguishable concentrations, maybe even 20 or more. Even from only four tastes, 10 levels give a minimum of 10,000 (10^4) distinct combinations.

In reality, cooks and manufacturers have to spend a great deal of time and money to get each combination right. This is because eaters and drinkers are familiar with the correct mixture of levels of tastes, however conscious or not of the specifics they are (or what investigators of ingestive behavior are aware of).

Tastes are the spice of life. They wake us thoroughly in the morning and can send us to bed happy at night. From birth, the sweet taste helps us to love our mothers. The bitter taste protected young children who explored outside the encampment during our species' nomadic period, helping us to survive near extinction and then to expand around the globe. The sharing of tasty drinks celebrates the heights and soothes the depths. Seeking comfort repeatedly from chocolate or fruit cake can become part of counterproductive coping strategy. Yet, the joys and satisfactions from tasty foods are also one of the happiest parts of regular daily life for many who live in richer countries.

12.6.7 AMOUNT OF TASTE, NOT JUST THE SORT OF TASTE

The first step toward understanding the roles of combinations of tastes in ingestion is to get away from the idea that the mixtures are just of the different tastes. This is not just an ordinary eater's naivety. The research literature is dominated by hypotheses and interpretations about interactions between saltiness or sweetness with bitterness or sourness, for example, or a category of taste with viscosity, aroma, color, or whatever. On the contrary, what matters to eaters and to chemosensory science is the particular level of each taste compound in the ingested material.

It follows inexorably that, like all good things, there can be too much of a nice taste. This can be very obvious at a given moment and quite easily rectified. Those of us who are used to unsweetened coffee can find the drink revolting when someone has added sugar without asking. We have come to find a moderate level of bitterness highly attractive alongside the aroma of coffee and perhaps a felt need for caffeine. Yet, even those of us who like strong coffee can find too much in a brew and may dilute it with hot water or even mask the taste with sugar or milk. For those who like lemonade, the taste of some acid is essential. Nevertheless, to make good lemonade, freshly squeezed lemon needs to be made less sour by adding water and not just sugar.

Ordinary eaters have learnt what levels work of the tastes in a familiar material. Unfortunately, so far, most scientists have not. From molecular neuroscience to sensory testing in industry, and even in multisensory psychology, all the effects of the taste of sweet, bitter, sour, salty, savory, or any of the rest are treated as though they are continuously increasing quantities. Yet, every effect of taste is tied to a particular amount of each taste and indeed of an aroma, a mouthfeel, a color, and so on.

Levels of stimuli are also neglected by theories of learning, including accounts of learnt combinations of stimuli. Theories of the recognition of objects have the same defect, even those invoking the idea of a specific prototype for each object. All these approaches treat stimuli as categories and not gradations.

12.6.8 WHICH LEVEL?

Every taste (and any other feature) needs to be scaled by how far it is above or below the learnt point for the combination it is in. That leaves a problem: how can distance from that standard level be measured? The answer lies with Weber's fraction, the half-discriminated disparity (HDF) of a tastant's concentrations detected by preference or some other response.

The fractional increase in stimulus levels that just made a difference in the response of interest (e.g., how pleasant or sweet) can be calculated from a linear regression through the pairs of stimulus and response levels observed during an individual's session, as can also the level in the standard used by the participant to make those responses (Torgerson 1958; McBride and Booth 1986; Conner et al. 1988a,b). The concentrations of a taste or odor compound or a mixture in fixed proportions can then be converted into a scale of a number of Weber fractions from the IP or familiar level.

Weber's fraction also solves the otherwise intractable problem of putting the concentrations of different compounds onto the same scale. Discriminative performance provides a common unit across and within tastes and all other sensed characteristics of a food or drink. Whatever the chemical structure of the sweetener, and whether a small or a large amount is needed to provide the usual sweetness of a particular mixture, the disparity of the mixture from the standard can be measured in the number of Weber's fractions.

Scaling based on Weber's fraction has been grossly neglected because of the preoccupation of psychophysicists since Fechner (1860) with formulating a mathematical law that covers all levels of stimulation (Stevens 1957). That is an impossible dream for two sorts of reason. The extreme limits cannot be in such a law because detecting the presence of a stimulus at low levels is a different task from discriminating between readily perceived levels (Laming 1985, 1986, 1987), and at high levels, the stimulus starts to saturate the receptors. A softer limit is that there is less experience of low and high levels of most stimuli than of the medium levels that commonly exist. Therefore, performance outside the familiar range is less likely to be precise or even just uniform.

The number of Weber's fractions from the most familiar or preferred level is the basic scale for a response to any stimulus. Since all these response/stimulus relationships use the same unit, they can interact with each other in a variety of ways within the mind (Booth and Freeman 1993). Hence, Weber's fraction is the key that unlocks the mental processing required to have chemosensory preferences and consequent effects of the chemical senses on nutrition.

12.7 COGNITIVE MECHANISMS THAT CONVERT SENSING INTO INGESTING

12.7.1 Causal Processes from Chemical Stimulation to Ingestive Movement

The rest of this chapter illustrates the experimental evidence for a mathematically precise account of the effects of perceived tastes and smells of foods and drinks on intended and involuntary consumption of selected items. The theory in its present stage of development is built up here piece by piece from quantitative evidence that has been published over the last three decades, plus some results in preparation for submission.

Central to the theory is the mathematical equivalence between the sensitivity of a response to differences in strength of a stimulus and the amount of influence that the stimulus has on the response. If preference responds to small variations in sweet taste, then sweet taste has a large influence on preference. In a more specifically psychological language, the salience of a feature of a food for a response is the same as the attention paid to that feature by that response.

In other words, psychology's long-standing measure of differential sensitivity, Weber's fraction, is the key to working out the causal processes by which tastes and smells produce selective ingestion. Central interactions between taste receptor afferents are well recognized. These are particularly evident in subadditivity between responses to components of experimental mixtures of taste compounds. Various mathematical models of such *mixture suppression* have been proposed from a widely used cosine function (Cain et al. 1995) to parallel versus fan interactions in the analysis of variance (De Graaf et al. 1987; McBride 1988, 1993; McBride and Finlay 1990). Yet, no specific mechanism has been proposed to justify either sort of calculation (see Schifferstein and Frijters 1993). In contrast, the concentrations of the taste compounds in the tested mixtures can be scaled on a number of discriminations from the standard in memory that was used by a response made to each sample. Then, the observed values of that response can be predicted from causal processes specified by exact arithmetic (Booth and Freeman 1993).

First, we consider the ubiquity of the phenomena that require scientific explanation.

12.7.2 MIXING IT

Perhaps the most important fact about the sense of taste is that identifiable tastes always come in combinations with each other in life. Of course, tastes in food and drink also go along with the other senses—aroma, color, shape, seen and felt texture, and so on. Some interactions between the senses can be amazing (Spence 2010). Yet, equally extraordinary interactions occur all the time within the sense of taste. Stimulation of one type of gustatory receptor is almost always combined with stimulation of another taste receptor type or even with two or three receptors.

These natural gustatory mixtures are very precise too. The tastes have to be balanced against each other, even when their overall strength is about right. Many eaters of fish and chips like to put their own salt and vinegar on the potato fries: their taste is not so nice when swamped in the sourness of vinegar or when made far too salty. Those who take sugar in coffee, with or without milk, are quite particular about both the strength of taste of the coffee and the number of spoonfuls of sugar. This is an example of three tastes too because coffee tastes sour as well as bitter. Take note the next time you have a drink made from ground coffee. What if it were too sour even if you like strong coffee? Tea can go with lemon, but coffee does not need it.

None of this has anything to do with aroma, color, crunchy sounds, or any other sense than taste, nor is it in the outer reaches of creative gastronomy or visual enough to matter in TV cooking competitions. It happens several times a day in everyone's life: talking often has to compete with taste for occupying the tongue.

These complexities of the sense of taste and their many roles in everyday living create challenges and opportunities for all sorts of cognitive processing, from physical information to social communication. Think of the mental mechanisms required to recognize each combination of tastes as appropriate to that food item and the dish it is in. Such cognitive science is way beyond the genetics and the neuroscience that deal with one taste at a time. Everyday taste cognition also flies well under the radar of the economics and the social anthropology of salt, sugar, oranges, chocolate, and coffee.

Yet, social and cognitive scientists generally consider tastes to be irrelevant to personal interaction, empathic perception, the acquisition of language, perception, memory, reasoning, and almost everything else of academic and practical interest. A cognitive psychologist has been heard to dismiss such matters as a trivial job for the hypothalamus. Yet, the taste pathways have much less influence on that region of the brain than on parts of the cortex relating to actions, expectancies, and percepts integrated across all the senses.

On the contrary, sensory science needs to join the mainstream of research into the cognitive processes in physical and social perception and action. Familiar mixtures of tastes are a good place to start. Tasting with the tongue is as deeply involved in human culture and language as other human capacity alleged to be *basic* and traditionally supposed to be wired into the brain by the genes. The neuroscience of the *basic emotions* expressed in the face has been forced to go beyond locating each emotion in its own bit of the brain.

Similarly, the question is no longer merely whether there are four or five (or more) *basic* tastes, each with its own type of receptor on the tongue and its own word in the English language. The whole idea of such labeled lines through the brain has broken down. Even a single nerve fiber going from the tongue to the brain can be activated by two or more types of taste receptor (Roper 2007). Indeed, a taste bud contains multiple receptor types that are coupled to an afferent nerve by the messengers between cells (Tomchik et al. 2007; Roper and Chaudhari 2009). Hence, even the first relay in the pathways for gustatory information through the brain lacks the information required to identify a compound that stimulates a single receptor type.

Rather, the approximation to a one-to-one relationship between the receptor type and verbal concept is a brilliantly flexible achievement by human societies in educating their youngsters into implicit understanding of the complex tastes of foods. We do not teach the meaning of *sweet* by giving some honey or sugar water to taste and saying the word. We use the word to warn a child that the fruit may not be ripe yet, for example, or to point out that no sugar is needed on the muesli because it contains raisins. The concept of sweetness emerges in such conversations, already defined by the contexts of its use (Wittgenstein 1953; Quine 1974). Sucrose is identified as sweet by the information from hT1R2 receptors interacting deeper in the brain with social and physical information gathered via other senses in the past as well as the present.

12.7.3 CONFIGURED IDEAL POINTS

12.7.3.1 Mixture Statistics

Even a mixture of molecules that all stimulate a single taste receptor type generates a severe scientific problem with enormous practical implications. There is no mechanistic theory in general use for mixtures having more than one taste. Until recently, experiments on interactions between tastes (or odors) used mixtures of single compounds that had not been experienced by the research participants before entering the laboratory. Mutual suppression of intensities was almost universally seen, which could be fitted to a theoretically unspecified angle in a cosine function (Cain et al. 1995). Intensification of intensity (synergy) was claimed in some special cases such as glutamate and ribonucleotides (Yamaguchi 1967).

When three or four arbitrarily chosen taste or odor compounds are mixed, the suppressive interactions become so strong that the components become difficult even to recognize (Laing et al. 2002). The compounds can only mask each other (Cain et al. 1995; Marshall et al. 2006). The masking gets worse if configural learning is prevented by training to attend to one of the compounds (Kurtz et al. 2009; Prescott and Murphy 2009).

The effect was reduced by familiarization with the mixtures, and so, it was suggested that learning to configure the separate tastes or smells could remove confusion among them (Laing et al. 2002). A major review of the literature on recognition of odors concluded that each profile of repeatedly stimulated receptors was stored in memory as a configuration that could be compared with subsequent mixtures of volatiles (Stevenson and Boakes 2003).

A theoretically cogent statistical theory of configural learning has been proposed (Pearce 1994, 2002). However, it has not been brought into use within research on the chemical senses. Norm-zeroed multiple discrimination theory provides a simple arithmetic of learnt configural stimuli (Booth and Freeman 1993). The remainder of this chapter is devoted to illustrating the analyses of data in accord with this quantitative mechanistic theory. The approach was first applied to mixtures of taste compounds. Indeed, it developed from work on variations of concentration of a single taste compound in a familiar context rather than in an unfamiliar pure solution (Booth et al. 1983). Contextual influences of various sorts have long been recognized in food research; indeed, they have sometimes been called cognitive effects (Davidson et al. 1999; Pfeiffer et al. 2006). Nevertheless, the concept of context has been vague and contextual effects poorly specified. Indeed, context has sometimes been dismissed as a nuisance variable.

12.7.3.2 Scientific Measurement of Context

The first measurement of the role of the chemical senses in preferences for familiar foods and drinks varied the concentration of a single taste compound—NaCl (Booth et al. 1983). The well-learnt contexts tested were plain white bread or tomato soup eaten by itself.

The strength of the taste of salt in each sample of bread or soup was rated relative to the individual eater's most preferred strength held in long-term memory. The key anchor phrase on the array of positions to choose as the response was *just right for me*. It is crucial that the participant is referred to a point on a linear array involving a single objective concept, such as an act of acceptance or the taste of salt.

Much research practice treats ordinary people as incapable of making such quantitative judgments on familiar matters. Hence, only a choice of boxes to tick is provided for agreement with one of the more or less complex phrases set against each box. Suitably chosen phrases can be arranged in a sequence of decreasing strength, e.g., from *like extremely* to *neither like nor dislike*, but the responses are then only ranks and not quantities. They represent only ranges of preference, of indeterminate width and hence unknown borders between ranges. The *just right* point was modified in that approach to a *just-about-right* range. The consequences have been disastrous for theoretical understanding of the cognitive approach and to the practical use of data on preferences, sensed characteristics, and marketed attributes (Booth and Shepherd 1988; Booth and Conner 1991, 2009).

In fact, anyone who watches TV talent shows is fully capable of constructing scores from 0 to 10 (with halves too and even decimal fractions). Percentages as well are readily handled by tennis fans examining champions' match performance of points—one on return of serve, and so on. Only two scores should be anchored because a third anchor is at risk of unequal spacing from the other two anchors. Then, unlabeled boxes, hatch marks on a line or a row of integers, can be provided for the response. The extraordinary procedure of measuring distances along an unstructured line is totally unnecessary (Bowman et al. 2004).

The theoretical zero point for discriminations by degree of preference is the most likely choice, i.e., a rating at the *just right* anchor point. However, the zero that the rater needs in order to make a genuinely quantitative judgment can be the absence of preference or of the characteristic being assessed. No sample should be presented that risks being rated close to zero preference or intensity, because that is liable to induce a floor effect and departure of the response/stimulus graph from linearity.

The concentrations of each taste compound varied and the ratings of closeness to its ideal level (or to the ideal version of the undescribed food) can then be fitted to the contextualized hyperbola (Figures 12.5 and 12.6). The key principle is that one peaked causal/discrimination relationship is always in the context of one or more other peaked response/stimulus functions. Since each response/stimulus relationship is linear in the number of Weber's fractions from the ideal or familiar point, the data points theoretically form an isosceles triangle, having the same slope (of opposite signs) on each side of the apex (Booth and Conner 1991). If two such triangles for the same response are set at right angles, with a single apex, the responses to the mixtures of two influences form a cone, with the data from each sample plotted at a point on its surface. Furthermore, if the variations in the level of one component are tested while the average of levels of the other influence being off the ideal or usual point, then the peaked function will be the surface of a cone on a vertical cut down the side of the cone away from the peak. The shape of this conic section is a hyperbola. Hence, the responses to a sensory influence should always be fitted to the formula for a hyperbola, $y^2/x^2 = 1$. When the context for each tested sample is near enough ideal in all respects, the fitted hyperbola will approximate to the isosceles triangle to which the limbs of the hyperbola asymptote. This calculation from the raw data gives functions like those in Figures 12.5 and 12.6 for sugar and acid in a fruit drink and for caffeine in coffee (other constituents of which taste sour as well as bitter).

The hyperbola for a single stimulus influencing preference follows from the mere presence of another taste. Alternatively, the whole context can be integrated into another single stimulus dimension. When these two dimensions are plotted at the right angle in the horizontal plane (x and z axes), with the response dimension plotted vertically (y axis), the result is a cone surface of data, even when there is no systematic variation in any element of the context. The mathematics follows independently of data on any other component of the mixture. For example, nothing needs to be known about other constituents of coffee in order for it to be correct to fit a hyperbola to responses to a coffee drink in which in caffeine levels were varied.

In this way, norm-zeroed discrimination scaling directly generates a mathematically exact theory of context (Booth and Freeman 1993). When one or more samples is close enough to the most preferred level, the peak of that hyperbola can be interpolated (as in the six individuals in Figure 12.6). The average distance of the whole context from ideal is then the distance from that rounded peak to the peak of the triangle formed by tangents to the hyperbola. The size of the defect is measured by the distance between the hyperbola and the triangle, either between the peaks in response units or horizontally in the number of Weber's fractions. A source of a defect in context can be sought by varying a suspected cause and interpolating its average levels in samples showing the defect into the scale of its influence on preference.

12.7.3.2.1   Interactions among Separate Influences

The cone is formed by preference responses to different levels of a single influential stimulus in any sort of context. If a second stimulus is varied independently of the first one, the cone provides a default model for a response that varies among those mixtures of the two distinct stimuli. For example, two compounds might stimulate distinct types of receptor (as in Figure 12.5) or two distinct profiles of multiple receptor types, such as bitter receptors or olfactory receptors.

The formula for the distance of the theoretically maximum response from the response to a mixture of two different sources of stimulation, at distances A and B, is $(A^2 + B^2)^{0.5}$ in accord with Pythagoras's theorem. This square root of the sum of squares extends to familiar mixtures of three, four, or more distinct stimuli, because the Pythagoras theorem is also valid over any number of dimensions (although such *hypercones* cannot be visualized. That is to say, the interactions among any number of influences on a response can be accommodated by this arithmetic.

12.7.3.3   Identical or Configured Influences

There are two ways in which distinct sources of stimulation can operate cognitively on a response on a single dimension (or, in terms of communication theory, transmit information from multiple input patterns to an output pattern over a single channel). One possibility is that the two stimuli may act on the same type of receptor. Hence, the information provided by that route cannot enable any response to distinguish between its sources. This unidimensional mental mechanism is used in this chapter to test if two taste compounds act on the same receptor. The discrimination distances simply add rather than act orthogonally.

An alternative is that learning creates a single dimension (or channel) from two stimuli that act on different receptor types, intramodally or intermodally (Booth 2013). Exposure to a particular mixture of distinct taste and/or odor compounds can set up a standard or norm in long-term memory in which those levels of the components are treated as a unity by the learnt response. In effect, the particular mixture becomes a new stimulus, distinct from any components of the mixture, although each component may retain control of a response distinct to it. The particular combination of levels becomes a unique configuration controlling the learnt response. When this emergent sensory influence comes from a binary mixture, it functions as a *third stimulus* to the response. This perceptual achievement is used in research into animal learning as the criterion of configuring among distinct sources of stimulation (Rescorla 1973).

Like any other learnt stimulus, departure of any component's level upward or downward from the learnt set of levels weakens the response. Such a test mixture has some dissimilarity from the configured mixture (Shepard 1958). This difference in performance on a combination of stimuli is the basis for a leading theory of less than perfect configuring (Pearce 1994), developed for categories of stimuli potentially having quantitative features (Pearce 2002; George and Pearce 2012).

The arithmetical formula predicting the response to such mixtures is changed by configural learning from the root sum of squares to straight summations of the discrimination distances from the norm, i.e., $(A + B)$ for a mixture of A and B (Booth and Freeman 1993). The same formula tests for a receptor type stimulated by two different compounds, even when one or both compounds also stimulate other types of receptor.

12.8 GUSTATORY CONFIGURATIONS IN INGESTION

12.8.1 BALANCE OF SWEET AND SOUR IN ORANGES

The taste of the flesh of a ripe orange is one of the best models for the study of gustation in real-life ingestive behavior. Peeled whole oranges are a widely consumed food. Juiced whole oranges are even more widely used as a drink, usually unmixed with other juices and without the addition of sugar or other materials. A long-life variant of fresh orange juice is made by condensation for dilution back to strength on use; that processing is liable to change the aroma but not the taste, texture, or color. Filtered condensate is made into a cordial (*orange squash* in the United Kingdom), which is popular among children after dilution to taste.

An orange-flavored drink, like orange soda without the carbonation, can be made by dissolving a mixture of orange-like coloring and aroma in mains water, adding fruit acid, table sugar and/or intense sweetener, and a clouding agent to replace fragments of orange. A still, clouded, orange-flavored drink, using sucrose and citric acid as tastants, is widely available in the United Kingdom from cold-drink vending machines. Frequent users can therefore be tested on a familiar sweet drink that is also sour at the balance of intensities expected of orange flavor.

In one series of experiments (Freeman et al. 1993), we sought evidence that sweet sugars act on one sort of taste receptor, whereas fruit acids stimulate another receptor type (or more than one). The only other evidence that different sugars act on the same taste receptor (now known to be oral hT1R2) used complex designs and calculations to uncover concentrations of pairs of sugars that could not be discriminated (Breslin et al. 1994, 1996). That approach is not applicable to mixtures of tastes or to single compounds that possess more than one taste, such as a sweet and bitter amino acid, or have any other sensory effect, such as the difference in osmotic pressure between equally sweet solutions of a monosaccharide and a disaccharide (Breslin et al. 1996).

In contrast, discrimination from the norm can readily pick out compounds that add stimulation to one type of receptor from different compounds (or the same compound) that stimulate another receptor additively. Illustrative findings are summarized in a graph calculated directly from the raw data gathered in an individual's session, assessing variants of the vended orange drink. In this experiment, we used quaternary mixtures close enough to the sweetness and sourness of the marketed drink to be within the region of constancy of Weber's fraction, halfway between perfect discrimination and random responding.

The learnt norm that the assessors were asked to use was the most preferred taste of the familiar drink. That is to say, an assessor was asked to judge where each sample was between being chosen every time and never being the choice. The mixtures were tailored to each assessor's range of tolerance as it became apparent from the first two or three samples, in order to avoid ratings close to either extreme.

12.8.2 Direct Stimulation of Preference

In one assessor, preferences in the second session were directly driven by stimulation of receptors specific to sugars or acids (Figure 12.8). If no concept of sweet or sour taste was activated, then these influences on preference could have been subconscious. In the cognitive processing, aware or unaware, that was most predictive of rated preference ($r^2 = 0.85$), distances from the norm of the levels of sucrose and fructose were added together (S1 + S2). In other words, the information from each of the sugars was transmitted over a single channel from the receptors in the mouth to the decision where to place the degree of preference for each sample between always and never choosing each variant of the drink.

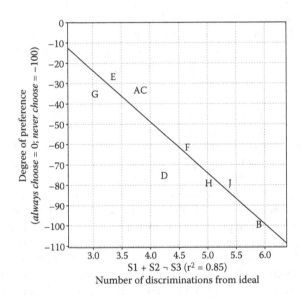

FIGURE 12.8 Cognitive integration (possibly unconscious) into initial ratings of closeness to most preferred quality (R1) for samples of a familiar orange-flavored drink (*always/never choose*: $r^2 = 0.85$) of the stimulation of one (+) type of taste receptor by sucrose (S1: 48% contribution) and fructose (S2: 41%) and of a different (¬) receptor type by citric acid (S3). Data point letters: sequence of presentation of samples, from A = 1st to J = 9th. Malic acid (S4) was also varied among the drink samples, but its stimulation was not integrated into preference by this assessor. Graphic output from a run of the recently programmed tool, Co-Pro2.29.

Stimulation from citric acid (S3) had an independent influence on preference (Figure 12.8). That is evidence that gustation depends on at least one receptor for acids, which is different from the receptor for sugars. No direct effect of malic acid (S4) on preference was seen in this most predictive model of the session's processing (Figure 12.8). Hence, this particular set of data happened to provide no test of the hypothesis that the two acids act on the same receptor.

Another assessor did provide such evidence in the third session on these quaternary mixtures (Figure 12.9b). The first session, however, again showed addition of the two sugars' distances from the norm with a separate effect of citric acid alone (Figure 12.9a).

12.8.3 SENSATIONS VERSUS THOUGHTS CONTROLLING PREFERENCE

In both these sessions with this participant (Figure 12.9), the effects of the taste compounds on preference were indirect. Indeed, they were mediated by processes even deeper in the mind than conceptualizing the stimulation (S/R), i.e., describing a feature of the drink.

The best account of the data from the first session was a set of S/R//R processes (Figure 12.9a). Such a conceptually modulated (//R) description (S/R) gives the meaning or intention of the modeled response—in this case, the degree of preference for each orange drink sample containing a tested mixture (R1). On this evidence, the session was dominated by two reasons for choosing a sample. One reason was a configuration summing (+) the closeness to an orange drink that is appropriately *sweet* (//R4), described as both sweet sucrose (S1/R4) and sweet fructose (S2/R4). A more minor reason was an appropriately *sour* taste (//R5) in sweet citric acid (S3/R4). This description of citric acid as sweet (S3/R4) rather than sour (S3/R5) could be interpreted as *unsweet* because the level of the acid can be recognized from its suppressive effect on the taste of sugars also included in a drink that is conceived overall as sweet.

In the third session (Figure 12.9b), there were three sorts of modulation of stimulation (S//) by a descriptive process (S/R), i.e., perceptual processes or sensations (S//S/R). The major taste sensation was a configuration (+) of two processes. The greater contribution came from the process of receptor stimulation by malic acid (S4) being described as sweet malic acid (S4/R4)—another case of recognition by suppression. The smaller contribution to the complex sensation was a process of describing citric acid (S3) as sour citric acid (S3/R5), i.e., perception of the acid as sour. There was a separate contribution from a simple sensation in which sucrose (S1) was described as the sourness of sucrose (S1/R5). This is the converse of the suppression (S3/S4) seen in the first session.

One of the remarkable aspects of this approach to measuring the determinants of preference is the diversity of cognitive hypotheses that compete as explanations of a modest amount of data from a single session with one individual, using only a total volume that is close to that usual for the drink. Norm-zeroed discrimination is a highly economical way of reading the mind, while the chemical senses are exerting their usual influence on ingestion. This fact in itself is evidence that these analyses get very close to what is actually going on as we eat and drink. Less precise

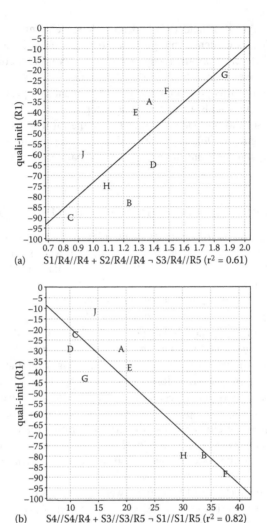

(a)   S1/R4//R4 + S2/R4//R4 ¬ S3/R4//R5 (r² = 0.61)

(b)   S4//S4/R4 + S3//S3/R5 ¬ S1//S1/R5 (r² = 0.82)

FIGURE 12.9 Preferences for variants of a familiar, orangey drink decided through complex meanings or sensations in the first and third sessions of one assessor. These cognitively integrating processes were objective achievements by the assessor, but they were also subjectively experienced, since they involved the concepts of *sweet* (R4) and *sour* (R5) that were used in other ratings of each sample for taste intensities. S1 = sucrose. S2 = fructose. S3 = citric acid. S4 = malic acid. Quali-initl (R1) = the first rating of each sample for its quality, at a freely selected point between the anchors *always choose* (0) and *never choose* (−100). In session 1 (panel a), the concept of sweetness gave meaning (//R4) to the description of each sugar as sweet (S1/R4 and S2/R4) within a single reaction (+), simultaneously with a different meaning (¬) of sourness (R4) to suppression of sweetness by citric acid (S3/R4). In session 3 (panel b), description (S/R) of malic acid (S4) as (un)sweet (R4) generated a sensation (S//S/R) from stimulation by malic acid (S//) that was the same (+) as a sensation in which citric acid stimulation was described as sour citric acid (S3/R5) alongside a separate sensation from stimulation by sucrose described as the sourness (suppression) of sucrose.

suggestions have recently been made from much more complex data. The ratios of components have been seen to be important to the combining of elements into a recognizable mixture (Jinks and Laing 2001). Weber's fractions of components have been found to affect the quality of the mixture (Le Berre et al. 2008).

12.8.4 MONOSODIUM GLUTAMATE: THE COMPLEX SAVORY TASTE

Another example of the power of norm-zeroed discrimination scaling within individuals exploited the approach's capacity to tackle the problem of a single chemical compound having multiple tastes. Monosodium glutamate (MSG) tastes both sweet and bitter, as do many amino acids. Since one of the two carboxylic acid moieties has not been neutralized, MSG also tastes sour. Its sodium content, of course, makes MSG taste salty as well. If concentrations of the five compounds, MSG, sucrose, caffeine, citric acid, and NaCl, are varied independently in a familiar glutamate-rich food, the assessor has the opportunity to show that MSG stimulates each of the four classic types of receptor by adding its discrimination distances from the norm to those of each of the other taste compounds. (Caffeine would not work in this design if MSG stimulated a different profile of the T2Rn [*bitter*] receptor types. Nevertheless, caffeine has a broad profile [Behrens et al. 2007] and can be tested because is widely used in coffee, tea, and other drinks.)

Such a four-dimensional discrimination model was found in pilot tests of mixtures in tomato and chicken soups (Freeman et al. 1993). That finding has been replicated and extended using mixtures of all five compounds in tomato juice (Booth et al. 2008, 2011a). The taste of a tomato is dominated by its large content of the monohydrogen glutamate ion in MSG. Tomatoes also contain some sodium ions, of course. Marketed tomato juice has a large amount of salt added. Evidence that the identical sodium ions from the chloride and glutamate salts act on the same receptor helps to validate the approach.

Different assessors added discrimination distances of MSG to the distances from the norm of different pairs or trios of the other four tastants (Booth et al. 2011a). Nevertheless, the four types of simple taste stimulated by MSG were covered across the set of assessors. That result is illustrated here for two overlapping trios and a different pair (Figure 12.10).

The component S4 + S2 + S1 in one session (Figure 12.10a) showed that information from citric acid (S4) and NaCl (NaCl:S2) was transmitted to the overall taste of tomato juice through the same channel as MSG (S1). The combining of MSG with NaCl validated this interpretation because the sodium ions from MSG and NaCl are, of course, identical and so must be undistinguishable. On that basis, the evidence from this session is that the acid moieties in the glutamate ion stimulate the same receptors as those in the (tricarboxylic) citric acid. That is unsurprising since both donate protons.

One session in another assessor (Figure 12.10b) had the component S5 + S1 + S4, where S5 is caffeine. Hence, MSG stimulates caffeine receptors as well as citric acid receptors. This session's data were fitted well by inclusion of a second component (S4 + S3), combining stimulation by citric acid and sucrose. The obvious explanation of this transmission of information from two types of taste receptors along the same

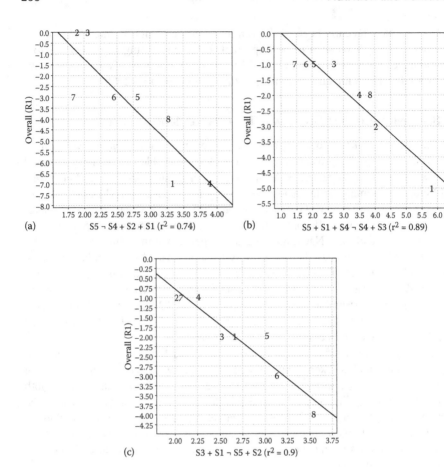

FIGURE 12.10 Three cases of stimulation by MSG of receptors for stimulants of a single taste (salty, sweet, sour, bitter). Data point integers: sequence of presentation of samples. R1 (*y* axis): overall similarity to tomato juice (0 = no difference). Cognitive model's number of half-discriminated fractions from familiar juice for each sample (*x* axis). S1: MSG. S2: NaCl. S3: sucrose. S4: citric acid. S5: caffeine. +: stimulation of receptors that are combined in the taste of MSG. ¬: stimulation of separate receptors. Data collected by Melanie Konle and Clare Wainwright.

channel is that they are both stimulated by glutamate. So, even though MSG itself was not included in this component, these data provide indirect evidence that MSG can taste both sour and sweet (Booth et al. 2011a).

The previous session in the same assessor (Figure 12.10c) combines stimulation by sucrose (S3) with MSG (S3 + S1). This is direct evidence that MSG stimulates the sugar receptor. A separate component summating stimulation from caffeine and NaCl would be explicable by MSG having a bitter taste as well as a salty one.

In short, the results of this experiment on mixtures of five taste compounds in a familiar drink show that norm-zeroed and contextualized discrimination scaling can identify concentrations of compounds that match exactly (are not discriminated from each other), even when one compound stimulates more than one type of a receptor. There is no need for tortuous cycles of testing for mismatches between a standard sample and the samples that try to mimic it exactly. Familiarity with the real-life item provides a standard in memory for judgments of any degree of dissimilarity from the experimental items. The resulting data provide not only Weber's fraction for each varied component but also its point of equality with that learnt norm.

12.8.5 AMINO ACID DETECTORS IN THE MOUTH AND BRAIN

The findings on MSG say nothing about the existence of a glutamate taste receptor on the human tongue (Li et al. 2002). The question they raise is whether such a receptor has been needed for human survival. Free and combined glutamate is a major source of nitrogen in the diet, but it is a nonessential (dispensable) amino acid. If we need a detector for the tastes of the amino acids that are essential to the diet (i.e., cannot be synthesized in the human body), then oral receptors specific to at least several of those are needed, such as methionine, creatine, leucine, or phenylalanine. There is (so far) no evidence for these.

In fact, the necessary detector has recently been identified, as long suspected, in the protein-synthesizing machinery of a specialized region in the forebrain. In pyriform cortex in rats, a local deficiency in one or more of the essential amino acids blocks transfer-ribonucleic acid (RNA) (Gietzen and Aja 2012). This creates an adverse neural effect, which rapidly conditions sensory aversion to a recently ingested novel food. In addition, a balanced supply of amino acids, restoring protein synthetic function, conditions preference to the most recent smell, taste, or flavor of food in rats (Booth and Simson 1971; Simson and Booth 1973; Booth 1974), sheep (Villalba and Provenza 1999), and people (Gibson et al. 1995).

Furthermore, the preference conditioned to any flavor by repletion of protein, or an essential amino acid, can become configured with the pyriform signal or some other effect specific to the depletion of essential amino acids. This learning process elaborates the selecting among foods into a protein appetite, i.e., an increase in sensory preference when in physiological need. Both rats (Gibson and Booth 1986; Baker et al. 1987; Booth and Baker 1990) and people (Gibson et al. 1995) learn a protein-specific appetite—that is, a learnt facilitation of ingestion by both the flavor and the state of need for protein, which have been followed by repair of that need.

The complex taste of glutamate may be a natural sensory component of the learnt appetite for protein (Gibson et al. 1995). Normal foods that are rich in good-quality protein (balanced in essential amino acids) often contain high levels of free glutamate and other amino acids. Hence, this distinctive sensory cue could be conditioned in combination with signals from lack of protein that can develop within a few hours after a protein-free breakfast (Gibson et al. 1995). Indeed, there is evidence that older people with low blood urea nitrogen may acquire a taste for hydrolyzed casein despite its bitterness and foul odor (Murphy and Withee 1987).

12.8.6 Savory Complex or a Fifth Simple Taste?

Presumably, the glutamate receptor on the human tongue has made it easier to recognize sources of protein. Glutamate is not an essential amino acid, but it is the most abundant component of proteins and occurs uncombined with other amino acids in the fluids of vegetables as well as meat and fish. However, most amino acids taste sweet and/or bitter, and those with two acid groups, like glutamic acid, taste sour as well. MSG stimulates all the other four types of taste receptor. Hence, it was proposed that those of us who think of the course of meat and vegetables in a main meal as savory transfer that concept to the complex mixture of tastes in the free glutamate ions and the sodium ions inherent in those foods (Freeman et al. 1993); that is, the taste of glutamate could create a learnt configural stimulus from mixtures of sugar, acid, and whatever type of bitter substance stimulates a profile of those receptors similar to that by this amino acid plus the salt that is there as well.

Such configural norms should allow better perceptual performance than does recognition of the components. That proved to be so for the savory taste of tomato juice (which has salt added to the juiced tomatoes). The Weber ratios of distances from the familiar mix of tastes that were achieved by ratings of how sweet, sour, bitter, and salty were better for the MSG in tomato juice than they were for added table sugar, fruit acid, caffeine, and salt.

12.8.7 All Sensory Vocabularies Are Learnt Social Names

Our tongues have receptors for the commonest amino acid, glutamic acid (with one of its acid groups ionized), as well as receptors for salt, sugar, acids, and a wide variety of poisons in plants. This finding has added some strength to the proposal that there is a fifth *basic taste*. Hitherto, that idea rested mainly on the ease with which the taste of MSG could be distinguished from the tastes of non-amino carboxylic acids, sugars, and bitter substances. However, all sorts of mixtures are readily distinguished from each other and from their components. If as much effort for MSG as for the tastes of seafood delicacies were put into trial-and-error matching of a natural taste mixture to an artificial mixture (Fuke and Konosu 1991), a taste indistinguishable from MSG could very likely be created. In any case, it is now clear that a theoretically appropriate approach enables matching mixtures to be interpolated from analyses of data from a single set of appropriately designed samples.

British English has long had the word *savory* for the vegetables and meats in which glutamate is at high levels, as well as the worldwide English names *salty*, *sweet* (or *sugary*), *sour* (or *acidic-tasting*), and *bitter* for stimulants of other types of gustatory receptor. The malleability of this cultural end of those alleged *labeled lines* has been neatly illustrated by a superb public responsibility marketing operation by the biggest manufacturer of the flavoring compound MSG. By promoting research into the taste of glutamate, the company in Japan has managed to displace the word *savory* in the English-speaking scientific community by a word they invented, *umami*, which is closely related to the Japanese word for delicious. How could there be a problem for consumers with a food additive that has its own receptor on the tongue with molecular genetics for the membrane protein? The MSG itself cannot be blamed if some cheap restaurants pour excessive amounts on their food or if some of their customers have bad reactions that they incorrectly attribute to the meal (Knibb et al. 1999; Knibb and Booth 2011).

12.8.8 QUANTITY OF MSG AND QUALITY OF A FOOD

It is in any case a fallacy to believe that the taste of glutamate makes a food more and more delicious as the anion's concentration increases without limit. As we have seen, for any familiar food or drink, each sensed constituent has a preference function that is peaked and not monotonic. Adding MSG does not automatically enhance flavor. The existing flavor is changed toward a generic savory flavor. For the flavor to remain the same but become stronger, the balance among all its component tastes must be maintained by any addition (Booth and Freeman 1993).

In other words, the learnt optimum strength of the taste based on the quantity of MSG, or a similarly tasting mixture in a familiar food, is complemented by the quality of the taste. The same applies to any complex taste and indeed to any odor, texture, color pattern, shape, etc. The quality of savory taste, or more specifically of the taste of an inherently MSG-rich food such as ripe tomatoes, is the closeness to the correctly balanced mixture of tastes, as implicitly remembered by the eater.

The top quality of the taste of MSG in a familiar brand of salted tomato juice beverage can be measured as the balance of IPs for each constituent of the matching mixture. The distribution of these most preferred (or most familiar) levels can be plotted in a histogram (as in Figure 12.7). The precision of each estimate is measured by Weber's fractions, with smaller fractions being better in differential acuity. The resulting ideal ranges enable the plotting of frequency polygons without bins (Figure 12.11). The central tendency or modal frequency for each taste compound's most accepted level gives the concentration that is balanced with the groupwide most prevalent IP for each of the other varied taste compounds.

The center of the modal count gives similar proportions by weight among the three tastants (log 1.1 to log 1.3, i.e., 12.6 to 20). The median IPs give proportions of sucrose 1.86 log mg/100 mL (with a very wide range), citric acid 1.43 log mg/100 mL, and caffeine 0.92 log mg/100 mL. The antilogarithms are 72:27:8.3 mg/100 mL—approximately 8:3:1. These proportions by weight represent the balance of stimulation by the glutamate that dominates the taste of tomatoes.

12.8.9 DIRECT ROUTE TO FOOD QUALITY

The exact calculation of each taste's (and any other sensed component's) number of discrimination units away from the learnt standard mixture should enable better eating on all fronts. Foods and drinks can be redesigned to provide better support for the healthier habits of eating and drinking. The suppliers of foods can increase the wealth available by more economical production and marketing. We can all become a little happier by enjoying the best-tasting foods and drinks.

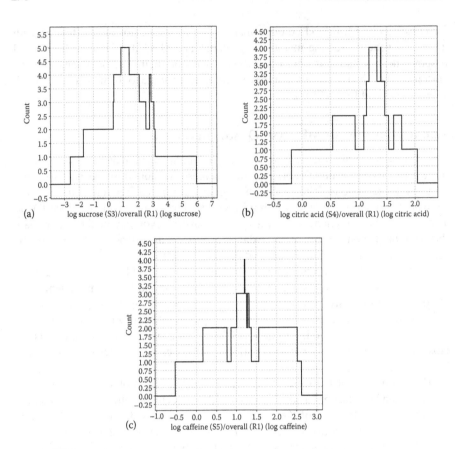

FIGURE 12.11   Frequency polygons of individuals' ideal concentrations ($\log_{10}$ mg/100 mL) of sucrose (a), citric acid (b), and caffeine (c) in tomato juice beverage. Each count is a horizontal line from one half-discriminated fraction below the IP to one HDF above.

12.9   OLFACTORY CONFIGURATIONS IN INGESTION

12.9.1   GOOD BALANCE AMONG COMPONENTS

The theory of quality illustrated previously for the complex savory taste in one food can be expressed diagrammatically. The example plotted here is of the concentrations of two odor compounds forming part of a quaternary mixture that simulates the aroma of fresh strawberries (Figure 12.12). One constituent is maltol, which has a sweetish smell, like a meringue. The other component in this two-dimensional illustration is ethyl acetoacetate. This compound by itself has a fruit-like aroma, but the smell is not readily identifiable with any familiar fruit.

The strength of the strawberry aroma in a test sample is on the 45° diagonal through the origin, which is each component's concentration at olfactory receptors in the strawberry norm in memory (Figure 12.12). The quality of the mixture, i.e., the balance of components, is the distance of the test sample along a perpendicular from the quantity diagonal. The off-aroma or lack of quality in the test sample is an excessively sweet

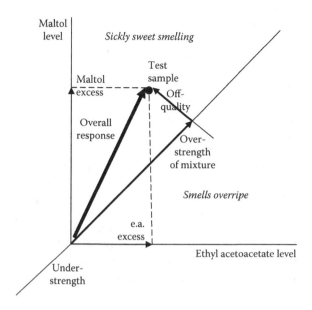

FIGURE 12.12 Strength-Quantity and Balance-Quality for maltol (*sweet*) and ethyl aceto-acetate (*fruity*) in the aroma of strawberries. (Redrawn from Booth, D.A., and R.P.J. Freeman, *Acta Psychologica*, 84:1–16, 1993, for two out of the four compounds in a mixture that can mimic the aroma of fresh strawberries.)

smell in the example plotted. If the imbalance were in the opposite direction, the off-quality could be an overripe smell or perhaps the hint of another fruit. These conceptualizations of defects in quality are objective in so far as an individual chooses words in accord with their successful use in the society speaking that language. That is, other appropriately acculturated assessors will agree with the verbal characterization.

The discrimination-scaled measure of marketed good quality or the personally preferred mixture of two sensed constituents provides a theoretical basis for the pragmatic ratio used, for example, for the sugar and cream in ice cream (Drewnowski and Greenwood 1983; Drewnowski et al. 1985).

12.9.2 AROMA OF FRESH STRAWBERRIES

Recognition of an odor is thought to be based on discrimination (Cain and Potts 1996). Yet, so far, there has been only one implementation for the olfaction of multisensory, multiconceptual cognition based on discrimination from a configural norm in memory (Booth and Freeman 1993). This example was the aroma of a ripe, dehulled strawberry (Kendal-Reed and Booth 1992a,b; Booth et al. 2010). The samples discriminated from that highly complex (and somewhat variable) natural mixture of volatiles were mixtures of just four odor compounds, each having its own assessor-named aroma note.

Four recognizable notes dominate the smell of a strawberry. Since we learn to label smells by their sources, each note is named after another object or sort of material. For a fruit, smells from the plant world are favored. The naming of an aroma as *sweet* probably arises from familiarity with caramelized, sugary foods. *Green* (or *leafy*) smell refers to the greenery on trees and bushes. *Fruity* is presumably a smell reminiscent of many species of fruit when ripe. The adjective *buttery* is a name learnt from the smell of that dairy product or from volatiles added to spreads based on vegetable oil in order to give a flavor said to be like that of butter.

The remarkable fact exploited by the experiments illustrated next is that compounds having odors similar to each of these four sorts of material, when mixed in the appropriate proportions, have an aroma that is hard to distinguish from that of fresh strawberries. The multireceptor profile of each compound (Polak 1973; Malnic et al. 1999) may compensate to some degree for deficiencies in the profiles of one or more of the other compounds because each is similar, but not identical, to a major volatile in the headspace from strawberries (Ulrich et al. 1997). The fruity compound in the tested quaternary mixture is an ester but with a sharper note than the esters predominant in strawberries. Similarly, the leafy green-smelling compound was a derivative of hexane (6-C) but not the compound dominant in strawberry itself. Maltol is formed when malts are roasted, and it smells of caramelized sugar. Diacetyl occurs in butter at low-enough levels to be characteristic of dairy fat rather than blatantly of its animal origin.

12.9.3 COGNITIVE ANALYSIS OF CONCENTRATIONS AND RATINGS

Ratings of the similarity of each test aroma to that of strawberries, and of the notes of each odorant in the mixture, need to be anchored on the smell of a real strawberry. Then, the perceived distance from the configural norm of the level of each odorant in a sample mixture can be put on a scale in units of discrimination (Weber's fraction; the HDF). Since all the distances are in that same unit, they can be combined algebraically without any assumptions about how concentrations of different compounds relate to each other or to the rated intensities under the different concepts (Booth and Freeman 1993).

There are two arithmetically simple possibilities (as stated above for taste mixtures). If two norm-zeroed discrimination functions are the same process (configured by learning about strawberries), then a sample's discrimination distances above or below the norm should add together, operating in the same cognitive dimension or over the same channel through the mind. If two of the odor compounds, the verbal concepts of notes, or the descriptions (concepts of compounds) are perceived as qualitatively different, then their norm-zeroed discriminations should be orthogonal, combining as the square root of the sum of the squares of the distances. As there were four odorants with a concept each, four-dimensional (4-d) models were tested. These calculations work if there are only three or two effective discriminations, or indeed just one. Similarly, the unidimensional (1-d) models had four components, but the additive formula works even if fewer than four inputs were discriminated. Poor discrimination (a weak influence) merely places all the samples close to the norm.

Regression from discrimination distance to rating of strawberriness (overall, strength or quality) was calculated for each sample for the odorant (an S), rating of a note (an R), and psychophysical function (an S/R). Those distances were summed into unidimensional integration (1-d) and were combined by the root sum of squares for multidimensional integration (4-d). Linear regression from distances to strawberriness scores gave the variance accounted for by each model (r^2; see the vertical axes in Figure 12.13).

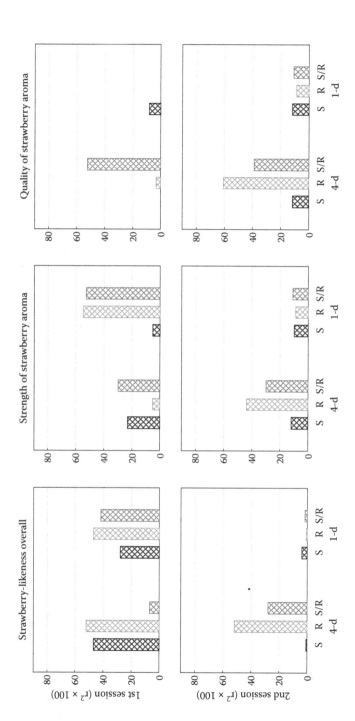

FIGURE 12.13 Cognitive processes integrating concentrations of four odor compounds into *strawberry* aroma. Each row of graphs comes from one session, from the first (top) to the fourth. Each mixture was rated first for overall similarity to the aroma of the fresh strawberry presented in the same way just before the mixture. Then, the strength of the mixture's strawberry aroma was rated and finally how the good the mixture was as the aroma of strawberry (see Figure 12.12). Both separate processing of up to four components (4-d) was calculated and also configuring into a single process (1-d). Discriminative predictors were calculated from the concentrations of stimuli directly (S) from the concept of strength and/or quality (R) or description of the stimulus in terms of that concept (S/R). (Case B in Booth, D.A. et al., *Appetite*, 55:738–741, 2010.)

(Continued)

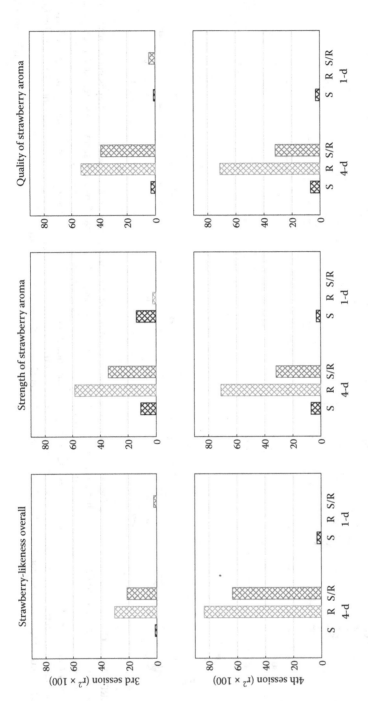

FIGURE 12.13 (CONTINUED) Cognitive processes integrating concentrations of four odor compounds into *strawberry* aroma. Each row of graphs comes from one session, from the first (top on the previous page) to the fourth. Each mixture was rated first for overall similarity to the aroma of the fresh strawberry presented in the same way just before the mixture. Then, the strength of the mixture's strawberry aroma was rated and finally how the good the mixture was as the aroma of strawberry (see Figure 12.12). Both separate processing of up to four components (4-d) was calculated and also configuring into a single process (1-d). Discriminative predictors were calculated from the concentrations of stimuli directly (S) from the concept of strength and/or quality (R) or description of the stimulus in terms of that concept (S/R). (Case B in Booth, D.A. et al., *Appetite*, 55:738–741, 2010.)

12.9.4 ANALYTICAL AND CONFIGURED NORMS

The assessor whose olfactory processing is summarized here assessed the overall strawberriness of the mixtures (left-hand column of four graphs, Figure 12.13) by use of the analytical concepts of sweet, leafy, fruity, and creamy throughout the four sessions—that is, four-dimensional processing, using the concepts alone (R) or in descriptions of the odorants (S/R). Nevertheless, 4-d stimulation (S) processing and 1-d conceptual (R) and descriptive (S/R) processing were almost equally as well evidenced in the first session. The analytical concepts rapidly gained in influence on the recognition of strawberry aroma in the tested mixtures, with the other processes dropping out, leaving solely the 4-d conceptual and descriptive processing in the fourth session (bottom left panel, Figure 12.13 continued). This finding is consistent with the view that practice with quantitative descriptive analysis interferes with configural perception, as might be mediated by immediate judgments of preference or familiarity (Barkat et al. 2012). Another factor that could have weakened the configuring is that at least two of the four analytical concepts—sweet and fruity—are likely to have been similar to the integrative concept of strawberry (Derby et al. 1996; Kay and Stopfer 2006).

Assessment of the strength of the strawberry aroma and the quality of the balance among odorants showed complementary learning. Judgments of strength were initially more configural (top middle panel, Figure 12.13). That is, the use of fresh strawberry as a standard set up a distinct holistic similarity among the concepts and descriptions. Nevertheless, as overall judgments became more analytical, strength was decided more by separate concepts. Unsurprisingly, the judgments of balance never used configural processing (right-hand column of four graphs, Figure 12.13). Analytical description dominated quality initially (top right panel, Figure 12.13), but conceptualization made an increasing contribution, resulting in a very similar pattern of processing of all three judgments by the fourth session (bottom right panel, Figure 12.13 continued).

Both strength and quality judgments were distinguished from overall judgments by the use of both analytical and configural processing of the olfactory stimulation (S processes). The contribution of direct stimulatory processing remained very small throughout, starting largest for strength (top middle panel, Figure 12.13). Yet, this stimulatory contribution was consistent throughout the three later sessions of both analytically and holistically decided judgments of strength and quality while never appearing in overall strawberriness.

The above results from one experiment with one person are, of course, merely illustrative. Nevertheless, they established the feasibility of person-by-person and situation-by-situation characterization of mediating cognitive processes in mixtures of odor compounds that come close enough to simulating a familiar aroma. Clearly, the ratios of concentrations presented are critical. If any one of them departs to a substantial extent from balance, the integrative and analytical tasks relative to the standard in memory may become impossible.

In addition, this approach provides a single solution for two major quantitative issues in olfaction (Booth and Freeman 1993; Booth 1995). One issue is the fundamental principles for measuring the quality of an odor (Wise et al. 2000). The traditional *difference tests* are not fully objective unless each sample's number of discriminations from the norm is estimated (Booth and Freeman 1993; Booth 1995). They are also far more laborious than is needed to detect differences, let alone to optimize quality. The other issue is how to specify the proportions of components in a mixture that can be configured into a familiar aroma (Jinks and Laing 2001; Le Berre et al. 2008) or taste, texture, color, etc. This too is achieved rapidly and objectively by scaling discrimination distances from the norm, as illustrated here and elsewhere (Booth et al. 1989, 2003a,b,c, 2010a,b, 2011a,b; Booth and Conner 1991; Booth and Freeman 1993). Furthermore, this solution to both problems is general to any sensory modality and indeed also to purely verbal or pictorial influences on preference.

12.9.5 FLAVOR

An obvious extension of this early work on tastants and odorants was to learnt configural norms of taste and odor in combination. Rated satiety to olfactory and visceral sensing has met the criterion for learnt configuring (Booth et al. 1994; Booth 2013). Configural integration of odor with taste occurs with sweetness at least (Prescott and Murphy 2009). Norm-zeroed discrimination analysis of performance before and after learning could advance associative theory in ways that categorical stimuli cannot do because they do not have intradimensional generalization gradients (Pearce 1994, 2002).

Particular levels of tastes and aromas (and colors) can be configured into the unique flavor of a food or drink. The collapse of New Coke, arguably the worst product development mistake ever made, was primarily excessive sweetness caused by poor methods of measuring ideal sweetness (Booth and Shepherd 1988), although the introduction of a new flavoring also played a part. Familiarity with a brand of cola (perhaps almost from weaning) establishes a highly precise memory of its taste and smell, as well as cooled temperature, level of fizz, and coloring.

It has recently begun to be recognized that the tastes and odors in familiar flavors do not add or multiply together (or suppress each other) in concentrations or in ratings but interact *cognitively* (Davidson et al. 1999). This fact invalidates long-standing claims to intensification of taste by odor or vice versa (Auvray and Spence 2008). However, discrimination-scaled data on configuring of taste and odor mixtures have yet to be published. The pilot analyses in the following indicate that the cognitively realistic approach could start to clear up the mess caused by inattention to the mental mechanisms of integration of inputs into ingestive output.

The concentrations in air of the volatile compounds in the peppermint flavoring of chewing gum were measured continuously in the breath in the nostrils that flows outward swallow by swallow. Menthone is a major contributor to the minty smell and so was taken as an indicator of concentrations across the profile of compounds measured by gas chromatography coupled with mass spectrometry. Sucrose concentration in saliva was measured every few seconds by the same technology (Davidson et al. 1999).

The sugar in a piece of gum begins to dissolve out quickly from the start of chewing. The gum (famously) becomes depleted within a few minutes. The steady decline in salivary sucrose concentration in contrast with a rise in menthone concentration is air in the mouth that goes into the nose up the back of the throat. This takes a minute or two to reach a peak and then declines somewhat more slowly. Hence, there is a set of menthone levels on either side of the peak that are essentially uncorrelated with the monotonic declining in sucrose levels. Rapidly repeated quantitative judgments of how *minty* the flavor currently is were used to construct a time-intensity profile.

Hence, the separate effects of sucrose and menthone stimulus levels on *minty* judgments can be measured. The various possible cognitive interactions between the descriptions of both sucrose and menthone as *minty* can be calculated to determine which of those hypotheses accounts for the greatest proportion of the variance in how *minty* the gum is said to be (Booth and Freeman 1993) at any moment around the time that the menthone levels in the nares reach their maximum.

Data for three sessions from different people are presented here. They illustrate the variety of cognitive processes that combine gustatory and olfactory information into the information conveyed by each individual's use in this context of society's objective verbal concept of a flavor. Sucrose and menthone were configured into *minty* in two of the three sessions but in very different ways. In one person (Figure 12.14), menthone provided the merest hint of flavor to the sucrose being dissolved out of the coating of the tablet of gum. Yet, in another set of data (Figure 12.15), menthone dominated the *minty* intensity while sucrose made a minor contribution, whereas the participant in Figure 12.16 responded the other way round, with menthone in a minor role. Nevertheless, all three analyses were dominated by configural processing, with signals from the two distinct modalities being transmitted over a single channel to the intensity of minty flavor. There was also some evidence than menthone was not a perfect match to the norm for *minty*. As well as the emergent *third stimulus* of configured menthone and sucrose, another aspect of menthone acted on its own (Figure 12.15). This may have been the parts of the olfactory receptor stimulation profile from menthone that most closely matched those of the whole spearmint aroma.

An alternative interpretation is that *minty* was not used to describe the volatiles of the spearmint flavoring in chewing gum, albeit cognitively modulated in strength by the taste of sucrose. It may have been used as a name for the candy imitated by gum (until it has lost its flavor). In that case, the norm in the memory that the word *mint* invoked would be the flavor of peppermint candy, which is overwhelmingly sweet. The normal balance of sweetness and peppermint aroma while sucking the candy was read from memory into the mixture of olfactory and gustatory stimuli presented as the volatilization of menthone from the chewing gum reached its peak. These, of course, are major practical issues for formulators of chewing gum for consumers' perceptions of quality. As in other areas of application of science, the most effective approach may be the measurement of what each user of the product is doing rather than statistical modeling of numbers collected from experts or customers without considering the mechanisms that generate the numbers.

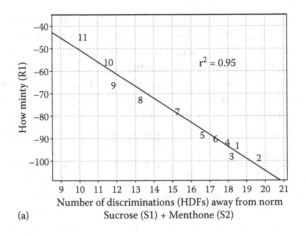

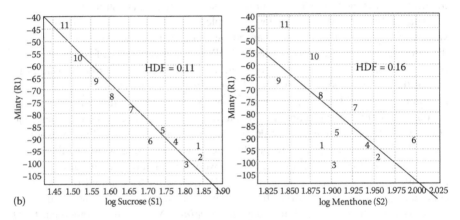

FIGURE 12.14 Best supported hypothesis of cognitive processing of sucrose taste and menthone aroma in intensity of *minty* around the peak release of menthone during chewing of a tablet of gum (a). Menthone and sucrose concentrations were configured into a single determinant (98% of r^2) of *minty*, but menthone made only a very slight contribution (1%), perhaps because of a less powerful effect, as measured by the greater half-discriminated fractions (in the two graphs of panel b). Data point numbers: sequence of concentrations delivered by chewing. (Raw data from GC-MS in this figure were kindly provided by Bob Davidson and Andy Taylor, University of Nottingham; see Davidson et al. 1999.)

12.9.6 FLAVORS OF CUISINES, NOT NUTRIENTS

It was well argued and pointed out long ago that flavors are not biologically determined but a cultural inheritance (Rozin 1973). Yet, it is still claimed that sweetness signals calories, saltiness signals sodium, fats have a taste, protein would not be recognized without a glutamate receptor, and aromas give emotional meaning to foods ahead of the material acquiring a culinary role in an individual's life. In fact, since the rise of agriculture, most of the energy in the human diet has come from grain

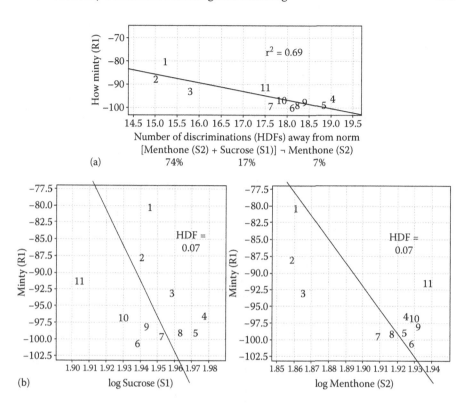

FIGURE 12.15 Best supported hypothesis of cognitive processing of *minty* intensity during the peak release of menthone from a chewed tablet of gum in an assessor who configured sucrose and menthone concentrations into an integrated flavor dominated by menthone and also had a separate small contribution from menthone alone (a). Nevertheless, both sucrose and menthone had a very weak influence on *minty*, and their concentrations were all a long way above ideal (b). Data point numbers: sequence of concentrations delivered by chewing. (Raw data from GC-MS in this figure were kindly provided by Bob Davidson and Andy Taylor, University of Nottingham; see Davidson et al. 1999.)

starch. Hunter-gatherer groups are most unlikely to have been rescued from extinction by honey from wild bees' nests. The ripening of fruit merely makes its energy content more digestible. Instead, it has been suggested that any selective pressure on the human sweet receptor could have arisen from its sensitivity to the free amino acids in milk countering bitterness in immunity promoting glycopeptides.

Also, as we saw at the start of this chapter (Sections 12.3.5 to 12.4.2), the human adult's appetite for sweetness, as for every other characteristic of a food, is learnt for each level (sometimes quite low) that is specific to a particular food habitually eaten (Conner et al. 1986, 1987). Such learning of preferences may be facilitated by hunger or a long-established norm of the hunger-reducing role of the flavored material (Irvine et al. 2013). The basic mechanism of glucose-conditioned sensory preference in naive rats can be configured with an internal state, but that signal can be from

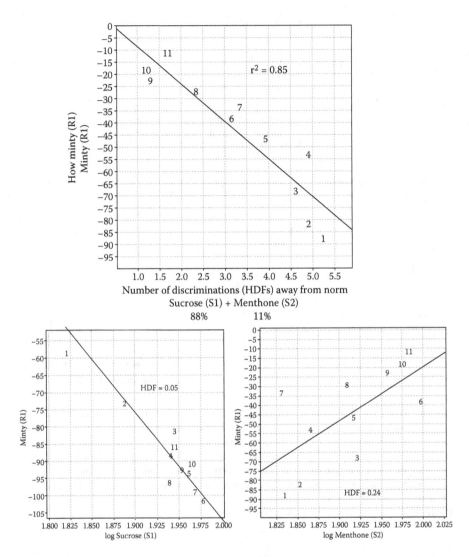

FIGURE 12.16 Best supported hypothesis of cognitive processing of *minty* intensity in an assessor who configured sucrose and menthone concentrations into *minty*. This integrated flavor was mostly the taste of sucrose (88%) but with a definite aroma of menthone (11%). The lower pair of graphs show that levels of sucrose were very well discriminated (Weber fraction of a mere 5%) but menthone levels not so well (24%). At this peak of release of menthone into the nares, all the sucrose concentrations on the tongue were above ideal for *minty* in gum, while all the concentrations of menthone in the nares were below ideal—albeit including levels very close to ideal in both cases. (Raw data from GC-MS in this figure were kindly provided by Bob Davidson and Andy Taylor, University of Nottingham; see Davidson et al. 1999.)

filling of the digestive tract with nonnutritive fluid, not necessarily a carbohydrate-specific deficit (Gibson and Booth 1989).

Similarly, as we saw in Section 12.4.11, there is no solid evidence for an innate appetite for sodium salts in human beings. Salt-deficient people may choose saltier foods (e.g., Leshem et al. 2008), but that could be a learnt appetite. Some selections of foods from the available cuisine may do better than others in rapidly repairing all the physiological components of a sodium deficit. That configural memory could produce the shift in sensory preferences when the signaled need for sodium recurs (see Booth 2013).

12.10 LONG-TERM EFFECTS OF TASTE ON NUTRITION

12.10.1 SALT AND STROKES

Long-term problems with too much taste are less obvious and may be hard to solve. For instance, we all need a little salt each day. Yet, that amount of sodium ions is far less than we consume from foods that we eat in quantity such as bread, pies, and biscuits. We do not think of pastry as a salty food, but a little salt is part of the character of a pie's crust and casing, and so the tradition continues of adding some to the dough. We may have a seriously salty item like a bag of potato crisps or a drink of tomato juice, or we may shake salt over the food on the plate. The result is that the body has to cope with a rush of salt during digestion of the meal. To keep sodium levels normal, water gets pushed into the blood, and its pressure goes up. That stretches the muscles in the walls of arteries, and so they get stronger. The result may be a persistently high pressure in the circulation, which is a danger to weaker blood vessels like those in the brain. Hence, there is an international problem with strokes to which lifetimes of salt intake have contributed.

How can we reduce the salt content of meals when eaters demand the levels of salt that they are accustomed to? The simplest answer in principle is to reduce the level in each food one step at a time, which is barely noticeable. Consumers who are interested can see what is happening in the information on the pack about nutrient contents. The changes should not be advertised as *healthier*, even though there is evidence to support that claim, because decades of poorly designed changes in sensed characteristics in the name of health has created the stereotype that healthy tastes bad and good-tasting food is unhealthy (Raghunathan et al. 2006).

There is so far no substitute for NaCl that gives its clean salty taste, even if it were safe and inexpensive enough for wide use. Substitutes (and amplifiers of the salty taste) found thus far have unfamiliar and therefore at least initially unpleasant side tastes. Hence, a substitute might work only in foods that already have other strong tastes that mask its side taste. Bland foods eaten in large amounts, such as bread, are therefore a serious problem for the search for substitutes. If there is not enough salt in bread to stop sodium ion levels in saliva being reduced, the unpleasant taste of distilled water can emerge, and the bread tastes like cardboard. Nevertheless, traditional levels are far above this minimum. Some people on a medically prescribed low-salt diet come to prefer a lower concentration of salt in a test food (Pangborn and Pecore 1982). Hence, if the salt level in bread were lowered by a barely detectable amount and consumers become familiar with the reduced level, they are all likely to come to prefer that level. After that, the level can be further lowered by a similar proportion. Such strategy requires accurate data on each consumer's most preferred level of salt in the food product to be adjusted. Individuals' IPs for salt in plain bread can be determined accurately from small amounts of data if the cognitive mechanisms of sensing are correctly exploited (Booth et al. 1983; Conner et al. 1988a). The frequency profile of IPs indicates that there could be no impact on sales from a reduction by 10%–15% (Figure 12.17). The most sensitive assessor who tolerated salt levels up to 2% would not have changed preference with a reduction of 10%–15%. The next lowest tolerance was for a reduction of approximately 20%. A few assessors found the saltiness of the plain bread very salient (narrow HDFs) and had IPs well above 2%. Pieces of bread without spread were tested, however, whereas these people would presumably have put a salty covering on their bread.

Lowering the salt content of bread happens to reduce costs in yeast as well as salt. Hence, major bakers in the United Kingdom were able to make year-on-year reductions in salt in the most popular brands of bread during the 1990s. The governmental regulatory agency then took advantage of this lead to persuade producers of other foods to reduce salt levels. Unfortunately, however, progress is limited in the United Kingdom, the United States of America, and other countries by failure

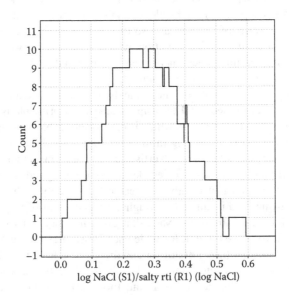

FIGURE 12.17 Directly observed prevalences of ideal ranges for salt in bread ($N = 15$). Each horizontal line begins at an assessor's IP minus one Weber fraction (HDF) and ends at an IP plus one HDF, excluding assessors with very wide HDFs. In these calculations, the determinant of preference was modeled as the cognitive process of describing NaCl as being *salty* in taste. rti: relative to ideal. log NaCl: $\log_{10}$ of grams of NaCl in 100 g of bread. (Reanalysis by CoPro2.29 of data presented in Booth, D.A. et al., *Appetite*, 4:301–312, 1983.)

to correct standard practice in sensory evaluation of consumer preferences. First, the set of food samples has to be designed to remove upward biases created by presenting unfamiliarly high concentrations (Riskey et al. 1979; Conner et al. 1987). Second, the rating and analyses of the data must measure each person's IP (*just right*), rather than degrading the data to a range that is broadly acceptable (*just about right*) and has indeterminate boundaries with categories unacceptably high and low (Booth and Conner 2009).

12.10.2 Sugar and Teeth

Sweetness has been posed as a problem for morality as well as for medicine (Rozin 1986). The only proven problem for physical health though is from leaving sugar repeatedly on the teeth at intervals of less than an hour. It is irrelevant how much sugar was eaten. Bacteria that are always in the mouth make acid from whatever little sugar is left. That softens the enamel. If it has no time to harden, rot sets in. A low level of fluoride slows the softening, but plainly, it is wise to wait at least an hour or two before having something else sugary after eating chocolate or cake, especially candy that sticks on the teeth. Health campaigners would help more by a focus on that risky pattern of actions instead of letting the scene be stolen by fulminations against sugar regardless of use.

If there is a connection between sweetness and a child's obesity, it is not sugar but a habit of eating lots of sugary food. Lots of starchy food is just as fattening and a diet of many fatty foods even more so. A growing child needs meals that are large and varied enough to go through to the next meal four or five times a day when the child concentrates just on eating and drinking and is given no more first course than is eaten up and leaves space for a little mildly tasting dessert. Foods supplied to children should not exploit the inborn attraction to sweet stuff.

Anyone who fears loss of control to intense pleasure should relax about sugar. The innate reflex to strong sweetness by itself has been suppressed by all the learning to like the moderate level of sweetness specific to each ordinary food and drink.

12.11   CONCLUSIONS

12.11.1 Mechanisms versus Tests

The state of the art remains reliant on group averaging of numbers taken from tests of meal sizes (weight of each food, total energy content, etc.), sensory descriptive analysis, ratings of appetite ("How much will you eat then?"; "How full are you now?"), modality-specified preferences (liking for taste, aroma, color, etc.), and so on, with or without statistical analyses that allows for redundancies among supposedly different measures. All of these approaches fail to address the basic scientific question: which stimuli actually control each (nonredundant) response?

It is logically impossible to start answering this question until potential influences on a response are measured, as well as the test response itself, whatever influence some investigators assume that it reflects. Those measurements of stimuli have to show that their levels vary independently of each other across the tested samples, because the effects caused by fully corelated variations cannot be separated, again as a matter of logic.

12.11.2 Chemosensory Influences on Nutrition

This chapter should have made crystal clear why it is fundamentally misconceived to try to measure the effects of sweetness on meal size, insulin resistance, or market share; of concentration of glutamate or added aroma on appetite in older people; or of genetic sensitivity to bitterness on food choices or rated preferences. Measurements of blood chemistry relate very poorly to the usual daily intake of the relevant nutrients. The chances of sensed chemical constituents of foods bearing a clear relation to nutritional health must be even more remote.

A single mechanism that varies the choice of each mouthful cannot be expected to bear on the intake of any nutrient. Even in the apparently most straightforward instance, the IPs for salt in various foods bear little relation to daily sodium intake (Shepherd 1988). As an absolute minimum, each individual's IP for the taste or aroma under investigation needs to be measured for each key food in a regular pattern of eating that has been shown to have the nutritional effect of interest.

Often, the potentially relevant foods or eating habits have yet to be measured in a way that identifies a mechanism for their effect. For example, the basic facts about fattening habits remain to be determined. If an individual maintains a change in frequency of a communally identified eating habit, how big is the step change in weight caused by that alteration in the rate of energy intake (Hall et al. 2011)? When an eating habit has been shown to be effective, then the question arises, which foods and drinks dominate that habit (Booth and Booth 2011; Booth and Nouwen 2011; Laguna-Camacho and Booth under review)? At that stage, measurement of sensory and other influences on choice can be used for scientific investigation of nutritional consequences.

There are feasible ways forward to understanding the roles of taste and smell in nutrition. Indeed, they have been available for several decades. As in genomics, neuroscience, individual development, or qualitative research, there is no alternative, even in the medium term, to publishing reports that relate the observations to the relevant known causal processes.

REFERENCES

Auvray, M., and C. Spence. 2008. The multisensory perception of flavour. *Consciousness and Cognition* 17:1016–1031.

Baker, B.J., D.A. Booth, J.P. Duggan, and E.L. Gibson. 1987. Protein appetite demonstrated: Learned specificity of protein-cue preference to protein need in adult rats. *Nutrition Research* 7:481–487.

Barkat, S., E. Le Berre, G. Coureaud, G. Sicard, and T. Thomas-Danguin. 2012. Perceptual blending in odor mixtures depends on the nature of odorants and human olfactory expertise. *Chemical Senses* 37:159–166.

Bartoshuk, L.M., V.B. Duffy, and I.J. Miller. 1994. PTC/PROP tasting: Anatomy, psychophysics and sex effects. *Physiology and Behavior* 56:1165–1171.

Beauchamp, G.K., and M. Moran. 1982. Dietary experience and sweet taste preference in human infants. *Appetite* 3:139–152.

Behrens, M., S. Foerster, F. Staehler, J.D. Raguse, and W. Meyerhof. 2007. Gustatory expression pattern of the human TAS2R bitter receptor gene family reveals a heterogenous population of bitter responsive taste receptor cells. *Journal of Neuroscience* 27:12630–12640.

Beidler, L.M. 1954. A theory of taste stimulation. *Journal of General Physiology* 38:133–139.

Berridge, K.C., and H.J. Grill. 1983. Alternating ingestive and aversive consummatory responses suggest a two-dimensional analysis of palatability in rats. *Behavioral Neuroscience* 97:563–573.

Berridge, K.C., and T.E. Robinson. 2003. Parsing reward. *Trends in Neuroscience* 26:507–513.

Berridge, K.C., I.L. Venier, and T.E. Robinson. 1989. Taste reactivity analysis of 6-hydroxy-dopamine-induced aphagia: Implications for arousal and anhedonia hypotheses of dopamine function. *Behavioral Neuroscience* 103:36–45.

Blundell, J.E., and A.J. Hill. 1986. Paradoxical effects of an intense sweetener (aspartame) on appetite. *Lancet* 8489:1092–1093.

Booth, D.A. 1972a. Conditioned satiety in the rat. *Journal of Comparative and Physiological Psychology* 81:457–471.

Booth, D.A. 1972b. Taste reactivity in satiated, ready to eat and starved rats. *Physiology and Behavior* 8:901–908.

Booth, D.A. 1974. Acquired sensory preferences for protein in diabetic and normal rats. *Physiological Psychology* 2:344–348.

Booth, D.A. 1976. Approaches to feeding control. In *Appetite and Food Intake*, ed. T. Silverstone, 417–478. West Berlin: Abakon Verlagsgesellschaft/Dahlem Konferenzen. Available at http://epapers.bham.ac.uk.

Booth, D.A. 1979. Metabolism and the control of feeding in man and animals. In *Chemical Influences on Behavior*, eds. K. Brown, and S.J. Cooper, pp. 79–134. London: Academic Press.

Booth, D.A. 1985. Food-conditioned eating preferences and aversions with interoceptive elements: Conditioned appetites and satieties. *Annals of the New York Academy of Sciences* 443:22–37.

Booth, D.A. 1988. Mechanisms from models—Actual effects from real life: The zero-calorie drink-break option. *Appetite* 11:94–102.

Booth, D.A. 1990. How not to think about immediate dietary and postingestial influences on appetites and satieties. *Appetite* 14:171–179.

Booth, D.A. 1991. Learned ingestive motivation and the pleasures of the palate. In *The Hedonics of Taste*, ed. R.C. Bolles, pp. 29–58. Hillsdale, NJ: Erlbaum.

Booth, D.A. 1994. *Psychology of Nutrition*. Bristol, PA: Taylor & Francis.

Booth, D.A. 1995. Cognitive processes in odorant mixture assessment. *Chemical Senses* 20:639–643.

Booth, D.A. 2005. Perceiving the texture of a food: Biomechanical and cognitive mechanisms and their measurement. In *Food Colloids: Interactions, Microstructure and Processing*, ed. E. Dickinson, pp. 339–355. Cambridge: Royal Society of Chemistry.

Booth, D.A. 2008. Physiological regulation through learnt control of appetites by contingencies among signals from external and internal environments. *Appetite* 51:433–441.

Booth, D.A. 2009a. Lines, dashed lines and "scale" ex-tricks. Objective measurements of appetite *versus* subjective tests of intake. *Appetite* 53:434–437.

Booth, D.A. 2009b. Learnt reduction in the size of a meal. Measurement of the sensory–gastric inhibition from conditioned satiety. *Appetite* 52:745–749.

Booth, D.A. 2013. Configuring of extero- and interoceptive senses in actions on food. *Multisensory Research* 26:123–142.

Booth, D.A., and B.J. Baker. 1990. dl-Fenfluramine challenge to nutrient-specific textural preference conditioned by concurrent presentation of two diets. *Behavioral Neuroscience* 104:226–229.

Booth, D.A., and P. Booth. 2011. Targeting cultural changes supportive of the healthiest life-style patterns. A biosocial evidence-base for prevention of obesity. *Appetite* 56:210–221.

Booth, D.A., and M.T. Conner. 1991. Characterisation and measurement of influences on food acceptability by analysis of choice differences: Theory and practice. *Food Quality & Preference* 2:75–85.

Booth, D.A., and M.T. Conner. 2009. Salt in bread. [Letter to the Editor]. *Journal of Food Science* 74:3:vii–viii.

Booth, D.A., and J.D. Davis. 1973. Gastrointestinal factors in the acquisition of oral sensory control of satiation. *Physiology and Behavior* 11:23–29.

Booth, D.A., and R.P.J. Freeman. 1993. Discriminative feature integration by individuals. *Acta Psychologica* 84:1–16.

Booth, D.A., and H.R. Kissileff. under review. Dissociation between visceral sources of infor-mation: Physiological signals of satiety from the stomach and beyond.

Booth, D.A., and N.E. Miller. 1969. Lateral hypothalamus mediated effects of a food signal on blood glucose concentration. *Physiology and Behavior* 4:1003–1009.

Booth, D.A., and A. Nouwen. 2011. Weight is controlled by eating patterns, not by foods or drugs. Reply to comments on "Satiety—No way to slim." *Appetite* 57:784–790.

Booth, D.A., and R. Shepherd. 1988. Sensory influences on food acceptance—The neglected approach to nutrition promotion. *BNF Nutrition Bulletin* 13:1:39–54.

Booth, D.A., and P.C. Simson. 1971. Food preferences acquired by association with variations in amino acid nutrition. *Quarterly Journal of Experimental Psychology* 23:135–145.

Booth, D.A., A.T. Campbell, and A. Chase. 1970a. Temporal bounds of postingestive glucose-induced satiety in man. *Nature* 228:1104–1105.

Booth, D.A., A. Chase, and A.T. Campbell. 1970b. Relative effectiveness of protein in the late stages of appetite suppression in man. *Physiology and Behavior* 5:1299–1302.

Booth, D.A., D. Lovett, and G.M. McSherry. 1972. Postingestive modulation of the sweetness preference gradient in the rat. *Journal of Comparative and Physiological Psychology* 78:485–512.

Booth, D.A., M. Lee, and C. McAleavey. 1976. Acquired sensory control of satiation in man. *British Journal of Psychology* 67:137–147.

Booth, D.A., P. Mather, and J. Fuller. 1982. Starch content of ordinary foods associatively conditions human appetite and satiation, indexed by intake and eating pleasantness of starch-paired flavours. *Appetite* 3:163–184.

Booth, D.A., A.L. Thompson, and B. Shahedian. 1983. A robust, brief measure of an indi-vidual's most preferred level of salt in an ordinary foodstuff. *Appetite* 4:301–312.

Booth, D.A., M.T. Conner, and E.L. Gibson. 1989. Measurement of food perception, food preference, and nutrient selection. *Annals of the New York Academy of Sciences* 561:226–242.

Booth, D.A., E.L. Gibson, A.M. Toase, and R.P.J. Freeman. 1994. Small objects of desire: The recognition of foods and drinks and its neural mechanisms. In *Appetite: Neural and Behavioral Bases*, eds. C.R. Legg, and D.A. Booth, pp. 98–126. Oxford: Oxford University Press.

Booth, D.A., T. Earl, and S. Mobini. 2003a. Perceptual channels for the texture of a food. *Appetite* 40:69–76.

Booth, D.A., S. Mobini, T. Earl, and C.J. Wainwright. 2003b. Consumer-specified instrumen-tal quality of short-dough cookie texture using penetrometry and break force. *Journal of Food Science: Sensory and Nutritive Qualities of Food* 68:382–387.

Booth, D.A., S. Mobini, T. Earl, and C.J. Wainwright. 2003c. Market-optimum instrumental values from individual consumers' discriminations of standard sensory quality of the texture of short-dough biscuits. *Journal of Food Quality* 26:425–439.

Booth, D.A., A.J. Blair, V.J. Lewis, and S.H. Baek. 2004. Patterns of eating and movement that best maintain reduction in overweight. *Appetite* 43:277–283.

Booth, D.A., M. Konle, and O. Sharpe. 2008. Taste of savoury foods does not need a fifth receptor type. *Appetite* 51:355.

Booth, D.A., S. Higgs, J. Schneider, and I. Klinkenberg. 2010a. Learned liking versus inborn delight. Can sweetness give sensual pleasure or is it just motivating? *Psychological Science* 21:1656–1663.

Booth, D.A., M.S. Kendal-Reed, and R.P.J. Freeman. 2010b. A strawberry by any other name would smell as sweet, green, fruity and buttery. Multisensory cognition of a food aroma. *Appetite* 55:738–741.

Booth, D.A., R.P.J. Freeman, M. Konle, C.J. Wainwright, and O. Sharpe. 2011a. Perception as interacting psychophysical functions. Could the configuring of features replace a specialised receptor? *Perception* 40:509–529.

Booth, D.A., G. O'Leary, L. Li, and S. Higgs. 2011b. Aversive viscerally referred states and thirst accompanying the sating of hunger motivation by rapid digestion of glucosaccharides. *Physiology and Behavior* 102:373–381.

Booth, D.A., O. Sharpe, and M.T. Conner. 2011c. Differential gustatory sensitivity to caffeine in normal use points to supertasters, tasters and non-tasters. *Chemosensory Perception* 4:154–169.

Booth, D.A., O. Sharpe, R.P.J. Freeman, and M.T. Conner. 2011d. Insight into sight, touch, taste and smell by multiple discriminations from norm. *Seeing and Perceiving* 24:485–511.

Booth, D.A., S. Jarvandi, and L. Thibault. 2012. Food after deprivation rewards the earlier eating. *Appetite* 59:790–795.

Bowman, S.J., D.A. Booth, R.G. Platts, and the UK Sjögren's Interest Group. 2004. Measurement of fatigue and discomfort in primary Sjögren's syndrome using a new questionnaire tool. *Rheumatology* 43:758–764.

Breslin, P.A.S., M.M. Gilmore, G.K. Beauchamp, and B.G. Green. 1993. Psychophysical evidence that oral astringency is a tactile sensation. *Chemical Senses* 18:405–417.

Breslin, P.A.S., S. Kemp, and G.K. Beauchamp. 1994. Single sweetness signal. *Nature* 369:447–448.

Breslin, P.A.S., G.K. Beauchamp, and E.N. Pugh. 1996. Monogeusia for fructose, glucose, sucrose and maltose. *Perception and Psychophysics* 58:327–341.

Cabanac, M. 1971. Physiological role of pleasure. *Science* 173:1103–1107.

Cabanac, M. 1979. Sensory pleasure. *Quarterly Review of Biology* 54:1–29.

Cabanac, M., and R. Duclaux. 1970a. Specificity of internal signals in producing satiety for taste stimuli. *Nature* 227:966–967.

Cabanac, M., and R. Duclaux. 1970b. Obesity: Absence of satiety aversion to sucrose. *Science* 168:496–497.

Cabanac, M., Y. Minaire, and E.R. Adair. 1968. Influence of internal factors on the pleasantness of a gustative sweet sensation. *Communications in Behavioral Biology* 1:77–82.

Cain, W.S., and B.C. Potts. 1996. Switch and bait: Probing the discriminative basis of odor identification via recognition memory. *Chemical Senses* 21:35–44.

Cain, W.S., F.T. Schiet, M.J. Olsson, and R.A. deWijk. 1995. Comparison of models of odor interaction. *Chemical Senses* 20:625–637.

Campbell, B.A., and F.D. Sheffield. 1953. Relation of random activity to food deprivation. *Journal of Comparative and Physiological Psychology* 46:320–322.

Chang, W.I., J.W. Chung, Y.K. Kim, S.C. Chung, and H.S. Kho. 2006. The relationship between phenylthiocarbamide (PTC) and 6-n-propylthiouracil (PROP) taster status and taste thresholds for sucrose and quinine. *Archives of Oral Biology* 51:427–432.

Chastrette, M., T. Thomas-Danguin, and E. Rallert. 1998. Modelling the human olfactory stimulus–response function. *Chemical Senses* 23:181–196.

Conner, M.T., and D.A. Booth. 1988. Preferred sweetness of a lime drink and preference for sweet over non-sweet foods, related to sex and reported age and body weight. *Appetite* 10:25–35.

Conner, M.T., A.V. Haddon, and D.A. Booth. 1986. Very rapid, precise measurement of effects of constituent variation on product acceptability: Consumer sweetness preferences in a lime drink. *Lebensmittel-Wissenschaft und -Technologie* 19:486–490.

Conner, M.T., D.G. Land, and D.A. Booth. 1987. Effects of stimulus range on judgments of sweetness intensity in a lime drink. *British Journal of Psychology* 78:357–364.

Conner, M.T., D.A. Booth, V.J. Clifton, and R.P. Griffiths. 1988a. Individualized optimization of the salt content of white bread for acceptability. *Journal of Food Science* 53:549–554.

Conner, M.T., A.V. Haddon, E.S. Pickering, and D.A. Booth. 1988b. Sweet tooth demonstrated: Individual differences in preference for both sweet foods and foods highly sweetened. *Journal of Applied Psychology* 73:275–280.

Conner, M.T., E.S. Pickering, R.J. Birkett, and D.A. Booth. 1994. Using an individualised attribute tolerance model in consumer acceptability tests. *Food Quality and Preference* 5:225–232.

Cowart, B.J., and G.K. Beauchamp. 1986. The importance of sensory context in young children's acceptance of salty tastes. *Child Development* 57:1034–1039.

Crook, C.K., and L.P. Lipsitt. 1976. Neonatal nutritive sucking: Effects of taste stimulation upon sucking rhythm and heart rate. *Child Development* 47:518–522.

Davidson, J.M., R.S.T. Linforth, T.A. Hollowood, and A.J. Taylor. 1999. Effect of sucrose on the perceived flavor intensity of chewing gum. *Journal of Agricultural and Food Chemistry* 47:4336–4340.

Davis, J.D. 1973. The effectiveness of some sugars in stimulating licking behavior in rat. *Physiology and Behavior* 11:39–45.

De Graaf, C., J.E.R. Frijters, and H.C.M. Van Trijp. 1987. Taste interaction between glucose and fructose assessed by functional measurement. *Perception and Psychophysics* 41:383–392.

Denton, D.A. 1982. *Hunger for Salt. An Anthropological, Physiological and Medical Analysis.* London: Springer.

Derby, C.D., M. Hutson, B.A. Livermore, and W.H. Lynn. 1996. Generalization among related complex odorant mixtures and their components: Analysis of olfactory perception in the spiny lobster. *Physiology and Behavior* 60:87–95.

Dessirier, J.M., C.T. Simons, M.I. Carstens, M. O'Mahony, and E. Carstens. 2000. Psychophysical and neurobiological evidence that the oral sensation elicited by carbonated water is of chemogenic origin. *Chemical Senses* 25:277–284.

Dethier, V.G. 1962. *To Know a Fly.* New York: McGraw-Hill.

Dibsdall, L., and D. Booth. 1996. Delayed physiological effects of fat and sugar on satiety for food. *Appetite* 27:272–273.

Dibsdall, L.A., and D.A. Booth. 2014. Physiological signals measured by food- and time-specific expected satiety. *Appetite* 83, 350 (abstract).

Dibsdall, L.A., C.J. Wainwright, N.W. Read, and D.A. Booth. 1996. How fats and carbohydrates in familiar foods contribute to everyday satiety by their sensory and physiological actions. *British Food Journal* 99:142–147.

Ditschun, T.L., and J.L. Guinard. 2004. Comparison of new and existing methods for the classification of individuals according to 6-*n*-propylthiouracil (PROP) taster status. *Journal of Sensory Studies* 19:149–170.

Drewnowski, A., and M.R.C. Greenwood. 1983. Cream and sugar: Human preference for high-fat foods. *Physiology and Behavior* 30:629–633.

Drewnowski, A., J.A. Grinker, and J. Hirsch. 1982. Obesity and flavour perception: Multidimensional scaling of soft drinks. *Appetite* 3:361–368.

Drewnowski, A., J.F. Brunzell, K. Sande, P.H. Iverius, and M.R.C. Greenwood. 1985. Sweet tooth reconsidered: Taste responsiveness in human obesity. *Physiology and Behavior* 35:617–622.

Duclaux, R., J. Feisthauer, and M. Cabanac. 1973. Effect of eating a meal on pleasantness of food and non-food odors in man. *Physiology and Behavior* 10:1029–1033.

Durlach, P.J., N.A. Elliman, and P.J. Rogers. 2002. Drinking while thirsty can lead to conditioned increases in consumption. *Appetite* 39:119–125.

Epstein, L.H., and J.J. Leddy. 2006. Food reinforcement. *Appetite* 46:22–25.

Fechner, G.T. 1860. *Elemente der Psychophysik, Volumes 1 & 2*. Leipzig: Breitkopf & Hartel. Translated 1966. *Elements of Psychophysics*, eds. H.E. Adler, D.H. Howes, and E.G. Boring. New York: Holt.

Freeman, R.P.J., N.J. Richardson, M.S. Kendal-Reed, and D.A. Booth. 1993. Bases of a cognitive technology for food quality. *British Food Journal* 95:9:37–44.

French, S.A., R.W. Jeffery, and D. Murray. 1999. Is dieting good for you? Prevalence, duration and associated weight and behaviour changes for specific weight loss strategies over four years in US adults. *International Journal of Obesity* 23:320–327.

Fuke, S., and S. Konosu. 1991. Taste-active components in some foods. A review of Japanese research. *Physiology and Behavior* 49:863–868.

Garcia, J., and R.A. Koelling. 1966. Relation of cue to consequence in avoidance learning. *Psychonomic Science* 4:123–124.

Garcia, J., D.J. Kimeldorf, and R.A. Koelling. 1955. Conditioned aversion to saccharin results from exposure to gamma radiation. *Science* 122:157–158.

Garcia, J., W.G. Hankins, and K.W. Rusiniak. 1974. Behavioral regulation of milieu interne in man and rat. *Science* 185:824–831.

George, D.N., and J.M. Pearce. 2012. A configural theory of attention and associative learning. *Learning and Behavior* 40:241–254.

Gibson, E.L., and D.A. Booth. 1986. Acquired protein appetite in rats: Dependence on a protein-specific need state. *Experientia* 42:1003–1004.

Gibson, E.L., and D.A. Booth. 1989. Dependence of carbohydrate-conditioned flavor preference on internal state in rats. *Learning and Motivation* 20:36–47.

Gibson, E.L., C.J. Wainwright, and D.A. Booth. 1995. Disguised protein in lunch after low-protein breakfast conditions food-flavor preferences dependent on recent lack of protein intake. *Physiology and Behavior* 58:363–371.

Gietzen, D.W., and S.M. Aja. 2012. The brain's response to an essential amino acid-deficient diet and the circuitous route to a better meal. *Molecular Neurobiology* 46:332–348.

Grill, H.J., and R. Norgren. 1978. The taste reactivity test. I. Mimetic responses to gustatory stimuli in neurologically normal rats. *Brain Research* 143:263–279.

Guidetti, M., M.T. Conner, A. Prestwich, and N. Cavazza. 2012. The transmission of attitudes towards food: Twofold specificity of similarities with parents and friends. *British Journal of Health Psychology* 17:346–361.

Hall, K.D., G. Sacks, D. Chandramohan et al. 2011. Quantification of the effect of energy imbalance on body weight. *Lancet* 378:826–837.

Harris, G., and D.A. Booth. 1987. Infants' preference for salt in food: Its dependence upon recent dietary experience. *Journal of Reproductive and Infant Psychology* 5:97–104.

Harris, G., A. Thomas, and D.A. Booth. 1991. Development of salt taste preference in infancy. *Developmental Psychology* 26:534–538.

Hill, A.J., L.D. Magson, and J.E. Blundell. 1984. Hunger and palatability: Tracking ratings of subjective experience before, during and after the consumption of preferred and less preferred food. *Appetite* 5:361–371.

Horne, J., J. Hayes, and H.T. Lawless. 2002. Turbidity as a measure of salivary protein reactions with astringent substances. *Chemical Senses* 27:653–659.

Hovland, C.I. 1937. The generalization of conditioned responses. I. The sensory generalization of conditioned cues with varying frequencies of tone. *Journal of General Psychology* 17:125–148.

Hull, C.L. 1947. The problem of primary stimulus generalization. *Psychological Review* 54:120–134.

Hunt, J.N., and J.D. Pathak. 1960. The osmotic effects of some simple molecules and ions on gastric emptying. *Journal of Physiology* 154:254–269.

Hunt, J.N., and D.F. Stubbs. 1975. Volume and energy contents of meals as determinants of gastric emptying. *Journal of Physiology* 245:209–225.

Irvine, M.A., J.M. Brunstrom, P. Gee, and P.J. Rogers. 2013. Increased familiarity with eating a food to fullness underlies increased expected satiety. *Appetite* 61:13–18.

Iwayama, K., and M. Eishima. 1997. Neonatal sucking behaviour and its development until 14 months. *Early Human Development* 47:1–9.

Jacobs, H.L. 1958. Studies on sugar preference. 1. The preference for glucose solutions and its modification by injections of insulin. *Journal of Comparative and Physiological Psychology* 51:304–310.

Jacobs, H.L. 1962. Some physical, metabolic, and sensory components in the appetite for glucose. *American Journal of Physiology* 203:1043–1054.

Jacobs, H.L., and K.N. Sharma. 1969. Taste versus calories: Sensory and metabolic signals in the control of food intake. *Annals of the New York Academy of Sciences* 157:1084–1112.

Jinks, A., and D.G. Laing. 2001. The analysis of odor mixtures by humans: Evidence for a configurational process. *Physiology and Behavior* 72:51–63.

Jones, L.V., D.R. Peryam, and L.L. Thurstone. 1955. Development of a scale for measuring soldiers' food preferences. *Food Research* 20:512–520.

Kay, L.M., and M. Stopfer. 2006. Information processing in the olfactory systems of insects and vertebrates. *Seminars in Cell Development Biology* 17:433–442.

Kelly, K.A. 1980. Gastric emptying of liquids and solids: Roles of proximal and distal stomach. *American Journal of Physiology* 239:2:G71–G76.

Kendal-Reed, M., and D.A. Booth. 1992a. Human odor perception by multidimensional discrimination from remembered patterns. *Chemical Senses* 17:5:649.

Kendal-Reed, M., and D.A. Booth. 1992b. Olfactory perception as receptor pattern recognition. *Chemical Senses* 17:6:848–849.

Kerkhof, I., D. Vansteenwegen, F. Baeyens, and D. Hermans. 2009. A picture–flavour paradigm for studying complex conditioning processes in food preference learning. *Appetite* 53:303–308.

Kissileff, H.R., D.A. Booth, J.C. Thornton, F.X. Pi-Sunyer, R.N. Pierson, and J. Lee. 2008. Human food intake is discriminatively sensitive to gastric signaling. *Appetite* 51:759.

Knibb, R.C., and D.A. Booth. 2011. Situation-specific cognitive behavioural self-therapy for erroneously suspected allergy or intolerance to a food. A short self-assessment tool. *Appetite* 57:439–442.

Knibb, R., D.A. Booth, A. Armstrong, R. Platts, A. Macdonald, and I.W. Booth. 1999. Episodic and semantic memory in reports of food intolerance. *Applied Cognitive Psychology* 13:451–464.

Krieckhaus, E.E., and G. Wolf. 1968. Acquisition of salt by rats. Interaction of innate mechanisms and latent learning. *Journal of Comparative and Physiological Psychology* 65:197–201.

Kurtz, A.J., H.T. Lawless, and T.E. Acree. 2009. Reference matching of dissimilar binary odour mixtures. *Chemosensory Perception* 2:186–194.

Laguna-Camacho, A., and D.A. Booth. under review. Step reduction in weight: The missing measure of the change in weight caused by change in a pattern of eating or exercise. Submitted on September 15, 2013.

Laing, D.G., C. Link, A.L. Jinks, and I. Hutchinson. 2002. The limited capacity of humans to identify the components of taste mixtures and taste–odour mixtures. *Perception* 31:617–635.

Laming, D. 1985. Some principles of sensory analysis. *Psychological Review* 92:462–485.

Laming, D.R.J. 1986. *Sensory Analysis*. London: Academic Press.

Laming, D. 1987. The discrimination of smell and taste compared with other senses. *Chemistry and Industry* 1:12–18.

Le Berre, E., N. Béno, C. Chabanet, P. Etiévant, and T. Thomas-Danguin. 2008. Just noticeable differences in component concentrations modify the odor quality of a blending mixture. *Chemical Senses* 33:389–395.

Le Magnen, J., and S. Tallon. 1966. La periodicité spontanée de la prise d'aliments ad libitum du rat blanc. *Journal de Physiologie* 58:323–349.

Leshem, M. 2009. The excess salt appetite of humans is not due to sodium loss in adulthood. *Physiology & Behavior* 98:3:331–337.

Leshem, M., A. Saadi, N. Alem, and K. Hendi. 2008. Enhanced salt appetite, diet and drinking in traditional Bedouin women in the Negev. *Appetite* 50:71–82.

Levin, B.E., A.A. Dunn-Meynell, and V.H. Routh. 1999. Brain glucose sensing and body energy homeostasis: Role in obesity and diabetes. *American Journal of Physiology— Regulatory, Integrative and Comparative Physiology* 276:R1223–R1231.

Li, X., L. Staszewski, H. Xu, K. Durick, M. Zoller, and E. Adler. 2002. Human receptors for sweet and umami taste. *Proceedings of the National Academy of Sciences, U.S.A.* 99:4692–4696.

Mace, O.J., N. Lister, E. Morgan et al. 2009. An energy supply network of nutrient absorption coordinated by calcium and T1R taste receptors in rat small intestine. *Journal of Physiology* 587:195–210.

Malnic, B., J. Hirono, T. Sato, and L.B. Buck. 1999. Combinatorial receptor codes for odors. *Cell* 96:713–723.

Marshall, K., D.G. Laing, A.L. Jinks, and I. Hutchinson. 2006. The capacity of humans to identify components in complex odor–taste mixtures. *Chemical Senses* 31:539–545.

Massei, G., and D.P. Cowan. 2002. Strength and persistence of conditioned taste aversion in rats: Evaluation of 11 potential compounds. *Applied Animal Behaviour Science* 75:249–260.

McBride, R.L. 1983. A JND-scale/category-scale convergence in taste. *Perception and Psychophysics* 34:77–83.

McBride, R.L. 1988. Taste reception of binary sugar mixtures: Psychophysical comparison of two models. *Perception and Psychophysics* 44:167–171.

McBride, R.L. 1993. Integration psychophysics: The use of functional measurement in the study of mixtures. *Chemical Senses* 18:83–92.

McBride, R.L., and D.A. Booth. 1986. Using classical psychophysics to determine ideal flavour intensity. *Journal of Food Technology* 21:775–780.

McBride, R.L., and D.C. Finlay. 1990. Perceptual integration of tertiary taste mixtures. *Perception and Psychophysics* 48:326–330.

McCleary, R.A. 1953. Taste and post-ingestion factors in specific-hunger behavior. *Journal of Comparative and Physiological Psychology* 46:411–421.

Mei, N. 1985. Intestinal chemosensitivity. *Physiological Reviews* 65:211–237.

Mei, N., and L. Garnier. 1986. Osmosensitive vagal receptors in the small intestine of the cat. *Journal of the Autonomic Nervous System* 16:159–170.

Meillon, S., A. Thomas, R. Havermans, L. Pénicaud, and L. Brondel. 2013. Sensory-specific satiety for a food is unaffected by the ad libitum intake of other foods during a meal. Is SSS subject to dishabituation? *Appetite* 63:112–118.

Murphy, C., and J. Withee. 1987. Age and biochemical status predict preference for casein hydrolysate. *Journals of Gerontology* 42:73–77.

Pain, J.F., and D.A. Booth. 1968. Toxiphobia to odors. *Psychonomic Science* 10:363–364.

Pangborn, R.M., and S.D. Pecore. 1982. Taste perception of sodium chloride in relation to dietary intake of salt. *American Journal of Clinical Nutrition* 35:510–520.

Pearce, J.M. 1994. Similarity and discrimination: A selective review and a connectionist model. *Psychological Review* 101:587–607.

Pearce, J.M. 2002. Evaluation and development of a connectionist theory of configural learning. *Animal Learning and Behavior* 30:73–95.

Pecina, S., and K.C. Berridge. 2005. Hedonic hot spot in nucleus accumbens shell: Where do mu-opioids cause increased hedonic impact of sweetness? *Journal of Neuroscience* 25:11777–11786.

Peryam, D.R., and N.F. Girardot. 1952. Advanced taste test method. *Food Engineering* 24: 7:58–61, 194.

Peryam, D.R., and J.G. Haynes. 1957. Prediction of soldiers' food preferences by laboratory methods. *Journal of Applied Psychology* 41:2–6.

Peryam, D.R., and F.J. Pilgrim. 1957. Hedonic scale method of measuring food preferences. *Food Technology* 11:9–14.

Pfaffmann, C. 1960. The pleasures of sensation. *Psychological Review* 67:253–268.

Pfaffmann, C. 1964. Taste, its sensory and motivating properties. *American Scientist* 52:187–206.

Pfaffmann, C., R. Norgren, and H.J. Grill. 1977. Sensory affect and motivation. *Annals of the New York Academy of Sciences* 290:18–34.

Pfeiffer, J.C., J. Hort, T.A. Hollowood, and A.J. Taylor. 2006. Taste–aroma interactions in a ternary system: A model of fruitiness perception in sucrose/acid solutions. *Perception and Psychophysics* 68:216–227.

Pliner, P. 1994. Development of measures of food neophobia in children. *Appetite* 23:147–163.

Polak, E. 1973. Multiple profile–multiple receptor site model for vertebrate olfaction. *Journal of Theoretical Biology* 40:469–484.

Prescott, J., and S. Murphy. 2009. Inhibition of perceptual and evaluative odour–taste learning by attention to the stimulus elements. *Quarterly Journal of Experimental Psychology* 62:2133–2140.

Quine, W.V. 1974. *The Roots of Reference*. Chicago: Open Court.

Raghunathan, R., R.W. Naylor, and W.D. Hoyer. 2006. The unhealthy = tasty intuition and its effects on taste inferences, enjoyment and choice of food products. *Journal of Marketing* 70:70–184.

Rescorla, R.A. 1973. Evidence for unique stimulus account of configural conditioning. *Journal of Comparative and Physiological Psychology* 85:331–338.

Richardson, N.J., and D.A. Booth. 1993. Multiple physical patterns in judgments of the creamy texture of milks and creams. *Acta Psychologica* 84:93–101.

Richardson, N.J., D.A. Booth, and N.L. Stanley. 1993. Effect of homogenization and fat content on oral perception of low and high viscosity model creams. *Journal of Sensory Studies* 8:133–143.

Riskey, D.R., A. Parducci, and G.K. Beauchamp. 1979. Effects of context in judgments of sweetness and pleasantness. *Perception and Psychophysics* 26:171–176.

Rolls, B.J., E.T. Rolls, E.A. Rowe, and K. Sweeney. 1981a. Sensory specific satiety in man. *Physiology and Behavior* 27:137–142.

Rolls, B.J., E.A. Rowe, E.T. Rolls, B. Kingston, A. Megson, and R. Gunary. 1981b. Variety in a meal enhances food intake in man. *Physiology and Behavior* 26:215–221.

Roper, S.D. 2007. Signal transduction and information processing in mammalian taste buds. *Pflügers Archiv—European Journal of Physiology* 454:759–776.

Roper, S.D., and N. Chaudhari. 2009. Processing umami and other tastes in mammalian taste buds. *Annals of the New York Academy of Sciences* 1170:60–65.

Rozin, E. 1973. *The Flavor-Principle Cookbook*. New York: Hawthorne Books.

Rozin, P. 1986. Sweetness, sensuality, sin, safety, and socialization: Some speculations. In *Sweetness*, ed. J. Dobbing, 99–109. London: Springer-Verlag.

Rozin, P. 1991. Family resemblance in food and other domains. The family paradox and the role of parental congruence. *Appetite* 16:92–103.

Rutter, M. (Ed.) 2008. *Genetic Effects on Environmental Vulnerability to Disease: State of the Art and Future Directions.* Chichester: Wiley-Blackwell.

Schifferstein, H.N.J., and J.E.R. Frijters. 1993. Perceptual integration in heterogeneous taste percepts. *Journal of Experimental Psychology—Human Perception and Performance* 19:661–675.

Schutz, H.G. 1965. A food action scale for measuring food acceptance. *Journal of Food Science* 30:365–374.

Sclafani, A. 1995. How preferences are learned: Laboratory animal models. *Proceedings of the Nutrition Society* 54:419–427.

Sclafani, A., and J.W. Nissenbaum. 1988. Robust conditioned flavor preference produced by intragastric starch infusions in rats. *American Journal of Physiology* 255:R672–R675.

Shankar, M.U., C.A. Levitan, J. Prescott, and C. Spence. 2009. The influence of color and label information on flavour perception. *Chemosensory Perception* 2:53–58.

Sheffield, F.D., and B.A. Campbell. 1954. The role of experience in the spontaneous activity of hungry rats. *Journal of Comparative and Physiological Psychology* 47:97–100.

Shepard, R.N. 1958. Stimulus and response generalization—Tests of a model relating generalization to distance in psychological space. *Journal of Experimental Psychology* 55:509–523.

Shepherd, R. 1988. Sensory influences on salt, sugar and fat intake. *Nutrition Research Reviews* 1:125–144.

Shepherd, R., C.A. Farleigh, and D.G. Land. 1984. Effects of stimulus context on preference judgments for salt. *Perception* 13:739–742.

Shuford, E.H. 1959. Palatability and osmotic pressure of glucose and sucrose solutions as determinants of intake. *Journal of Comparative and Physiological Psychology* 52:150–153.

Simson, P.C., and D.A. Booth. 1973. Olfactory conditioning by association with histidine-free or balanced amino acid loads. *Quarterly Journal of Experimental Psychology* 25:354–359.

Smith, M.H. 1966. Effect of hypertonic preloads on concurrent eating and drinking. *Journal of Comparative and Physiological Psychology* 61:338–341.

Smith, M., and M. Duffy. 1957. Some physiological factors that regulate eating behavior. *Journal of Comparative and Physiological Psychology* 50:601–608.

Spence, C. 2010. The multisensory perception of flavour. *The Psychologist* 23:720–723.

Stein, L.J., B.J. Cowart, and G.K. Beauchamp. 2012. The development of salty taste acceptance is related to dietary experience in human infants: A prospective study. *American Journal of Clinical Nutrition* 95:123–129.

Steiner, J. 1977. Facial expressions of the neonate infant indicating the hedonics of food-related chemical stimuli. In *Taste and Development. The Genesis of Sweet Preference*, ed. J.M. Weiffenbach, pp. 173–189. Bethesda, MD: U.S. Department of Health, Education and Welfare.

Steiner, J.E., D. Glaser, M.E. Hawilo, and K.C. Berridge. 2001. Comparative expression of hedonic impact: Affective reactions to taste by human infants and other primates. *Neuroscience and Biobehavioral Reviews* 25:53–74.

Stevens, S.S. 1957. On the psychophysical law. *Psychological Review* 64:153–181.

Stevenson, R.J., and R.A. Boakes. 2003. A mnemonic theory of odor perception. *Psychological Review* 110:340–364.

Stevenson, R.J., R.A. Boakes, and J. Prescott. 1998. Changes in odor sweetness resulting from implicit learning of a simultaneous odor–sweetness association. *Learning and Motivation* 29:113–132.

Stroud, S., and D. Booth. 1999. Improved questionnaire assessment of PROP foods' bitterness, predictive of aversions and preferences. *Appetite* 32:293.

Tatzer, E., M.T. Schubert, W. Timischl, and G. Simbruner. 1985. Discrimination of taste and preference for sweet in premature babies. *Early Human Development* 12:23–30.

Tepper, B.J., Y. Koelliker, L. Zhao et al. 2008. Variation in the bitter-taste receptor gene TAS2R38, and adiposity in a genetically isolated population in Southern Italy. *Obesity* 16:2289–2295.

Thompson, D.A., and R.G. Campbell. 1977. Hunger in humans induced by 2-deoxy-D-glucose: Glucoprivic control of taste preference and food intake. *Science* 198:1065–1068.

Thompson, D.A., H.R. Moskowitz, and R.G. Campbell. 1976. Effects of body weight and food intake on pleasantness ratings for a sweet stimulus. *Journal of Applied Physiology* 41:77–83.

Tomchik, S.M., S. Berg, J.W. Kim, N. Chaudhari, and S.D. Roper. 2007. Breadth of tuning and taste coding in mammalian taste buds. *Journal of Neuroscience* 27:10840–10848.

Torgerson, W.S. 1958. *Theory and Methods of Scaling.* New York: John Wiley.

Ulrich, D., E. Hoberg, A. Rapp, and S. Kecke. 1997. Analysis of strawberry flavour—Discrimination of aroma types by quantification of volatile compounds. *Zeitschrift für Lebensmittel-Untersuchung und -Forschung* 205:218–223.

Valenstein, E.S., V.C. Cox, and J.W. Kakolewski. 1967. Polydipsia elicited by the synergistic action of a saccharin and glucose solution. *Science* 157:552–554.

van Aken, G.A. 2010. Modelling texture perception by soft epithelial surfaces. *Soft Matter* 6:826–834.

Verendeev, A., and A.L. Riley. 2012. Conditioned taste aversion and drugs of abuse. History and interpretation. *Neuroscience and Biobehavioral Reviews* 36:2193–2205.

Vickers, Z.M. 1984. Crispness vs. crunchiness—A difference in pitch. *Journal of Texture Studies* 15:157–163.

Villalba, J.J., and F.D. Provenza. 1999. Nutrient-specific preferences by lambs conditioned with intraruminal infusions of starch, casein, and water. *Journal of Animal Science* 77:378–387.

Wansink, B., G. Bascoul, and G.T. Chen. 2006. The sweet tooth hypothesis: How fruit consumption relates to snack consumption. *Appetite* 47:107–110.

Weber, E.H. 1843. *De pulsu, resorptione, auditu et tactu.* Translated 1996 On the pulse, breathing, hearing and touch. In *On the Tactile Senses*, eds. H.E. Ross, and D.J. Murray, pp. 23–136. Hove, UK: Psychology Press.

Wise, P.M., M.J. Olsson, and W.S. Cain. 2000. Quantification of odor quality. *Chemical Senses* 25:429–443.

Witherley, S.A., and R.M. Pangborn. 1980. Gustatory responses and eating duration of obese and lean adults. *Appetite* 1:53–63.

Wittgenstein, L. 1953. *Philosophical Investigations.* Oxford: Basil Blackwell.

Yamaguchi, S. 1967. The synergistic taste effect of monosodium glutamate and disodium 5′-inosinate. *Journal of Food Science* 32:473–478.

Yeomans, M.R., and S. Mobini. 2006. Hunger alters the expression of acquired hedonic but not sensory qualities of food-paired odors in humans. *Journal of Experimental Psychology. Animal Behavior Processes* 32:460–466.

Yeomans, M.R., and T. Symes. 1999. Individual differences in the use of pleasantness and palatability ratings. *Appetite* 32:382–394.

Yeomans, M.R., A. Jackson, M.D. Lee, J. Nesic, and P.J. Durlach. 2000. Expression of flavour preferences conditioned by caffeine is dependent on caffeine deprivation state. *Psychopharmacology* 150:208–215.

Yeomans, M.R., S. Mobini, T.D. Elliman, H.C. Walker, and R.J. Stevenson. 2006. Hedonic and sensory characteristics of odors conditioned by pairing with tastants in humans. *Journal of Experimental Psychology. Animal Behavior Processes* 32:215–228.

13 Review of Chemosensation for Weight Loss

Darin D. Dougherty

CONTENTS

13.1 Hedonically Aversive Odors and Tastes 295
13.2 Hedonically Positive Odors 298
13.3 Hedonically Positive Tastes 300
References...305

While virtually unknown during this age of diets and bariatric surgery, the concept that chemosensory stimuli may mediate satiety has existed for decades at least. As opposed to allesthesia from secondary effects of ingestion (stretch receptors in stomach, change in insulin, or metabolic effect), chemosensory-mediated satiety occurs even before ingestion and absorption. This has been shown with both high-fat or high-carbohydrate liquid meals, which when infused directly into the stomach or into the small intestine had less appetite suppression effects than when provided orally (Cecil et al. 1998a,b); whereas when a chemosensory stimulus is sniffed or mandibulated without deglutination, satiety is produced (Chapelot and Louis-Sylvestre 2008).

For the purpose of this review, I will discuss the use of odorants and tastants or both.

Over the last century, the concept of using chemosensory stimuli to induce weight loss has been extensively explored and can be categorized into three phases: hedonically aversive odors, hedonically pleasant odors, and hedonically pleasant tastants.

13.1 HEDONICALLY AVERSIVE ODORS AND TASTES

Initially, smells and tastants were employed as a form of aversive stimuli as a part of classical avoidance conditioning. As far back as 1924, a case study described the successful use of vinegar in a child to establish food aversion (Moss 1924).

Joseph Wolpe, a luminary of classical conditioning, is noted in the mid-1950s in a study whereby he applied *vile-smelling* asafetida to the nostrils in two cases of obesity (Wolpe 1969). This would be paired with concurrent handling, smelling, and tasting hedonically positive foods. The results suggested a temporary control of overeating in one, while the other achieved lasting control with *a sylph-like* figure (Wolpe 1969).

Later, butyric acid, a noxious odor, was employed as aversive stimuli for behavioral treatment of a 29-year-old woman (Kennedy and Foreyt 1968). After 22 weeks, she had lost 30 lb. from the starting weight of 322 lb. Despite such positive results, for two reasons, the clinical utility of such an approach remains doubtful. One has to do with habituation to the unpleasant odor. To avoid this, the author suggested that eight different unpleasant odors be employed as part of the deconditioning phase, which requires a laborious, user-unfriendly apparatus consisting of a turret of eight tubes. Secondly, for many, compliance may be a problem. Their subject, who required 9 days of hospitalization to undergo aversive conditioning treatment, noted the unpleasant nature of the experience, "S was strongly affected by the gas; she became ill a number of times during the sessions and vomited once" (Kennedy and Foreyt 1968, p. 575). It would be doubtful that most patients would readily tolerate such side effects. Furthermore, it is unclear how much weight was lost during the 9 days of hospitalization with forced restriction to a 1000 cal/day diet.

These same authors extended their work with aversion therapy (Foreyt and Kennedy 1971). In each therapy session, six of seven malodors in various combinations were employed including butyric acid, pure skunk oil, trimethylamine, pyridine, diisopropylamine, benzylamine, and methyl sulfide.

After 9 weeks, six overweight subjects lost 13.3 lb. as opposed to 1 lb. among the six control subjects. After 4 months, the weight loss averaged 9.2 lb. in the treatment group as opposed to 1.3-lb. weight gain in the control group. While significant weight loss was seen, it remains unclear if the odorants were the origin of this. Unlike control subjects, treatment subjects were weighed in at each treatment session and maintained food diaries, which were extensively discussed. Both of these actions could have acted to motivate for further weight loss by focusing attention on the food that they ate as well as promoting the Rosenthal effect of positive experimental results not due to treatment but rather as a result of trying to please the experimenter (Rosenthal 1966; Hirsch et al. 2007).

Another treatment component that could have acted independently of the odors was the therapy. Aversive conditioning was applied 15 times per session, with each session lasting half an hour. Subjects underwent three sessions per week for 1 month followed by biweekly sessions for 5 weeks for a total of 11 h of therapy time. The authors even recognized that this therapy may have been the motivation for weight loss in the treatment group.

> Even though the conditioning may have been successful to some degree with each of the SS except perhaps E5, it certainly was not the only factor involved in the weight loss. Without question, the experimenter–patient relationship was vital in achieving the initial weight loss. E formed positive relationships with each of the six SS. He talked with them at length, was quite interested in them and listened to their daily problems, their troubles with their children, husbands, and school work. He insisted that they lose weight; he checked their food lists thoroughly during each session and told them repeatedly that they were to stop eating certain foods. This relationship cannot be overemphasized as being crucial in the initial period. (Foreyt and Kennedy 1971, p. 33)

Further confounding the active treatment was the addition of a 1000–1300 cal restrictive diet in the active group, which, if adhered to, would surely have had some influence on the weight loss. Moreover, practical application of such a program would be prohibitive. Twenty-two hours of psychotherapy would be cost-prohibitive and, in today's market, would exceed approximately $6000 or almost $700 per pound lost.

The use of mephitic aroma of hydrogen sulfide (H_2S) for covert sensitization was performed on two morbidly overweight subjects (308 and over 400 lb.) (Ashem et al. 1972). Images of food were conjured and presented with aversive odor and active imagery of rotten eggs; vomit; pus; bronchial discharge; or dirt on food, vomit, and unclean dishes for each subject, respectively. Twenty-minute treatment sessions were administered twice a day for 3 days, followed by three times weekly for the course of the trial. After 8 weeks, although having lost 40 lb., the first subject refused further treatment. The second subject lost 60 lb. in 12 weeks, became noncompliant, and 4 months later, had regained 50 of the 60 lb. Concurrent treatment may have acted as one mechanism of action in addition to the aversive odors.

While compliance was an issue, this study again suggested that chemosensory manipulation may have a role in weight management.

The use of malodorous valeric acid as a form of assisted covert sensitization was described in a 27-year-old female *compulsive eater* (Maletzky 1973). In this approach, after relaxation training, the subject was told to imagine chocolate goodies that she had just eaten, infested with lice and maggots. Coincident with this, the smell of valeric acid was released, inducing nausea and gagging. After 10 sessions, she no longer ate chocolate, and, at 7 months, continued weight loss was noted. While the exact weight loss remains unclear, this provides further suggestion of the role of chemosensation and weight loss.

Self-managed aversion therapy with cigarette smoke aroma was reported in a 24-year-old "attractive, but extremely obese, graduate student" (Morganstern 1974). With 18 weekly sensitization sessions, she was taught to self-administer a malodor–food pairing: "Before swallowing the candy she was told to take one long 'drag' on the cigarette and to immediate spit out the food, exclaiming at the same time, 'even this junk makes me sick' " (Morganstern 1974, p. 256–257). This approach resulted in a 41-lb. weight loss in 18 weeks. The author suggested that self-inhalation of other noxious odors warranted investigation. This study changes the locus of control from experimenter treater to self-administration of an odor.

In trying to ferret out the mechanism of action, a further study of aversive odorant conditioning was undertaken (Frohwirth and Foreyt 1978). In this trial, 12 subjects received olfactory aversion two times per week for 10 weeks with the same malodor used in a previous successful aversive treatment study (benzylamine, butyric acid, etc.) (Kennedy and Foreyt 1968). Twelve placebo group subjects received one of four pleasant odors during the treatment sessions including sandalwood, rose, lemon, or orange. Fourteen who were on a waiting list for the study served as the control subjects. After 10 and 20 weeks, there was no significant difference in the weight loss groups, thus calling into question the validity of using noisome odors to induce weight loss.

Another investigation into the use of olfactory aversive conditioning in overeating failed to display significance (Cole and Bond 1983). Four noxious odors were used, one per week, to avoid habituation: benzylamine, pyridine, butyric acid, and trimethylamine. After 1 month of treatment, the active group lost 4.7 lb., the attention–placebo group lost 3.6 lb., and the nontreatment control lost 0.5 lb. However, 2 months after treatment was completed, there was no significant difference, and all had regained the weight that they had lost. Such results were the death knell for the use of aversive odors as a treatment paradigm in weight loss, ushering in the next phase of hedonically positive odors for weight loss.

13.2 HEDONICALLY POSITIVE ODORS

Possibly hedonically pleasant odors could induce satiety and thus weight loss. Early studies examined the opposite: could food odors stimulate appetite, in particular, in those in need of greater nutrition, i.e., the elderly?

In attempting to answer this question, 16 nursing home residents underwent exposure to 27 different food odors prior to eating for 5 weeks as compared to the no-treatment control group (Brouillette and White 1991). No statistically significant effect, either enhancement or inhibition of calorie intake, was found. Given the elderly's poor olfactory ability, these results are not unexpected. While a negative study, its relevance to younger, normosmic, overweight subjects is tenuous.

The use of hedonically positive odors as a weight loss tool was suggested as early as 1982 by Engen (1982). He suggested using a nasal spray of an odor with a short-term adaptation effect, thus reducing any olfactory stimuli from the ingestion of food and the subsequent inhibition of desire to eat the food.

Just sniffing a food odor for the same duration as would be required to eat the actual food induced both a decrease in hedonics toward that food and a decreased desire to eat the food (Rolls and Rolls 1997).

A series of studies by Hirsch highlighted the possibility of using hedonically positive food odors for weight loss. In a double-blind crossover study of sniffing 2-acetylpyridine (the smell of Fritos), 105 volunteers, at least 10 lb. overweight adults under age 65, were assessed (Hirsch and Dougherty 1993). They were instructed to inhale in each nostril three times whenever hungry. Of the 46 (47%) who completed 2 weeks active followed by 2 weeks placebo (or vice versa), an average weight loss with the active odorant was 1.49 lb. versus a placebo of 1.10 lb. Subdividing those with normal olfactory ability on olfactory testing, the average weight loss was 2.78 lb. on the active treatment, and, further subdividing those into who had positive hedonics toward the odor, the average weight loss was 3 lb.

While very suggestive of the effect of odorants on weight loss, this study suffered from the serious limitations of duration and subject size. The study only lasted 2 weeks on the active arm, a duration of insufficient length to overcome any yo-yo effect of weight loss. Moreover, the subject size that completed the study was low. If one assumed that the dropout rate reflected those in whom the odorant was ineffective, the true active agent, normosmic hedonically positive weight loss could be calculated to be approximately 1.3 lb. Such ambiguity prompted further investigation. This time, a sequence of food odors—banana, green apple, and peppermint—were administered (Hirsch and Gomez 1995).

Of the 3193 subjects who were at least 10 lb. overweight who completed the study, the average initial weight was 217 lb. and the average weight loss was 4.7 lb. or 2% of body weight per month over the course of the 6-month study. A direct correlation was found among the frequency of the inhalation of odors and loss (18–288 sniffs per day), hedonics toward the odorant, and olfactory ability with weight loss. Despite its positive results, this study could be faulted for its lack of a control group and being motivation dependent (Ostman et al. 2004).

These criticisms were partially answered by a 4-month double-blinded random-ized control study that used banana, apple, and peppermint as its active odorant and a scented placebo control (Mayer et al. 1999). Eighty subjects, who were at least 10 lb. overweight, were equally divided between the active and placebo groups. Subjects were instructed to sniff a different scent each day on a rotating basis three times in each nostril 5 min before and immediately prior to eating. Those in the active group lost 19 lb. in 4 months as compared to a 4-lb. weight loss in the placebo group. Appetite reduction, a mechanism of action, was demonstrated on 30 additional sub-jects who were induced to experience a state of hunger with presentation of the olfac-tory and visual stimuli of a slice of pizza (Mayer et al. 1999). They then inhaled these three scents as prescribed and rated their hunger levels. The odors blunted their appetite by 35% at 1 min and 49% at 5 min as compared to no reduction with a placebo inhaler. This significant response suggests that the odors' method of action was reduction in appetite, which then induced weight loss.

The hedonic nature of the odor may be more important than the relative food quality of the odor. Among the 90 subjects aged 18–35, the pleasant aroma of either chocolate or baby powder reduced hunger possibly through their promotion of posi-tive affect (Knasko 1995). It has been suggested that the mechanism of action of odors' mediated weight loss is through affective manipulation and thus alleviation of emotional eating (Martin 1992). If so, other affective nonfood modulating odors may have similar effects. In Hirsch's pilot study, this was not found to be the case (Hirsch, personal communication, 2012); however, given the plethora of unexamined odors, other possibilities warrant further investigation.

In the animal model, validating the use of food odors in weight loss is seen in the Wistar rat (Shen et al. 2005). Exposure to the scent of grapefruit oil for 15 min, three times per week, served to reduce food intake and body weight. This mechanism was hypothesized to be due to the autonomic nervous system stimulation inducing enhanced lipolysis and secondary reduction in appetite. Such a mechanism has not been explored in humans.

Bridging the gap between taste and smell, the use of retronasal aroma in sati-ety was explored. This issue was addressed in a double-blind, placebo-controlled, randomized crossover study of 27 healthy subjects with a body mass index (BMI) ranging from 19 to 37 kg/m^2 (Ruijschop et al. 2008). Concurrent with inhalation of a retronasal strawberry aroma, subjects consumed a sweetened milk drink. Compared to consumption of the sweetened milk without the retronasal aroma, subjects demonstrated a significant decrease in desire to consume sweet foods (not savory foods).

This effect was attributed to *sensory-related satiation* (Ruijschop et al. 2008, p. 1146), ultimately implying an expansion of the concept of sensory-specific satiety, from a single food to a whole category of foods, "a generalization over sweet products... a larger band width" (Ruijschop et al. 2008, p. 1146). They conclude that "perceived satiation can thus be increased by altering the extent of aroma release [from food]" (Ruijschop et al. 2008, p. 1146) and encourage the "development of foods that contain triggers that are able to induce or increase the feeling of satiation,... [with] ...application...for...people who are participating in a weight loss program..." (Ruijschop et al. 2008, p. 1147). That retronasal sweet aroma could affect satiety was also demonstrated with presentation of a multicomponent strawberry odorant in a single-blind, placebo-controlled, random crossover design. In 21 female and 20 male normal-weight subjects, a suction catheter was inserted 9 cm through the lower meatus of the lower right nasal cavity to provide retronasal stimulation (Ruijschop et al. 2010). Through this tube, a 15-component strawberry aroma was delivered coincident with the consumption of a strawberry yogurt. Satiety was demonstrated with a visual analog scale. Ratings revealed enhanced sense of fullness with the multicomponent aroma. The author suggested, "Satiation-enhancing effects may be explained by increased sensory stimulation" (Gould 1947, p. 982).

13.3 HEDONICALLY POSITIVE TASTES

The use of tastants extended the concept of use of smells for weight loss. Parallel to Engen's hypothesis (Engen 1982) that olfactory adaptation or anesthesia would reduce appetite or consumption by reducing the food's retronasal olfactory sensation and thus the hedonics of eating, a series of investigations assessed the effect of anesthetizing or inhibiting taste as a treatment modality for weight loss. In the late 1940s, such an approach was instituted along with a variety of flavorants to enhance taste (retronasal smell). These are described in more detail later in this review (Gould 1947, 1950).

The use of anesthetic benzocaine, 1/15 g, in the form of a gum, to be chewed before meals and whenever hungry as an inhibitor to taste, was described over half a century ago (Plotz 1958). Of 50 overweight or obese patients (12–102 lb. excess weight), over a 10-week period, 90% (45) lost *satisfactory* weight. Average weight loss was 2.3 lb./week for the first and 0.33 and 1.8 lb./week for the remaining time. Of 35 patients on a control commercial chewing gum, only 18% (6) lost *satisfactory* weight. While these results suggest that the anesthetic has an impact, how much was due to the other sensory components of the gum remains unclear. (The gum was flavored with eugenol, oils of wintergreen, anise, peppermint, and cinnamon.) The 18% with weight loss in the commercial gum control arm is also worthy of consideration in light of the study by Hirsch et al. (2011) to be discussed later.

Substantial literature supports the concept that intense tastes or flavors can induce satiety. Epidemiological data support this: a greater spicy food preference is associated with lower adiposity (Sullivan et al. 2007). That tastes and flavors, in the absence of ingestion, indicate a chemosensory mechanism for such weight loss is a logical extension.

Maximizing chemosensory experience in the absence of ingestion, without swallowing, subjects chewed and expectorated out the food bolus. Despite the absence of ingestion, hedonic reduction toward the food was noted (Rolls and Rolls 1997).

Julis and Mattes (2007, pp. 167–168) presciently predicted "...an approach to reduce eating frequency without subsequently increasing energy intake at other eating events could be an effective means to moderate or eliminate positive energy balance. A food item that would provide high oral satiety with minimal calories would be ideal."

One paradigm for delivering chemosensory stimuli in the absence of ingestion is the mandibulation of gum. As a preload, mucilage manducation for 10 min prior to a meal of Japanese noodles reduced consumption compared to the absence of chewing gum (Sakata 1995).

Chewing of sweet gum for 15 min every hour for 3 h induced satiety and reduced intake of sweet snacks (Hetherington 2005). Chewing sweet-flavored gum reduced the desire to eat sweet (but not salty) snacks, reduced energy intake by 36 cal, and increased fullness ratings (Hetherington and Boyland 2007).

Similar findings of chewing sweet-flavored, sugar-free gum as an inducer of satiety were demonstrated in 10 boys and 10 girls in response to mandibulating 11 different gum flavors including spearmint, cinnamon, bubble mint, peppermint, sweet mint, strawberry, watermelon, and wintermint (Hirsch et al. 2011). Mandibulating without ingestion of these gums induced satiety equivalent to that of eating 110 cal of white bread. Similarly, mandibulation of sugar-free apple pie-flavored gum induced satiety equal to ingestion of 100 kcal of pumpkin pie, suggesting that a sensory component of desserts without consumption could be of value as an approach for weight reduction (Hirsch et al. 2012). Successfully providing enhanced chemosensory experience of taste with minimal effect of ingestion as a treatment for obesity was demonstrated over half a century ago. Gould (1950) reported a series of 568 cases of obesity. Eighty percent had their appetite controlled with use of aromatic flavoring extracts including powdered ginger, licorice, oils of anise, wintergreen, coriander, and cloves, combined with 1/20 gain of benzocaine along with a single reducing diet. From this study, it remains unclear how much of the weight loss was due to the tastes, the benzocaine, or the reducing diet. However, Gould suggests that it was not the benzocaine alone that was the active agent: the tastants alone in the lozenge caused anorexia in 40%. This demonstrates weight loss in response to taste stimulation.

Dissolving the same agent on the tongue whenever hungry or 15–20 min prior to eating in 100 obese hypertensive patients induced a diminished appetite after 5–7 days (Gould 1950) and, along with a low-carbohydrate, low-fat diet, induced a 2 lb./week weight loss over 11 weeks. Even though after several months, one-third began to gain weight again, such substantial weight loss suggested that the tastants may have efficacy in weight management.

Benzocaine in this instance, while possibly reducing taste, would have had no appreciable effect on retronasal smell, which is the probable mechanism of action of the lozenges.

Using the physiological synesthesia of smell representing taste through retronasal olfaction, the use of hedonically pleasant tastants was introduced for weight loss. Initially designed to intensify the flavor of food, the mechanism was to affect sensory-specific satiety, or satiety set point, for the specific food eaten. Thus, almost an infinite number of tastants had to be utilized, corresponding with the exact foods eaten. In the 1980s, the approach was championed by Schiffman (1986) who postulated that since the obese want more flavors from their food and have a higher flavor set point, such flavor enhancers would increase the sensory impact of food and thus change the eating habits and lead to weight reduction. She noted that overweight children, as young as 4 years old, required more flavor for satiety than normal-weight children. She reported that the obese require more bites per day of 20 different foods for induction of satiety compared to normal weight. This was especially true for the high-sensory-impact foods: sweet, chewy, creamy, spicy, fried, and chocolate. She found that when artificial apple flavor was added to applesauce, overweight subjects reduced their consumption of the applesauce. A similar reduction was seen when cheese flavor was added to macaroni and cheese, tomato flavor to tomato juice, tuna flavor to tuna salad, and bacon flavor to green vegetables. She concluded that the overweight can be satisfied with less volume if they receive the taste and odor that they like (corresponding to the taste and flavor of the food that they were eating). In a 2-week study of overweight subjects on a 1000 cal/day diet, two methods of such an approach were evaluated. Eleven subjects underwent food flavor amplification with noncaloric food-specific products. Fourteen sprayed chocolate and vanilla on the tongue, and 17 served as the control. While the control group lost an average of 3.5 lb., the flavor-amplified group lost 4.6 lb. and the tongue spray group lost 4.3 lb., both significant compared to the control group. She suggested that, "The most effective... strategy described for producing satiety is the introduction of noncaloric flavors into the diet by amplification of table food..." (Schiffman 1986, pp. 44N–44P). She presciently concluded, "Flavor enhancers, flavor sprays, and changes in eating habits that increase the sensory impact obtained from food are helpful aids in dieting" (Schiffman 1986, p. 44R).

Schiffman (1996, p. 8) summarizes, "Addition of a variety of intense noncaloric flavors to food can reduce intake in the short run because people think that they have eaten more food...that is we can fool the body to some extent with additional flavor." In another article, she continues, "...taste and smell signals sustain and terminate ingestion and hence play a major role in the quantity of food eaten and the size of the meals... taste sensations induce feelings of satiety" (Schiffman and Graham 2000, p. S54).

While demonstrating the efficacy of tastants for weight loss, practical application of such a program would be difficult, since it would require a specific tastant for each different food flavor consumed (Schiffman and Graham 2000).

Similar satiety effects of specific tastants sprinkled on corresponding specific foods was not found in the elderly (Schiffman and Warwick 1993). Rather, the elderly increased food consumption when flavor is enhanced, statistically significant for mushroom gravy, peas and carrots, and maple syrup. Schiffman (2000) similarly did not find that flavor enhancers induced weight loss; rather, they enhanced appetite in the elderly especially those with taste and smell disturbances. Amplification of flavor has even been found to have contrary effects depending upon age: increased consumption in the elderly and reduction in the young (Griep et al. 1997).

The lack of efficacy for flavor intensifiers in the elderly is not surprising given their overall impaired olfactory ability and thus taste (which is perceived as retronasal smell).

Since one-half of those over 65 and three-fourths of those over 80 have an impaired sense of smell (Doty et al. 1984), it is not surprising that smell- and flavor-enhanced foods would not demonstrate significant sensory-specific satiety effects. Furthermore, if it did ameliorate appetite, the mechanism would need to be called into question, for if the subjects are anosmic and ageusic, how could chemosensory stimuli cause a change?

Subsequent studies began to address the possibility of sensory-generalized satiety of using a single flavor to generalize to more than just a specific food. These have revolved around sweet tastes for all sweet foods and salty tastes for all salty foods. Anecdotally, it has been observed that a single sweet flavor could act to satisfy the desire for sweet foods and savory flavor for salty foods. Winters (1989, p. 109) observed, "A dash of cinnamon or allspice can increase the perception of sweetness, or lemon or basil could help cut the desire for more salt...."

The possibility that introduction of noncaloric sweet taste to food could induce weight loss was examined with the artificial sweetener aspartame. In 12 men and 12 women normal-weight, nondieting volunteers, the ingestion of aspartame artificial sweetener added to breakfast cereal significantly diminished hunger 2 h later, as compared to ingestion of plain or even sucrose-sweetened cereal (Mattes 1990). These results suggest that a noncaloric, sweet taste, when added to a traditionally sweet food, can enhance induction of satiety to a greater degree than sugar itself.

In a 12-week study of 59 obese subjects, comparing diet alone to diet and aspartame-sweetened food, no significant effect was seen in men (Kanders et al. 1988). However, in women, 16.5 lb. was lost in the aspartame group compared to 12.8 lb. in the control group, a significant difference. The authors suggested that diet compliance was enhanced by the aspartame and that "...the hedonic component of satiety can be exploited with a modest intake of aspartame to achieve compliance to a hypocaloric dietary program that includes modest amounts of desserts and other sweets" (Kanders et al. 1988, p. 82).

Not all studies found a similar aspartame-induced weight loss. Compared to doing nothing or chewing unsweetened gum, subjects chewing aspartame-sweetened gum reported an increase in hunger (Tordoff and Alleva 1990). They suggested that "...the desire to eat was increased by sweet sensation of the oral cavity" (Tordoff and Alleva 1990, p. 558).

Extending findings from aspartame to other foods, the increased flavor of tea resulted in less consumption than weak tea possibly through sensory-specific satiety (Vickers and Holton 1998).

In a combined sensory, high-fat and high-carbohydrate breakfast enhanced with vanilla and aspartame was found to be more satiating than nutritionally identical bland meals, made even blander by subjects wearing nose clips during consumption (Warwick et al. 1993). Sensory enhancement increased satiety in high-fat, high-carbohydrate, and both high-fat and high-carbohydrate meals. This satiating effect began almost immediately and lasted at least 5 h. The author suggests that in the traditional weight loss diet, there is a relative sensory deficit. Such oral sensory deprivation further reduces the likelihood of success of such diets. Complicating the picture, the oral sensory-induced satiety to fat has been postulated to be at least partially on an unconscious basis (French and Robinson 2003).

Expanding this chemosensory integration concept to both smell and taste, Hirsch performed studies looking at the use of flavored sprinkles, dichotomized as to savory or sweet. The sprinkles were provided, two per month, in a specific order, and flavors were changed every month to avoid habituation. After determining the primary taste sensation of the food (savory or sweet), subjects were instructed to sprinkle salty or sweet tastants on all that they consumed corresponding to the primary taste of the food. Tastant combinations were cheddar cheese and cocoa, onion and spearmint, horseradish and banana, ranch and strawberry, taco and raspberry, and parmesan and malt. Of the 108 overweight subjects (BMI 30) who enrolled, 92 completed the study, losing an average of 5.6 lb./month. The control group of 100 traditional diet program enrollees gained an average of 1.1 lb. during the course of the study (Hirsch and Gallant-Shean 2003), suggesting efficacy of the approach.

Hirsch performed a larger study of 2437 overweight or obese subjects over a 6-month period sprinkling the same crystals prior to mandibulation (Hirsch 2008, 2009). The 6-month period was completed by 1436 subjects (59%). The average weight loss was 30.5 lb. as compared to 100 nontreatment control subjects who lost an average of 2 lb. With sensitivity analysis, assuming all dropouts gained the most of the control group (13 lb.), the average weight loss would be 12 lb. over the 6 months, which is not an unsubstantial amount. While subjects were instructed not to change their diet or exercise programs, as weight was disappearing, many described becoming more social, going out more, and thus adding a covert increase in activity. This may have led to further weight loss than due to tastants alone and induced a positive snowball effect of weight loss leading to exercise leading to weight loss. The exact mechanism of action remains unclear. While sensory-generalized satiety is likely, monotony effect and attention effects are reasonable alternative explanations.

Validation that oral sensory (smell and taste) satisfaction precipitated meal termination was demonstrated in 40 non-obese females (Poothullil 2009). In this condition, two high-energy isoenergetic (high fat or high sugar) rice puddings were consumed to the point when the taste of the pudding was no longer pleasing. When a hedonic change in taste was the determinant for meal cessation, there was 24.1 g less intake. Poothullil (2009, p. 29) concludes, "During intake, taste perception, combined with olfaction, produces enjoyment but also produces sensory feedback that leads to satisfaction and meal termination," adding "...This suggests that taste satisfaction could be a mechanism that is used to reduce food intake" (Poothullil 2009, p. 33).

Further support for this came by way of impact of tastants as stimuli for retronasal olfactory perception through the oral pharynx (Ruijschop et al. 2009). Thirty subjects consumed nine different food products: strawberry milkshake, banana custard, raspberry pudding, cheese crackers, milk, dark chocolate, Gouda cheese—young and aged—, and *wine gum* candy. The level of retronasal aroma for each subject for each food was determined, and post-ingestion ad libitum food consumption was recorded. A negative trend between the extent of retronasal aroma release and the amount of food consumed was observed. The author suggested that "...neural brain activation, to a food odor sensed retronasally signals the perception of food, which is hypothesized to be related to satiation.... Limited extent of retronasal aroma release may result in less sensory stimulation, which in turn may lead to decreased feelings of satiation and increased food intake" (Ruijschop et al. 2009, p. 401). They proposed,

Examples of applications could be the development of food products with an increase of after-taste, an increase or lingering of aroma release via flavor delivery systems or encapsulation technology, or the development of long chewable food structures in beverages that evoke substantial oral processing and an increase in transit time in the oral cavity. These applications may lead to a more efficient retro-nasal aroma release and sensory stimulation, which in turn may affect satiation and food intake behavior. (Ruijschop et al. 2009, p. 402)

The concept that retronasal aroma coincident with ingestion acts to reduce consumption was further validated through investigation into the size of bites (deWijk et al. 2009). When a higher intensity of retronasal aroma of cream was presented, the bite size of vanilla custard shrank. deWijk et al. (2009, p. A38) observed,

Higher aroma intensities resulted in smaller bite sizes, which demonstrate that bite size control is sensitive to food sensations that vary from bite to bite, even at aroma concentrations below or near perception threshold. This result suggests a rapid feedback mechanism in which the aroma is perceived during the filling of the mouth, and where the outcome of this evaluation is used to determine the bite.

Since a smaller bite size of foods is more satiating than a larger bite size, this also suggests that the use of food with intensified aromas added may be of relevance for weight management (deWijk et al. 2009). Such cross-modal influence of smell on taste and flavor perception was demonstrated on 30 subjects consuming cheese while presented with salty aromas of cheese or sardines (Lawrence et al. 2009). Unlike the aroma of carrots, these salty aromas enhanced the perceived saltiness of the cheese and confirmed that concurrent savory aroma may have an expanded or generalized influence on other nonspecific, sensory-savory foods as with sensory-generalized satiety.

Based on the extensive literature cited in this review, future weight loss approaches utilizing chemosensory modification should be subject to further investigation.

REFERENCES

Ashem, B., E. Poser, and P. Trudell. 1972. The use of covert sensitization in the treatment of overeating. In *Advances in Behavior Therapy; Proceedings of the Conference*, eds. R.D. Rubin, H. Fensterheim, J.D. Henderson, and L.P. Ullman, pp. 97–103. New York: Academic Press.

Brouillette, M.E., and L.W. White. 1991. The effects of olfactory stimulation on the appetites of nursing home residents. *Physical and Occupational Therapy in Geriatrics* 10:1:1–13.

Cecil, J.E., K. Castiglione, S. French, J. Francis, and N.W. Read. 1998a. The effects of intragastric infusions of macronutrients on ingestion and satiety. *Appetite* 30:65–77.

Cecil, J.E., J. Francis, and N.W. Read. 1998b. Relative contributions of intestinal, gastric, orosensory influences and information to changes in appetite induced by the same liquid meal. *Appetite* 31:377–390.

Chapelot, D., and J. Louis-Sylvestre. 2008. The role of orosensory factors in eating behavior as observed in humans. In *Appetite and Food Intake*, eds. R.B.S. Harris and R.E. Mattes, pp. 133–161. Boca Raton, FL: CRC Press.

Cole, A.D., and N.W. Bond. 1983. Olfactory aversion conditioning and overeating: A review and some data. *Perceptual and Motor Skills* 57:667–678.

deWijk, R.A., I.A. Polet, and J.H. Bult. 2009. Bitesize is affected by food aroma presented at sub- or peri threshold concentrations. *Chemical Senses* 34:7:A38.

Doty, R.L., P. Shaman, S.L. Applebaum, R. Gilberson, L. Sikorski, and L. Rosenberg. 1984. Smell identification ability: Changes with age. *Science* 226:1441–1443.

Engen, T. 1982. *The Perception of Odors*. New York: Academic Press.

Foreyt, J.P., and W.A. Kennedy. 1971. Treatment of overweight by aversion therapy. *Behavior Research & Therapy* 9:29–34.

French, S., and T. Robinson. 2003. Fats and food intake. *Current Opinion in Clinical Nutrition and Metabolic Care* 6:629–634.

Frohwirth, R.A., and J.P. Foreyt. 1978. Aversive conditioning treatment of overweight. *Behavior Therapy* 9:861–872.

Gould, W.L. 1947. On the use of a medicament to reduce the appetite in the treatment of the obese and other conditions. *New York Journal of Medicine* 47:981–983.

Gould, W.L. 1950. Obesity and hypertension: The importance of a safe compound to control appetite. *N.C. Medical Journal* 11:327–334.

Griep, M.I., T.F. Mets, and D.L. Massart. 1997. Different effects of flavor amplification of nutrient-dense foods on preference and consumption in young and elderly subjects. *Food Quality and Preference* 8:2:151–156.

Hetherington, M. 2005. Potential role for chewing in satiety and appetite control. [Abstract]. *American Dietetic Association Annual Meeting*.

Hetherington, M.M., and E. Boyland. 2007. Short-term effects of chewing gum on snack intake and appetite. *Appetite* 48:397–401.

Hirsch, A.R. 2008. Use of gustatory stimuli to facilitate weight loss. [Abstract] *1st International Conference on Advance Technologies & Treatment for Diabetes (ATTD)*, Prague, Czech Republic.

Hirsch, A.R. 2009. Chemosensory disorders. In *Food and Nutrients in Disease Management*, ed. I. Kohlstadt, Ch. 3, pp. 43–60. Boca Raton, FL: CRC Press.

Hirsch, A.R., and D.D. Dougherty. 1993. Inhalation of 2-acetylpyridine for weight reduction. *Chemical Senses* 18:5:113.

Hirsch, A.R., and M.B. Gallant-Shean. 2003. Use of tastants to facilitate weight loss. *Chemical Senses* 28:A124.

Hirsch, A.R., and R. Gomez. 1995. Weight reduction through inhalation of odorants. *Journal of Neurologic and Orthopaedic Medicine and Surgery* 16:28–31.

Hirsch, A.R., J. Li, A. Kao, M. Hayes, M. Choe, and Y. Lu. 2007. Effect of television viewing on sensory-specific satiety: Are Leno and Letterman obesogenic? [Abstract] *89th Annual Meeting Endocrine Society*.

Hirsch, A.R., M.O. Soto, and J.W. Hirsch. 2011. The relative satiety value of chewing gum in American children. *Chemical Senses* 36:9:843.

Hirsch, J.W., S.R. Aiello, and A.R. Hirsch. 2012. Relative satiety value of candy and gum: Potential therapies for childhood obesity. *Journal of Obesity and Weight Loss Therapy* 2:1–8.

Julis, R.A., and R.D. Mattes. 2007. Influence of sweetened chewing gum on appetite, meal patterning and energy intake. *Appetite* 48:167–175.

Kanders, B.S., P.T. Lavin, M.B. Kowalchuk, I. Greenberg, and G.L. Blackburn. 1988. An evaluation of the effect of aspartame on weight loss. *Appetite* 11:73–84.

Kennedy, W.A., and J.P. Foreyt. 1968. Control of eating behavior in an obese patient by avoidance conditioning. *Psychological Reports* 22:571–576.

Knasko, S.C. 1995. Pleasant odors and congruency: Effects on approach behavior. *Chemical Senses* 20:479–487.

Lawrence, G., M. Pegoud, J. Busch, C. Salles, and T. Thomas-Danguin T. 2009. Cross-modal interactions: Way to counterbalance salt reduction in solid foods? *Chemical Senses* 34:E43.

Maletzky, B.M. 1973. "Assisted" covert sensitization: A preliminary report. *Behavior Therapy* 4:117–119.

Martin, G.N. 1992. The effects of odour on illness. Can smell be used to eliminate bulimia? Paper presented at the *Research Discussion Seminar, Department of Psychiatry,* University of Birmingham, UK as referenced in: Martin, G.N. 1996. Olfactory remediation: Current evidence and possible applications. *Social Science & Medicine* 43(1):63–70.

Mattes, R. 1990. Effects of aspartame and sucrose on hunger and energy intake in humans. *Physiology & Behavior* 47:1037–1044.

Mayer, S.N., R.S. Davidson, and C.B. Hensley. 1999. The role of specific olfactory stimulation in appetite suppression and weight loss. *Journal of Advancement in Medicine* 12:1:13–21.

Morganstern, K.P. 1974. Cigarette smoke as a noxious stimulus in self-managed aversion therapy for compulsive eating: Technique and case illustration. *Behavior Therapy* 5:255–260.

Moss, F.A. 1924. Note on building likes and dislikes in children. *Journal of Experimental Psychology* 7:475–478.

Ostman, J., M. Britton, and E. Jonsson. 2004. *Treating and Preventing Obesity.* Weinheim: Wiley-VCH Verlag.

Plotz, M. 1958. Obesity. *Medical Times* 86(7):860–863.

Poothullil, J.M. 2009. Meal termination using oral sensory satisfaction: A study in non-obese women. *Nutritional Neuroscience* 12(1):28–34.

Rolls, E.T., and J.H. Rolls. 1997. Olfactory sensory-specific satiety in humans. *Physiology & Behavior* 61(3):461–473.

Rosenthal, R. 1966. *Experimenter Effects in Behavioral Research.* New York: Appleton.

Ruijschop, R.M., A.E.M. Boelrijk, J.A. deRu, C. deGraaf, and M.S. Westerterp-Plantenga. 2008. Effects of retro-nasal aroma release on satiation. *British Journal of Nutrition* 99:1140–1148.

Ruijschop, R.M., M.J.M. Burgering, M.A. Jacobs, and A.E.M. Boelrijk. 2009. Retro-nasal aroma release depends on both subject and product differences: A link to food intake regulation? *Chemical Senses* 34:395–403.

Ruijschop, R.M., A.E.M. Boelrijk, M.J.M. Burgering, C. deGraff, and S. Westerterp-Plantenga. 2010. Acute effects of complexity in aroma composition on satiation and food intake. *Chemical Senses* 35:91–108.

Sakata, T. 1995. A very-low-calorie conventional Japanese diet: Its implications for prevention of obesity. *Obesity Research* 3:233s–239s.

Schiffman, S.S. 1986. The use of flavor to enhance efficacy of reducing diets. *Hospital Practice* 21:44H–44R.

Schiffman, S.S. 1996. The potential use of odor for weight loss and weight maintenance. *The Aromachology* V:2:2, 8.

Schiffman, S.S. 2000. Intensification of sensory properties of foods for the elderly. *Journal of Nutrition* 130:927S–930S.

Schiffman, S.S., and B.G. Graham. 2000. Taste and smell perception affect appetite and immunity in the elderly. *European Journal of Clinical Nutrition* 54(3):S54–S63.

Schiffman, S.S., and Z.S. Warwick. 1993. Effect of flavor enhancement of foods for the elderly on nutritional status: Food intake, biochemical indices, and anthropometric measures. *Physiology & Behavior* 53:395–402.

Shen, J., A. Niijima, M. Tanida, Y. Horii, K. Maeda, and K. Nagai. 2005. Olfactory stimulation with scent of grapefruit oil affects autonomic nerves, lipolysis and appetite in rats. *Neuroscience Letters* 380:289–294.

Sullivan, B., J.E. Hayes, P.D. Faghri, and V.B. Duffy. 2007. Connecting diet and disease risk via food preference. *Chemical Senses* 32:A97.

Tordoff, M.G., and A.M. Alleva. 1990. Oral stimulation with aspartame increases hunger. *Physiology & Behavior* 47:555–559.

Vickers, Z., and E. Holton. 1998. A comparison of taste test ratings, repeated consumption, and postconsumption ratings of different strengths of iced tea. *Journal of Sensory Studies* 13:199–212.

Warwick, Z.S., W.G. Hall, T.N. Pappas, and S.S. Schiffman. 1993. Taste and smell sensations enhance the satiating effect of both a high-carbohydrate and a high-fat meal in humans. *Physiology & Behavior* 53:553–563.

Winters, R.K.V. 1989. Adapting the environment to age-related sensory losses. *Journal of the American Academy of Nurse Practitioners* 1(4):106–111.

Wolpe, J. 1969. *The Practice of Behavior Therapy*. Elmsford, NY: Pergamon Press.

14 Chemosensation to Enhance Nutritional Intake in Cancer Patients

Cheryl A. Bacon and Veronica Sanchez Varela

CONTENTS

14.1 Chemosensory Alterations in Cancer Patients 309
14.2 Assessment of Chemosensory Alterations in Cancer Patients 310
14.3 Dietary and Food Delivery Modifications for Managing Chemosensory
      Alterations in Cancer Patients 312
14.4 Additional Strategies for Managing Chemosensory Alterations in
      Cancer Patients 316
      14.4.1 Pharmacological Interventions 316
      14.4.2 Psychosocial Interventions 317
14.5 Limitations and Future Directions 319
References 320

14.1 CHEMOSENSORY ALTERATIONS IN CANCER PATIENTS

Chemosensory dysfunctions, most notably alterations in taste or smell, are common in individuals undergoing cancer treatment, with prevalence rates that can reach up to 90% (Wickham et al. 1999; Ravasco 2005; Brisbois et al. 2006; Hong et al. 2009). Chemosensory alterations reported by cancer patients can be generally classified into three main categories: changes in taste acuity, changes in taste quality, and changes in olfaction (Farmer et al. 2009; Hong et al. 2009; Brisbois et al. 2011). More specifically, cancer patients may experience hypogeusia (diminished sense of taste), hyposmia (diminished sense of smell), ageusia (complete loss of taste), or anosmia (complete loss of smell). Changes in taste acuity are often reported by cancer patients in the form of an increase in the threshold for taste perception, and frequently, reported taste quality alterations are perceptions of metallic or bitter taste for both food and liquids. Smell alterations are less frequently reported by cancer patients and include reports of smells being unpleasant or different. Studies on chemosensory alterations are limited in number, sample size, and overall methodological approach. However, cancer patients appear to experience taste and smell alterations both jointly and independently, and studies document a highly variable array of alterations. For example, a study of 192 advanced cancer patients found that 60% reported both taste and smell alterations, while 26% reported taste alterations only, and 3% reported olfactory alterations only. A number of these patients reported an increase in the threshold for taste acuity, while others experienced a decrease in threshold values for some tastes such as bitterness; some cancer patients might experience a mixed pattern of changes with some sensations becoming stronger and others weaker (Brisbois et al. 2011).

Suggested mechanisms of chemosensory alterations in cancer patients include damages in sensory receptor cells and neural activity, most likely secondary to cancer and treatment type. These damages, nevertheless, provide only a partial understanding of the etiology of taste and smell changes experienced by cancer patients. Factors such as micronutrient deficiencies, infections, poor oral hygiene, smoking, mucositis, and dry mouth are also likely contributors to perceived changes in taste and smell (Brisbois et al. 2006; Farmer et al. 2009; Hong et al. 2009; McLaughlin and Mahon 2012). Regardless of the degree of taste or smell alterations, cancer patients often experience highly detrimental side effects derived from these chemosensory dysfunctions. The senses of taste and smell together generate *flavor*, and chemosensory alterations have been found to correlate with a decreased energy intake, decreased appetite, anorexia, early satiety, nausea, and poor quality of life (DeWys et al. 1980; Cunningham and Bell 2000; Vigano et al. 2000; Capra et al. 2001; Hutton et al. 2007; Farmer et al. 2009; Hong et al. 2009; Brisbois et al. 2011). Hutton et al. (2007) collected data on self-reported taste and smell abnormalities from advanced cancer patients who were at least 2 months in the postcancer treatment. Patients were grouped by severity of chemosensory abnormality scores: absent, mild, moderate, and severe. The researchers found that those with severe chemosensory scores consumed significantly less calories (900–1100 less calories per day) than patients with milder or no chemosensory alterations. This type of inadequate nutrition, when prolonged, can lead to malnutrition, which is the second most common comorbid diagnosis in individuals with cancer (Buzby 1990; Smith and Souba 2001) accounting for 20% of all cancer deaths (Ottery 1997). In spite of the high prevalence, distressing quality, and detrimental side effects of chemosensory alterations experienced by cancer patients, changes in taste and smell are often unaddressed (Brisbois et al. 2006; Hopkinson 2010). To address this issue, this chapter aims at familiarizing clinicians with published studies and clinical information relevant to the assessment of chemosensory alterations in oncology patients and recommendations for intervention.

14.2 ASSESSMENT OF CHEMOSENSORY ALTERATIONS IN CANCER PATIENTS

Timely assessment of the presence and severity of chemosensory alterations is a crucial first step in adequately addressing the consequences of taste and smell changes in cancer patients. As such, it is imperative that an integrative approach to cancer care should include a systematic way to identify cancer patients who experience chemosensory alterations and are at risk for malnutrition, and to initiate referrals to registered dietitians, mental health providers, pharmacists, and other appropriately trained professionals for further assessment and intervention.

The literature reflects two possible different mechanisms for the assessment of chemosensory alterations in cancer patients. The first mechanism includes threshold testing, which consists of a clinical evaluation of taste acuity for the five basic tastes (Wismer 2008). In threshold tasting, patients are provided with a series of samples of tastes in various concentrations (from the weakest to the strongest) to determine which concentration is needed for the proper identification of each particular taste. Threshold testing offers a methodologically strong mechanism of identification of chemosensory alterations in research studies; however, threshold testing is impractical for use in clinical settings. A second mechanism of assessing whether patients are experiencing chemosensory alterations is the utilization of self-report instruments, a method that could be more easily implemented in a clinical setting. An example of a self-report tool is Heald et al.'s (1998) Taste and Smell Survey, a nine-item questionnaire originally developed to evaluate chemosensory function in patients with AIDS and that has been adapted for use in cancer patients (Hutton et al. 2007; Brisbois et al. 2011). Another tool, the ChemoSensory Questionnaire (CSQ) (Goldberg et al. 2005), is a brief, eight-item survey that provides a rapid assessment of the presence of chemosensory alterations while minimizing patient and provider burden. These tools are brief and easy to implement during a patient assessment and may provide prompt identification of cancer patients experiencing chemosensory alterations and who are therefore at risk for distress and inadequate nutrition.

In general, chemosensory alterations may be best assessed through a combination of objective and open-ended questions in order to more adequately inform the need for further referrals for evaluation and intervention. Open-ended questions such as "Are things too salty/bitter/sweet/sour?"; "How have your senses of taste and smell changed during treatment?"; "Do you have a complete lack of taste?"; "Do you have a diminished sense of taste?"; and "How did foods use to taste, and how do they taste now?" are particularly useful when starting the conversation about chemosensory alterations and designing adequate interventions. After gaining a better understanding of the patient's primary complaint, dietary suggestions can be provided to help patients manage specific chemosensory alterations. Additionally, it is important to gather information on the patients' food preferences and typical eating behaviors. The use of a 3-day dietary food record is a valid and reliable method to estimate a patient's dietary intake (Bruera et al. 1986; Gibson 1990).

Registered dietitians can further assess cancer patients experiencing chemosensory alterations and who are at increased risk for malnutrition. Examples of assessment instruments utilized by registered dietitians for this purpose include the Malnutrition Universal Screening Tool (Stratton et al. 2004), the Nutritional Risk Screening–2000 (Kondrup et al. 2003), the Mini Nutritional Assessment (Nestle Nutrition 2013), the scored Patient-Generated Subjective Global Assessment (PG-SGA) (Bauer et al. 2003), and the Malnutrition Screening Tool (Ferguson et al. 1999). The PG-SGA has been validated for use within the oncology patient population (Bauer et al. 2003), consists of a complete list of common nutrition-related side effects, and allows for patient input; however, the professional must be specifically trained to use this tool. The Malnutrition Screening Tool is brief and user-friendly, and no special training is required for its administration (Kim et al. 2011). Regardless of the screening method used, nutrition assessment should be conducted by a registered dietitian who is trained to also evaluate the patient's past medical/surgical history, diet history, anthropometric data, and biochemical data and to make appropriate recommendations for intervention based on the results of the assessment (Elliott et al. 2006).

Chemosensory alterations can also have a significant impact on one's quality of life given the emotional distress associated with drastic unintentional weight loss and chemosensory barriers to food intake (Hutton et al. 2007). At the same time, psychological distress itself can affect food intake and weight. Anxiety and depression are prevalent in cancer patients, and their diagnostic criteria involve appetite disturbances, nausea, and involuntary weight loss (American Psychiatric Association 2013), which are symptoms also secondary to chemosensory alterations. Therefore, in order to provide optimal care to cancer patients who experience taste and smell changes and are at risk for malnutrition, the implementation of a multidisciplinary approach that includes a psychosocial assessment to rule out and/or address psychological factors that may also be affecting food intake is recommended. Psychological screening therefore can assist in ruling out contributing factors, other than possible chemosensory alterations, to low caloric intake, weight loss, and food hedonics and to guide intervention.

Validated instruments for psychosocial distress screening are available and can be utilized in inpatient and outpatient oncology settings. These instruments are usually designed to be administered, scored, and interpreted by trained mental health professionals. However, nursing staff and other medical providers could receive training in administering some of these instruments and in referring to appropriate resources for intervention. Examples of these instruments include the Patient Health Questionnaire (PHQ) (Spitzer et al. 1999), the Hospital Anxiety and Depression Scale (Zigmond and Snaith 1983), and the Brief Symptom Inventory (Derogatis and Melisaratos 1983). Many of these psychological assessment instruments include questions regarding appetite disruption and anhedonia, which could be influenced by chemosensory alterations especially if food and meals are a resource for patient's socialization or pleasure.

14.3 DIETARY AND FOOD DELIVERY MODIFICATIONS FOR MANAGING CHEMOSENSORY ALTERATIONS IN CANCER PATIENTS

Cancer patients, who are identified as experiencing changes in taste and smell, and especially those who are at increased risk for malnutrition and other detrimental side effects derived from these changes, should be referred to a registered dietitian for further assessment and intervention. Registered dietitians can provide cancer patients with appropriate nutritional information relevant to improving the effect of chemosensory alterations. Research suggests that cancer patients could also benefit from receiving instruction on how to utilize flavor enhancement products when preparing their meals (Schiffman et al. 2007). In a study of 107 elderly breast and lung cancer patients receiving active adjuvant or palliative chemotherapy, patients were randomized to receive nutritional information, chemosensory instruction and flavor enhancement products, or just nutritional information. The effect of each intervention on the patients' chemosensory experience, nutritional status, functional status, immune status, and quality of life was measured. In this study, both threshold testing and self-report instruments were used to measure chemosensory alterations, and data were collected at baseline, 1, 3, and 8 months after starting chemotherapy. Patients in the experimental group (information/instruction + flavor enhancement) received 13 different flavor enhancers (bacon, beef, pork, roasted chicken, roasted carrot, roasted onion, mushroom, roasted red bell pepper, roasted garlic, blueberry, raspberry, apple, and strawberry) and were taught how to incorporate these flavor enhancers into their meals. Authors found that patients in the experimental group obtained higher nutritional assessment scores when using the Mini Nutrition Assessment tool and experienced a significant improvement in physical function as measured by the European Organization for Research and Treatment of Cancer Quality of Life Questionnaire. Although there were no improvements in the mean caloric intake (in fact, there was a decline in caloric intake in both groups), functional status, immune status, or quality of life between the two groups, these results are promising as they suggest increased benefit for patients who receive more in-depth and versatile instructions on how to implement dietary modifications.

Table 14.1 summarizes common dietary and food delivery/preparation modifications and strategies for commonly reported taste and smell alterations. However, there is a scarcity of research examining the effectiveness of these recommendations on addressing chemosensory alterations in cancer patients and improving nutritional intake. Therefore, many of the recommendations discussed here are based on clinical practice and anecdotal accounts. Regardless of the type of altered taste, good mouth care is also critical. Dry mouth can be a consequence of cancer treatments and can result in an increased sense of altered taste. Saliva helps regulate the proliferation of bacteria inside the mouth, and these bacteria can contribute to bad taste. Diligent mouth care helps restore normal bacterial balance inside the mouth, and rinsing the mouth before meals to clear away excess bacteria, and after meals to reduce *aftertaste*, can be helpful in moderating taste changes. Commercial nonalcohol-based mouthwashes are available and may be recommended. There are also common kitchen items that can be used as *natural* mouthwashes such as mixing ½ teaspoon of salt and ½ teaspoon of baking soda in 1 cup of warm water and swishing and spitting before and after meals (Cancer.net 2014). If dry mouth is contributing to altered taste, in addition to good oral mouth care, stimulating saliva production during meals by adding tart foods (e.g., lemon, vinegar) can also help enhance flavor; keeping foods moist with gravies or sauces and avoiding caffeine, as this can exacerbate dry mouth, can also be helpful (Elliott et al. 2006).

The use of *Synsepalum dulcificum*, also known as *miracle fruit*, has received some attention as an alternative method to combat chemosensory alterations, in particular, taste changes, in cancer patients. *S. dulcificum* contains a natural protein, miraculin, that when consumed in conjunction with other foods masks certain tastes for a short duration of time, making otherwise unpleasant foods more palatable. A small pilot study examined the effect of *S. dulcificum* in cancer patients, where a total of eight patients took turns receiving the miracle fruit or a placebo (dried cranberries) for 2 weeks at a time (Wilken and Satiroff 2012). Patients were instructed to consume the fruit immediately before their meal and to keep a 28-day food diary

TABLE 14.1
Dietary and Food Delivery Modifications for Commonly Reported Taste and Smell Alterations

Type of Taste Alteration	Suggested Dietary Intervention
Salty taste (i.e., foods taste too salty/ decreased threshold for salty foods)	Limit salty foods and foods with added salt. Do not add salt during the cooking process or after meal preparation. Add sugar or artificial sweetener to salty foods.
Bitter taste	Try room-temperature or cold foods. Limit coffee.
Sweet taste	Limit sweet foods and foods with added sugar. Add salt, lemon, lime, or vinegar to sweet foods. Add instant, decaffeinated coffee powder to sweet foods.
Sour taste	Limit sour and tart foods such as citrus fruits.
Lack of taste (ageusia)	Experiment with stronger flavors such as spices and marinades. Consume foods with high moisture or water content; add sauces or gravies to moisten foods.
Bad taste (dysgeusia)	Avoid strong flavors and spices. Choose bland/unseasoned foods such as baked chicken, potatoes, pasta, and rice.
Metallic taste	Limit red meat and other foods high in iron; experiment with other high-protein food choices such as eggs, poultry, fish, beans, and soy. Use plastic utensils instead of metal; avoid consuming foods from metal cans; avoid cooking in an iron skillet.
Bad or distorted smell	Choose colder foods (sandwiches, salads, fruits, and cheeses) that are less aromatic. Open the windows and use the exhaust fan when cooking; open containers away from patient's face.

Source: Elliott, L. et al., *The Clinical Guide to Oncology Nutrition, 2nd Edition*, Chicago: American Dietetic Association, 2006; Cancer.net. Taste changes. Available at http://www.cancer.net/all-about-cancer/treating-cancer/managing-side-effects/taste-changes (accessed June 24, 2014).

recording whether typical foods consumed tasted the same, worse, or better than previously experienced. Although the sample size was small, the results were promising in that all the participants reported an improvement in taste with the miracle fruit, stating that most foods tasted sweeter compared to their previous complaints of foods tasting bitter, dry, or metallic.

Direct dietary modifications may not be sufficient to see an impact on increasing calorie and protein intake in patients with taste and smell alterations. In a clinical setting, the method of meal delivery should also be considered as a contributing factor to inadequate nutrition in these patients. The typical style of meal delivery within an inpatient hospital setting is called the *traditional method*. With this method, patients are usually requested to select which foods they would like to consume in advance, sometimes up to 24 h before that meal is scheduled to be delivered. However, cancer patients may experience side effects from treatment, including a variety of chemosensory alterations that fluctuate in severity from day to day. Therefore, a more flexible meal service, such as the *room service* method—in which patients select their meal shortly before it is served (commonly 45–60 min)—may allow patients to select preferences and food amounts that sound appealing to them at that particular time. A study by Piertsma et al. (2003) found that a bedside food cart service, in which a food cart is brought up to the patient care unit and patients are allowed to select the food type and amount, resulted in significant improvements in patients' satisfaction. The authors in this study did not evaluate whether this method of meal delivery resulted in increased caloric intake at meal times, and therefore, further investigation on nutritional outcomes using this delivery method is needed particularly in the adult patient population. Williams et al. (1998) conducted a similar study in pediatric oncology patients evaluating both patient satisfaction and change in caloric intake after implementation of an *on-demand* or room service meal delivery style, and reported a statistically significant 28% increase in caloric intake. Investigators also reported a 30% increase in patient satisfaction; however, details were not provided on whether this increase was statistically significant.

When alterations in smell may be contributing to altered taste and flavor, the food delivery method can be particularly impactful. In clinical settings and hospitals, meals are often delivered in dense containers for the purpose of holding foods at desirable temperatures. However, these dense containers tend to also concentrate and merge odors, intensifying the aroma of foods. When patients lift the container lid, the concentrated strong smell may become offensive and turn the patient off from eating. Strategies for helping patients overcome this particular barrier include opening the lid away from the face and in a *Pac-Man*-like manner, allowing for the odor to slowly escape from under the lid and away from the patient. Patients could also ask the person delivering the tray to remove the lid prior to bringing the tray in the room or setting the tray on the opposite side of the room and removing the lid. Serving and consuming meals utilizing paper and plastic plates and utensils, rather than metallic or ceramic, may also allow odors to escape prior to reaching the patient's room and thus making the food smells less intense and more appealing.

Not all facilities have the resources needed to offer a variety of prepared meals, convert their method of meal delivery to room service, or accommodate to specific delivery requirements by patients. In such cases, a simpler approach in which patients are provided with the alternative of choosing fortified meals and between-meal snacks might be adequate. Although not specific to oncology patients affected by chemosensory disorders, Gall et al. (1998) provide evidence that female and male orthopedic inpatients and elderly female inpatients who are offered fortified snacks at meals and between-meal snacks (such as soups fortified with dry skim milk powder, cake, or cheese sandwich) significantly increased their caloric intake by 17.5% compared to a control group of patients that were not offered these options. It is important to note that in Gall et al.'s study, patients were not encouraged to consume these fortified and between-meal snacks; rather, it was the patients' decision to choose this option at meal times.

14.4   ADDITIONAL STRATEGIES FOR MANAGING CHEMOSENSORY ALTERATIONS IN CANCER PATIENTS

Nutrition advice alone may not be sufficient to significantly improve energy intake or impact weight gain (Baldwin et al. 2012) in cancer patients who struggle with chemosensory alterations. A multidisciplinary approach that considers pharmacological therapies and psychosocial factors, in addition to nutrition counseling, may be optimal to address the consequences of cancer-related taste and smell changes.

14.4.1   PHARMACOLOGICAL INTERVENTIONS

While certain pharmacological agents have been evaluated on their effectiveness to improve appetite and increase caloric intake in the cancer population, few studies have evaluated the direct impact that an agent had on improving taste and smell disturbances. One study focused on the potential effects of delta-9-tetrahydrocannabinol in improving chemosensory alterations. Delta-9-tetrahydrocannabinol, or Marinol, was used in a pilot study conducted by Brisbois et al. (2011), in which patients were randomized to receive 2.5 mg of Marinol per day (for the first 3 days, increased to 2.5 mg twice a day on day 4) or placebo over an 18-day period. Patients in this study must have previously reported disturbances in taste and smell as well as decreases in appetite. The authors found statistically significant improvements in chemosensory experiences in the intervention group compared to the placebo group. In addition, patients in the intervention group reported that *food tastes better* significantly more often compared to those in the placebo group. Of note, although appetite was significantly improved from baseline in the intervention group compared to the placebo group, both groups experienced similar increases in caloric intake.

Certain chemotherapy regimens have been found to alter zinc metabolism and result in carbonic anhydrase VI deficiency in cancer patients (Henkin et al. 1999). Subsequently, patients with carbonic anhydrase VI deficiency have been found to uniformly exhibit chemosensory alterations. Earlier studies had showed promise with zinc supplementation improving taste perceptions (Fong and Newberne 1978; Prasad et al. 1997; Bakan et al. 1998; Ripamonti et al. 1998). However, more recent randomized, controlled studies have failed to demonstrate the same benefit. In a double-blind, placebo-controlled, randomized clinical trial, Lyckholm et al. (2012) provided 220 mg oral zinc sulfate twice daily to patients who had reported taste or smell changes since starting chemotherapy, but were unable to find statistically significant differences between the placebo and intervention groups. Similarly, Haylard et al. (2007) randomized patients receiving radiation therapy to the head and neck to either 45 mg of oral zinc sulfate three times a day or a placebo. Investigators did not find any significant improvements in taste alterations in either group.

Adequate salivary flow is essential for taste perception (Norris et al. 1984; Christensen et al. 1987). Additionally, since digestion begins within the mouth, enzymes present within the saliva contribute to the texture of a food and thus taste perception (Heinzerling et al. 2008). Investigators have demonstrated that modifying salivary flow rate can alter the perceived intensity of sourness and saltiness in a group of healthy individuals but had no impact on sweetness and bitterness (Heinzerling et al. 2011). Unfortunately, to our knowledge, no clinical trials have demonstrated the beneficial effects of administering artificial saliva on significantly improving taste perception in cancer patients.

14.4.2 PSYCHOSOCIAL INTERVENTIONS

Psychiatrists, psychologists, and other mental health providers who work with cancer patients could play a critical role in addressing the impact of chemosensory alterations in patients' quality of life. This role may range from providing patients and their families with education about the relationship among chemosensory alterations, family dynamics, and quality of life to implementing prevention and treatment interventions for the development of food aversions. Eating meals is a behavior that tends to surpass for humans its basic purpose of life sustenance. Peoples' eating behaviors are influenced not only by taste and smell but also by past experiences with certain foods; preferences; and beliefs related to the contents of foods, health, and personal characteristics such as sex and weight (Scalera 2002; Bernhardson et al. 2012; Boltong and Keast 2012). In addition, meals are often related to family, social, and cultural events, and as such, certain foods and eating habits may possess deeply entrenched meanings. It is commonplace to listen to cancer patients report "I am not hungry, and food does not taste good, but am forcing myself to eat and keeping it down." Following reports such as this, there is a valuable opportunity for providers to inquire further about the patient's cognitive and emotional processes linked to food and eating. Patients could benefit from empathic and curious listening, as well as from normalization of their experience by providing them with information regarding treatment-related chemosensory and appetite changes (Hopkinson 2010). Family members and caregivers are also likely to play an important role in the manner in which cancer patients process the impact of chemosensory and appetite changes during treatment. For instance, patients may feel too poorly to eat and reject foods that are prepared or provided by a caregiver. This kind of scenario, along with other similar ones, may pose a particular challenge to the patients–caregivers' dynamic, making food intake (or lack thereof) a source of contention. Therefore, information about common patient responses to treatment-related chemosensory alterations and appetite changes should also be provided to family members and friends of patients whenever possible. In addition to psycho-education, cancer patients who are experiencing chemosensory or appetite problems but are somehow managing to ingest any amount of food could benefit from the encouragement, praise, and support of caregivers and staff to continue their efforts. Patients sometimes *anchor* their unpleasant experiences with food in the adequate belief that chemosensory alterations are likely temporary, and the staff can offer reassurance that these changes are likely to improve in time.

For a number of patients, however, the emotional distress brought about by chemosensory alterations and treatment-related side effects can be greatly exacerbated by the development of food aversions. Food aversions are a learned response, or a type of Pavlovian conditioning, through which a stimulus (in this case, food) that was previously neutral or even desired becomes powerfully unpleasant or aversive. Moreover, a learned response to taste or food aversion could generalize to other similar tastes and greatly influence and limit patients' choices of food and liquids. In the particular case of cancer, the use of chemotherapeutic agents and irradiation to the gastrointestinal tract might produce taste aversions even when patients do not report changes in taste. Cancer patients may be particularly vulnerable to developing aversions to foods and liquids that are consumed right before receiving chemotherapy or radiation, and over time, patients may extend this association to stimuli other than cancer therapies such as hospital sights or smells (Scalera 2002).

Because taste aversions are a learned behavior, both a preventative and interventional approach can be helpful to cancer patients. Although the research is rather scarce, prevention interventions include psycho-education relevant to the development of food aversions and strategies to avoid their development. One strategy is to recommend that a patient eat a small meal several hours prior to receiving cancer therapy (rather than immediately preceding therapy) and to avoid foods that are high in protein or that are considered favorites (thus avoiding the development of food aversion toward a particularly nutritious or favored meal) (Scalera 2002; Jatoi 2010). Also, research suggests that patients could intentionally consume a food that is strong in flavor but that lacks nutritional value or personal meaning as a type of *scapegoat* strategy. Broberg and Bernstein (1987) examined the effectiveness of utilizing the scapegoat strategy in preventing the development of food aversions by conducting a small study among pediatric cancer patients. The patients in this study either consumed a coconut/root beer-flavored candy before chemotherapy infusion or received no intervention, and it was found that patients who received the candy were less likely to develop a taste aversion from the next meal item consumed than those who did not receive the strong-flavored candy. Cognitive manipulation of nausea expectancies related to cancer treatment also appears to be a predictor of actual nausea in cancer patients. Nausea expectancies are often rooted on past experiences and learned behaviors and influence the development of taste and food aversions. However, these expectancies can also be driven by factors such as information regarding treatment-related side effects and clinicians and other patients' accounts. In a pilot study of 74 breast cancer patients, Roscoe et al. (2010) found that targeted expectancy manipulation interventions (expectancy-neutral versus expectancy-enhancing printed and audio information relevant to the efficacy of acupressure bands in reducing treatment-related nausea) improved the control of nausea in patients who had high nausea expectancies prior to receiving treatment. Conversely, patients who initially had low nausea expectancies experienced a lessening of control over their nausea when they were exposed to an expectancy-enhancing intervention. Although these results are still considered exploratory, investigators demonstrated that targeted manipulation of expectancies could have a powerful bidirectional effect on the development of nausea (and arguably food aversions) in cancer patients.

For patients who have already developed a taste aversion, behavioral strategies should help reverse this learned process. Systematic desensitization, originally proposed by psychiatrist Joseph Wolpe, is a behavioral intervention commonly utilized by mental health professionals when helping cancer patients alter an aversive reaction to otherwise neutral stimuli (in this case, food) that has been linked with unpleasant side effects of cancer treatments (such as nausea) (Redd et al. 2001; Lofti-Jam et al. 2008). In systematic desensitization, the trained clinician develops with the patient a hierarchy of aversive stimuli (from least aversive to most aversive) and gradually introduces these events while the patient is in a calm and relaxed state. The introduction of the aversive stimuli can be done *in vivo* (where the actual stimulus is presented to the patient) or imagined (by asking the patient to evoke the stimulus through memory). Repeated exposure to the aversive stimulus during a calm and relaxed state eventually leads the aversion to cease or become extinct. Systematic desensitization is a strategy that requires careful planning and execution and should only be performed by trained professionals.

14.5 LIMITATIONS AND FUTURE DIRECTIONS

The goal in this chapter has been to familiarize health-care professionals with the most up-to-date relevant methods of assessment of chemosensory alterations in oncology patients and recommendations for intervention to ultimately improve nutritional intake. A number of assessment instruments are available to promptly identify patients who struggle with chemosensory alterations and are therefore at risk for malnutrition and for experiencing poor quality of life. For patients who are experiencing chemosensory alterations as a result of cancer and its treatments, adequate intervention should include an interdisciplinary approach of registered dietitians, pharmacology, and mental health providers. A number of nutritional, pharmacological, and psychosocial interventions have been studied. However, limitations in the literature are apparent and demand further attention. A wide range of chemosensory alterations are found across studies, likely due to differences in methodology and patient populations, and intervention studies have often been conducted with small sample sizes making generalization implausible. Noticeably, there is a lack of evidence on whether the recommended strategies for intervention to improve chemosensory alterations and nutritional intake in cancer patients are effective, and therefore a large number of these recommendations continue to be based on clinical expertise and anecdotal accounts. These limitations are not uncommon to clinical research. However, considering the apparent high prevalence of chemosensory alterations in cancer patients, and the equally high likelihood that these issues tend to remain unaddressed in spite of the grave detrimental effects of these alterations on patients' physical and mental recovery from treatment, it is imperative that the scientific community commit a larger effort to the systematic study of adequate assessment strategies and interventions to address chemosensory alterations and improve nutritional intake in this population. More specifically, future studies should examine whether the commonly recommended strategies for addressing chemosensory alterations in cancer patients reviewed in this chapter are, in fact, effective in improving taste and smell changes, whether targeted interventions are more effective in improving certain outcomes based on the type of cancer and treatment, and whether these interventions ultimately improve cancer patients' nutritional intake and prevent malnutrition.

REFERENCES

American Psychiatric Association. 2013. *Diagnostic and Statistical Manual of Mental Disorders 5 (DSM-5).* Arlington, VA: American Psychiatric Publishing.

Bakan, N., E. Bakan, M. Suerdem, and M.R. Yiğitoğlu. 1998. Serum zinc and angiotensin-converting enzyme levels in patients with lung cancer. *BioFactors* 2:177–178.

Baldwin, C., A. Spiro, R. Ahern, and P.W. Emery. 2012. Oral nutritional interventions in malnourished patients with cancer: A systematic review and meta-analysis. *J Natl Cancer Inst* 104:1–15.

Bauer, J., S. Capra, and M. Ferguson. 2003. Use of the scored Patient-Generated Subjective Global Assessment (PG-SGA) and its association with quality of life in ambulatory patients receiving radiotherapy. *Eur J Clin Nutr* 57:305–309.

Bernhardson, B., K. Olson, V.E. Baracos, and W.V. Wismer. 2012. Reframing eating during chemotherapy in cancer patients with chemosensory alterations. *Eur J Oncol Nurs* 16:483–490.

Boltong, A., and R. Keast. 2012. The influence of chemotherapy on taste perception and food hedonics: A systematic review. *Cancer Treat Rev* 38:152–163.

Brisbois, T.D., J.L. Hutton, V.E. Baracos, and W.V. Wismer. 2006. Taste and smell abnormalities as an independent cause of failure of food intake in patients with advanced cancer—An argument for the application of sensory science. *J Palliat Care* 22:111–114.

Brisbois, T.D., I.H. deCock, S.M. Watanabe et al. 2011. Delta-9-tetrahydrocannabinol may palliate altered chemosensory perception in cancer patients: Results of a randomized, double-blind, placebo-controlled pilot trial. *Ann Oncol* 22:2086–2093.

Broberg, D.J., and I. Bernstein. 1987. Candy as a scapegoat in the prevention of food aversions in children receiving chemotherapy. *Cancer* 60:2344–2347.

Bruera, E., S. Chadwich, L. Cowan et al. 1986. Caloric assessment of advanced cancer patients: Comparison of three methods. *Cancer Treat Rep* 70:981–983.

Buzby, K.M. 1990. Overview: Screening, assessing and monitoring. In *Nutrition Management of the Cancer Patient*, ed. A.S. Bloch, pp. 3–23. Rockville, MD: Aspen Publishers.

Cancer.net. Taste changes. Available at http://www.cancer.net/all-about-cancer/treating-cancer/managing-side-effects/taste-changes (accessed June 24, 2014).

Capra, S., M. Ferguson, and K. Ried. 2001. Cancer: Impact of nutrition intervention outcome—Nutrition issues for patients. *Nutrition* 17:769–772.

Christensen, C.M., J.G. Brand, and E. Malammue. 1987. Salivary changes in solution pH—A source of individual differences in sour taste perception. *Physiol Behav* 40:221–227.

Cunningham, R.S., and R. Bell. 2000. Nutrition in cancer: An overview. *Semin Oncol Nurs* 16:90–98.

Derogatis, L., and N. Melisaratos. 1983. The Brief Symptom Inventory: An introductory report. *Psychol Med* 13:595–605.

DeWys, W.D., D. Begg, P.T. Lavin et al. 1980. Prognostic effect of weight loss prior to chemotherapy in cancer patients. *Am J Med* 69:491–497.

Elliott, L., L.L. Molseed, P.D. McCallum, and B. Grant. 2006. *The Clinical Guide to Oncology Nutrition, 2nd Edition.* Chicago: American Dietetic Association.

Farmer, M.N., R.S. Raddin, and J.D. Roberts. 2009. The relationship between taste, olfaction, and nutrition in the cancer population. *J Support Oncol* 7:70–72.

Ferguson, M., S. Capra, J. Bauer, and M. Banks. 1999. Development of a valid and reliable malnutrition screening tool for adult acute hospital patients. *Nutrition* 15:458–464.

Fong, L.Y., and P.M. Newberne. 1978. Nitrosobenzylmethylamine, zinc deficiency and oesophageal cancer. *IARC Sci Publ* 19:503–513.

Gall, M.J., G.K. Grimble, N.J. Reeve, and S.J. Thomas. 1998. Effect of providing fortified meals and between-meal snacks on energy and protein intake of hospital patients. *Clin Nutr* 17:259–264.

Gibson, R. 1990. *Principles of Nutritional Assessment*. Oxford: Oxford University Press.

Goldberg, A.N., J.A. Shea, D.A. Deems, and R.L. Doty. 2005. A chemosensory questionnaire for patients treated for cancer of the head and neck. *Laryngoscope* 115:2077–2086.

Haylard, M.Y., A. Jatoi, J.A. Sloan et al. 2007. Does zinc sulfate prevent therapy-induced taste alterations in head and neck cancer patients? Results of phase III double-blind, placebo-controlled trial from the North Central Cancer Treatment Group (N01C4). *Int J Radiat Oncol Biol Phys* 67:1318–1322.

Heald, A.E., C.F. Pieper, and S.S. Schiffman. 1998. Taste and smell complaints in HIV-infected patients. *AIDS* 12:1667–1674.

Heinzerling, C.I., G. Smit, and E. Dransfield. 2008. Modeling oral conditions and thickness perception of a start product. *Int Dairy J* 18:867–873.

Heinzerling, C.I., M. Stieger, J. Bult, and G. Smit. 2011. Individually modified saliva delivery changes the perceived intensity of saltiness and sourness. *Chem Percept* 4:145–153.

Henkin, R.I., B.M. Martin, and R.P. Adarwal. 1999. Decreased parotid saliva gustin/carbonic anhydrase VI secretion: An enzyme disorder manifested by gustatory and olfactory dysfunction. *Am J Med Sci* 318:380–391.

Hong, J.H., P. Omur-Ozbeck, B.T. Stanek et al. 2009. Taste and odor abnormalities in cancer patients. *J Support Oncol* 7:58–65.

Hopkinson, J.B. 2010. The emotional aspects of cancer anorexia. *Curr Opin Support Palliat Care* 4:254–258.

Hutton, J.L., V.E. Baracos, and W.V. Wismer. 2007. Chemosensory dysfunction is a primary factor in the evolution of declining nutrition status and quality of life in patients with advanced cancer. *J Pain Symptom Manage* 33:156–165.

Jatoi, A. 2010. Cancer chemotherapy: With or without food? *Support Care Cancer* 18:S13–S16.

Kim, J.Y., G.A. Wie, Y.A. Cho et al. 2011. Development and validation of a nutrition screening tool for hospitalized cancer patients. *Clin Nutr* 30:724–729.

Kondrup, J., H.H. Rasmussen, O. Hamberg, Z. Stanga, and Ad Hoc ESPEN Working Group. 2003. Nutritional risk screening (NRS-2002): A new method based on an analysis of controlled clinical trials. *Clin Nutr* 22:321–336.

Lotfi-Jam, K., M. Carey, M. Jefford, P. Schofield, C. Charleson, and S. Aranda. 2008. Nonpharmacologic strategies for managing common chemotherapy adverse effects: A systematic review. *J Clin Oncol* 26:5618–5629.

Lyckholm, L., S.P. Heddinger, G. Parker et al. 2012. A randomized, placebo controlled trial of oral zinc for chemotherapy-related taste and smell disorders. *J Pain Palliat Care Pharmacother* 26:111–114.

McLaughlin, L., and S.M. Mahon. 2012. Understanding taste dysfunction in patients with cancer. *Clin J Oncol Nurs* 16:171–178.

Nestle Nutrition. 2013. User's Guide to Completing the Mini Nutritional Assessment (MNA). Available at http://www.mna-elderly.com/ (accessed December 24, 2014).

Norris, M.B., A.C. Nobel, and R.M. Pangborn. 1984. Human saliva and taste responses to acids varying in anions, titratable acidity, and pH. *Physiol Behav* 32:237–244.

Ottery, F.D. 1997. Nutritional oncology: A proactive, integrated approach to the cancer patient. In *Nutrition Support: Theory and Therapeutics*, eds. S.A. Shikora, and G.L. Blackburn, pp. 395–409. New York: Chapman & Hall.

Piertsma, P., S. Folett-Bick, B. Wilkinson, N. Guebert, K. Fisher, and J. Pereira. 2003. A bedside food cart as an alternate food service for acute and palliative oncological patients. *Support Care Cancer* 11:611–614.

Prasad, A.S., J. Kaplan, F.W. Beck et al. 1997. Trace elements in head and neck cancer patients: Zinc status and immunologic functions. *Otolaryngol Head Neck Surg* 116: 624–629.

Ravasco, P. 2005. Aspects of taste and compliance in patients with cancer. *Eur J Oncol Nurs* 9:S84–S91.

Redd, W.H., G.H. Montgomery, and K.N. DuHamel. 2001. Behavioral intervention for cancer treatment side effects. *J Natl Cancer Inst* 93:810–823.

Ripamonti, C., Z. Ernesto, C. Brunelli et al. 1998. A randomized, controlled clinical trial to evaluate the effects of zinc sulfate on cancer patients with taste alterations caused by head and neck irradiation. *Cancer* 82:1938–1945.

Roscoe, J.A., M. O'Neill, P. Jean-Pierre et al. 2010. An exploratory study on the effects of an expectancy manipulation on chemotherapy-related nausea. *J Pain Symptom Manage* 40:379–390.

Scalera, G. 2002. Effects of conditioned food aversions on nutritional behavior in humans. *Nutr Neurosci* 5:159–188.

Schiffman, S.S., E.A. Sattely-Miller, E.L. Taylor et al. 2007. Combination of flavor enhancement and chemosensory education improves nutritional status in older cancer patients. *J Nutr Health Aging* 11:439–454.

Smith, S.J., and W.W. Souba. 2001. Nutrition support. In *Cancer Principles and Practice of Oncology*, eds. V.T. DeVita, S. Helman, and S.A. Rosenberg, pp. 3012–3032. Philadelphia: Lippincott Williams and Wilkins.

Spitzer, R.L., K. Kroenke, and J.B. Williams. 1999. Validation and utility of a self-report version of PRIME-MD: The PHQ primary care study. Primary Care Evaluation of Mental Disorders. Patient Health Questionnaire. *JAMA* 282:1737–1744.

Stratton, R.J., A. Hackston, D. Longmore et al. 2004. Malnutrition in hospital outpatient and inpatients: Prevalence, concurrent validity and ease of use of the "Malnutrition Universal Screening Tool" ("MUST") for adult. *Br J Nutr* 92:799–808.

Vigano, A., E. Bruera, G.S. Jhangri, S.C. Newman, A.L. Fields, and M.E. Suarez-Almazor. 2000. Clinical survival predictors in patients with advanced cancer. *Arch Intern Med* 160:861–868.

Wickham, R.S., M. Rehwaldt, C. Kefer et al. 1999. Taste changes experienced by patients receiving chemotherapy. *Oncol Nurs Forum* 26:697–706.

Wilken, M.K., and B.A. Satiroff. 2012. Pilot study of "miracle fruit" to improve food palatability for patients receiving chemotherapy. *Clin Journal Oncol Nurs* 16:E173–E177.

Williams, R., K. Virtue, and A. Adkins. 1998. Room service improves patient food intake and satisfaction with hospital food. *J Pediatr Oncol Nurs* 15:183–189.

Wismer, W.V. 2008. Assessing alterations in taste and their impact on cancer care. *Curr Opin Support Palliat Care* 2:282–287.

Zigmond, A.S., and R.P. Snaith. 1983. The hospital anxiety and depression scale. *Acta Psychiatr Scand* 67:361–370.

Index

Page numbers followed by f and t indicate figures and tables, respectively.

A

Acceptance, 246–247
  curve for sodium, 90
  food
    BMI and, 117
    long-term impairment of, 211–212
    glucose, NST and, 91, 92f, 94f
    IP for bitterness of caffeine, 236, 237f, 238f
    maltodextrin-averted taste-distension, 233f
    osmotically reduced facilitation of, 233–234
    preference and, 250–251
    reduced, 249
    reflexive, 86
    rejection behavior *vs.*, 87, 88, 223
    of sweet taste, 228, 228f, 230
    umami term, 17
Acetylcholine, 28, 39, 46
2-Acetylpyridine, 298
Acoustics, nutrition and, 203–206
Acute alcohol intoxication, 34t
A.D. Little Inc., 14
Adaptation
  olfactory/gustatory, sensory-specific satiety
    and, 213–214
  sensory, 69
Adenoidectomy, 36
Age-related hearing impairment, waist
    circumference and, 205
Aging, chemosensory disorders and, 30–36,
    31t–35t. *See also* Elderly population
Ajinomoto, 13
Alcohol, 68, 109, 194
  acute alcohol intoxication, 34t
  beer, 161, 163, 164, 170
  consumption, background music in, 204, 205
  on olfaction, 40
  static pressure on tongue, 198
  thiamine deficiency and, 42
  wine, 70, 144, 151, 168, 170, 197, 204, 205
Alcohol Sniff Test (AST), 45–46, 45f
Alertness, olfaction role, 75
Allergic rhinitis, 31t
Alliesthesia, post-ingestive negative, 210
Allyl isothiocyanate, 176
Alterations, chemosensory
  in cancer patients, 309–310
    additional strategies, managing, 316–319

    assessment, 310–312
    dietary and food delivery modifications,
      managing, 312–315, 314t
    limitations and future directions, 319
Altered eating habits, patients' awareness, 50, 51t
Aluminosilicates, 40
Alzheimer's disease, 39–40
  type, senile dementia of, 32t, 46
American Chemical Society, 19
Amino acid detectors, in mouth and brain, 267
Amoebiasis, 39–40
Amygdala, 67
Amyotrophic lateral sclerosis, 33t
Anatomy
  gustatory functional, 83–86
    central taste system, 84–86. *See also*
      Central taste system
    peripheral nerves, 84
    receptors, 83–84. *See also* Receptors,
      taste
  olfactory, 66–67
  smell, 27–29, 28f
Anesthesia, oral, 124–125
Anorexia, sensory-specific satiety and, 214
Anosmia, 36–37, 42
  steroid-dependent, 36
  temporary, 41
Antidepressants, 75
Anxiety, 42, 86, 312
Appearance, 194–195
  diners' perception of food and, 150
  food, lighting on, 151
  insular neurons and, 86
  refreshing, 146, 164
  textures and, 194
  visual, 139, 170
Appetite
  capsaicin on, 176, 177t–181t, 188t
  capsiate on, 185t–187t, 188t
  conditioned, for caffeine, 236
  for food, hunger, 247–248
  ingestive, food preference responses and,
    246
  missing IP, 246–247
  model, saccharin preference as, 224–225
  in older people, glutamate/added aroma,
    284
  ratings, words for, 248–249

Aromas, 68–69
added, on appetite in older people, 284
of fresh strawberries, 271–272
Aspartame, 214, 303
Assessment
chemosensory alterations in cancer patients,
310–312
olfaction, 44–46, 45f
Assimilation, food expectations and, 168
Associative reward, words for, 252
AST (Alcohol Sniff Test), 45–46, 45f
Astringency, 197
Atmospheric pressure-sensitive paroxysmal
unilateral phantosmia, 31t
Auditory system, nutrition and, 203–206
Aversion
conditioned taste, 229
food, cancer patients and, 317–319
hedonically, odors and tastes, 295–298
Awareness, patients
of altered eating habits, 50, 51t

B

Balances
maltol and ethyl acetoacetate, 270–271, 271f
of sweet and sour in oranges, 261–262
Bartoshuk, Linda, 16–17
Baylis, Leslie L., 18
Beer, color, 161, 163, 164, 170
Benzocaine, 300–301
Bernard, Claude, 209
Beverages
black tea, 214
colors, 143–147, 160, 163. See also Color
correspondences
cues to flavor–aroma identity, 144
cues to flavor–aroma intensity, 144–146
cues to other sensations, 146–147
hedonically positive/negative, 167–168
preference development for bitter, 236, 237,
238
quinine, 167–168
sensory-specific satiety of, 214
seven7UP, 167–168, 171
sip size, 195
sugary, 20–22
thirst-quenching, 147, 163
viscosity, 196
Bieber, Justin, 204
Biles, yellow and black, 6
Bite size, 195–196
Bitterness
cabbage, 9
caffeine, IP for, 236, 237f–238f
Galen's concepts, 3–10
levels, learnt likings for, 235–236

preference development for foods and drinks,
236, 237, 238
thiourea, 113
On Black Bile, 4, 6
Black tea, 214
Blood urea nitrogen, older people with low, 267
BMS (burning mouth syndrome), 124
Body mass index (BMI)
food acceptance and, 117
Bonito, 11, 13
Boring, Edwin, 17
Brain, amino acid detectors in, 267
Breast feeding, sweetness and, 226, 227
Brightness, defined, 143
Burn, 197–198
Burning mouth syndrome (BMS), 124
Butyric acid, 296

C

Cabbage, bitterness, 9
Cacosmia, 38
Cadmium, 87
Caffeine
for chemosensory disorders, 47
conditioned appetite for, 236
IP for bitterness of, 236, 237f–238f
Calcium inhibitors, intranasal
for chemosensory disorder, 48–49
Cancer, elderly patients and, 74
Cancer patients, chemosensation in, 309–319
chemosensory alterations, 309–319
additional strategies for managing,
316–319
assessment, 310–312
dietary and food delivery modifications
for managing, 312–315, 314t
limitations and future directions, 319
Cannon, Walter B., 209
Capsaicin
burn, 198
chili and, 176, 182, 183
obesity/overweight and, 183–184
red hot pepper, 176, 182–184
on thermogenesis and appetite, 176,
177t–181t, 182–184, 188t
in weight loss management, 189
in Western diet, 184, 189
Capsiate, on thermogenesis and appetite,
185t–187t, 188t
Carbidopa, on olfaction, 39
Carbohydrates
red hot pepper and, 182–183
somatic contexts of sweet preference,
231–234, 232f, 233f
Carbonic anhydrase VI deficiency, 316
Central nucleus of amygdala (CNA), 86

Central pathway dysfunction, 32t
Central sensation, 248
Central taste system, 84–86
    NST, 84, 85f
    primary taste cortex, 84–86, 85f
    thalamic taste area, 84
CH-19, 183–184
Chaudhari, Nirupa, 18
Chemesthesis, thermogenesis and, 175–189. *See also* Thermogenesis
Chemical senses, 82
Chemical signals, in retronasal olfaction, 67–68
Chemical stimulation, to ingestive movement, 255–256
Chemical taste thresholds, 106–107
Chemosensation
    in cancer patients, 309–319
        alterations. *See* Chemosensory alterations
    color correspondences in, 139–153. *See also* Color correspondences
    defined, 65
    food and, 74–75
    response to, 73–74
    for weight loss, 295–305
        hedonically aversive odors and tastes, 295–298
        hedonically positive odors, 298–300
        hedonically positive tastes, 300–305
        overview, 295
Chemosenses, impact, 1
Chemosensory alterations, in cancer patients, 309–319
    additional strategies for managing, 316–319
    limitations and future directions, 319
    pharmacological interventions, 316–317
    psychosocial interventions, 317–319
    assessment, 310–312
    dietary and food delivery modifications for managing, 312–315, 314t
    limitations and future directions, 319
Chemosensory disorders, 25–52
    anatomy and pathophysiology, 27–43
        neurotransmitters, smell mediators, 29
        smell, 27–29, 28f
        taste, physiology, 30
    epidemiology, 26–27
    etiologies, 30–43
        aging, 30–36, 31t–35t
        Alzheimer's disease, 39–40
        diagnoses with olfactory impairment, 42–43
        endocrine disorders, 36–37
        meningiomas, 37
        nasal obstruction, 36
        nutritional deficiencies, 41–42
        Parkinson's disease, 38–39
        temporal lobe lesions, 37–38

        thalamic and hypothalamic lesions, 38
        toxic agents, 40
        trauma, 41
        viral hepatitis, 36
    overview, 26
    patient evaluation, 43–46
        assessing olfaction, 44–46, 45f
    treatment, 46–51
        caffeine, 47
        chiropractic manipulation, 50
        intranasal calcium inhibitors, 48–49
        patients' awareness of altered eating habits, 50, 51t
        pentoxifylline, 48
        phosphatidylcholine, 46–47
        prednisone, 49
        sniff therapy, 49
        theophylline, 49
        thiamine, 47
        vitamin A, 47
        zinc, 47–48
Chemosensory influences, 223–284
    cognitive mechanisms, convert sensing into ingesting, 255–261
        chemical stimulation to ingestive movement, processes, 255–256
        configured IP, 257–261. *See also* Configured IP
        mixing, 256–257
    gustatory configurations in ingestion, 261–270
        amino acid detectors in mouth and brain, 267
        direct route to food quality, 269
        direct stimulation of preference, 262–263, 262f
        MSG, complex savory taste, 265–267, 266f
        MSG quantity, quality of food and, 269, 270f
        savory complex/fifth simple taste, 268
        sensations *vs.* thoughts controlling preference, 263–265, 264f
        sensory vocabularies, 268–269
        sweet and sour in oranges, balances, 261–262
    ingestive behavior, basic theory, 223–224
    missing IP, 240–249
        energy intakes and appetite ratings, words for, 248–249
        family paradox, 245–246
        food preferences and obesity, 241–245. *See also* Obesity, food preferences and
        food preferences and PROP genetics, 241
        group-averaged scores for preference, 240–241
        hunger, appetite for food, 247–248

ingestive appetite and food preference
responses, 246
preference/appetite, 246–247
sensations/sensed characteristics, 246
olfactory configurations in ingestion,
270–281
analytical and configured norms, 275–276
aroma of fresh strawberries, 271–272
balances among components, 270–271,
271f
cognitive analysis of concentrations and
ratings, 272, 273f–274f
flavors, 276–281, 278f, 279f, 280f
overview, 223
sweetness level, excitation and inhibition of
ingestion, 224–230
conditioned taste aversion, 229
conditioned taste preference, 229–230
learnt preferences for, 227–229, 228f
reflex-ingestive movements to sweet taste,
227
saccharin preference as appetite model,
224–225
sensory motivation without pleasure/
reward, 227
solutions, ingestive responses to,
225–226, 226f
sweetness level, learnt peak of preference for,
230–240
conditioned appetite for caffeine, 236
development for bitter foods and drinks,
236, 237, 238
evidence, human sensory preferences, 234
facilitation by sensory factor, 234–235,
235f
human preference for salt taste, 239–240
IP for bitterness of caffeine, 236,
237f–238f
likings for bitterness levels, 235–236
most preferred strength, 230–231
PROP and, 238–239
somatic contexts of, 231–234, 232f, 233f
strengths of taste, 230
tastes, smells, colors, and textures, 240
taste on nutrition, long-term effects, 281–283
salt and strokes, 281–283, 282f
sugar and teeth, 283
words for intensities and preferences,
250–255
amount of tastes, 254
combinations of tastes, roles, 254
different taste, food, 253
food preferences, 250
intensities, gustatory and olfactory, 250
motivating stimulus/associative reward,
252
pleasant vs. pleasurable, 250–251

stimulus levels, 254–255
strength of influence, 252–253
ChemoSensory Questionnaire (CSQ), 311
Chemosensory satiety, 74–75
Chen, Joyce, 20
Chewing gum, 276–277, 278f, 279f, 280f
on sensory-specific satiety, 214
Chiang, Connie, 19–20
Children, diet for, 211–212
Chili, capsaicin and, 176, 182, 183
Chiropractic manipulation, for chemosensory
disorders, 50
Chorda tympani (CT), 119
Chorda tympani anesthetization, 72
CIELAB color space, 143
Circumvallate papillae, 30, 83
Citric acid, stimulation from, 263
Clinical correlates, localized taste loss,
122–125
anesthesia in evaluation, 124–125
oral disinhibition, 123–124
Clinical evaluation, oral anesthesia in, 124–125
Clinical testing, retronasal smell, 70–73, 70f
Clomiphene, 37
CNA (central nucleus of amygdala), 86
CNI (cranial nerve I)
assessment, 44
disorder, 31t
Coca-Cola, 21
Cognitive analysis, of concentrations and ratings,
272, 273f–274f
Cognitively impaired normosmic elderly, 212
Cognitive mechanisms, convert sensing into
ingesting, 255–261
chemical stimulation to ingestive movement,
processes, 255–256
configured IP, 257–261
identical/configured influences,
260–261
mixture statistics, 257–258
scientific measurement of context,
258–260
mixing, 256–257
Cognitive mediation, chemosensory influences
on, 223–284. See also Chemosensory
influences
Colon cancer, risk factors for, 110–111
Color(s)
defined, 142
flavor intensity and, 161–162
food identification and, 160–161
freshness and, 140, 146–147
liking and, 161
packaging, 140, 141, 142
preferences for specific level of sweetness,
240
refreshment and, 163–164

Color correspondences, 139–153
  cross-modal, 141–142
  food/beverages, 143–147, 160, 163
    cues to flavor–aroma identity, 144
    cues to flavor–aroma intensity, 144–146
    cues to other sensations, 146–147
  fundamental importance, 139–142
  future research directions, 152–153
  individual differences in, 151–152
  interim summary, 148–149
  overview, 139–142
  of packaging, 147–148, 148f
  perception, basics, 142–143
  surroundings/environment, 151
  tableware, 149–151
Columella variant, of glossopharyngeal
    neuralgia, 34t
Complex partial seizures, 32t
Concentrations, cognitive analysis, 272,
    273f–274f
Conditioned appetite, for caffeine, 236
Conditioned taste aversion (CTA), 89, 229
Conditioned taste preference, 229–230
Configured influences, 260–261
Configured IP, 257–261
  identical/configured influences, 260–261
  mixture statistics, 257–258
  scientific measurement of context, 258–260
    separate influences, interactions, 260
Congenital adrenal hyperplasia, 37
Congruency, 205–206
Constipation, cause, 6
Consumption, music-induced enhanced, 204–205
Control, gustatory
  of eating, 87–94
    enduring changes, 88–89
    momentary changes, 90–94, 92f, 94f
    taste system, organization, 87–88
    transient changes, 90
Correspondences, color, 139–153. *See also* Color
    correspondences
Cortex
  primary taste, 84–86, 85f
    ingestive, 85
    insular, 84–85, 85f, 86
    OFC, 83, 86, 91, 93, 213
Cranial nerve I (CNI)
  assessment, 44
  disorder, 31t
Crispiness, 203
Crocker, E. C., 14–15, 20
Cross-modal correspondences, 141–142
Cross-modal interaction, food odors in, 196–197
Cross-modality matching, 110
Crunchiness, 203
Crystal Pepsi, 161
CSQ (ChemoSensory Questionnaire), 311

CT (chorda tympani), 119
CTA (conditioned taste aversion), 89, 229
Cuisines, flavors, 278, 279, 281
Culinary Institute of America, 166
Culinary presentations, 165–167
Cultivated leeks, 7

D

D-amphetamine, 38
Da-Nippon Chemical, 13
Decomposition, of food, 164
Delta-9-tetrahydrocannabinol, 316
Delwiche, Jennine, 19
Dementia, senile
  of Alzheimer's type, 32t, 46
Depression, 312
Detectors, amino acid
  in mouth and brain, 267
Diet
  American, 11, 14, 19, 20, 90
  amino acids in, 267
  balanced, 103
  based on satiety index, 215
  beverages, weight gain and, 196
  for children, 211–212
  compliance, aspartame and, 303
  design, satiety value of food, 213
  Galen's observations on, 1, 3–10
  late twentieth-century, 20–22
  liquid, 194
  major components, 87
  nitrogen source in, 267
  noncaloric flavors in, 302
  reducing, benzocaine and, 301
  restrictive, 297
  salt level in, 281–282
  sugar in, 20–22
  unbalanced, 36
  varied, for infants, 211
  weight loss, 303
  Western, capsaicin in, 184, 189
Dietary fat, tactile sensations from, 124
Dietary intake, 196
Dietary modifications, for managing
    chemosensory alterations, 312–315,
    314t
Dietary patterns, 26, 223
Dietary red pepper, on energy metabolism,
    182–184
Dietary restriction, sodium, 90
Diet-induced thermogenesis, in rats, 176
Dietitians, registered, 311, 312, 319
Diffuse brain dysfunction, 32t
Direct scaling, of suprathreshold intensity,
    108–119
  magnitude estimation, 108–109

oral sensory differences, labeled scales,
    113–119, 114f
  GIS, 117, 119
  gLMS, 116–119, 118f
  intensity labels, properties, 113–115
  invalid comparisons, consequences,
    115–116, 115f
oral sensory differences, magnitude
    matching, 109–113
  genetic factors in variation, 111–112
  overview, 110–111
  taster status classification, 112–113
Direct stimulation, of preferences, 262–263, 262f
Dirhinous inhalation, 27
Disinhibition, oral, 123–124
Dopamine, 28, 29
Drinks/drinking
  chemosensory influences on, 223–284. *See
    also* Chemosensory influences
  colors, 139–153. *See also* Color
    correspondences
  preference development for bitter, 236, 237,
    238
On Drugs, 5
Dufresne, Wyle, 170
Dysgeusia, 36, 37, 42, 123
Dysosmia, 38, 42
Dysthymia, 32t

E

Eating, 17
  altered habits, patients' awareness and, 50, 51t
  animal, 6
  behaviors, 317
    extrasomatic acoustics on, 203–204
  chemosensory influences on, 223–284. *See
    also* Chemosensory influences
  food color and, 161
  frequency, 245, 301
  gustatory control, 87–94
    enduring changes in taste, 88–89
    momentary changes in taste, 90–94, 92f,
      94f
    taste system, organization, 87–88
    transient changes in taste, 90
  illness by, 7
  motivational aspects, 86
  music-induced enhanced consumption,
    204–205
  obesity and, 245
  olfactory aversive conditioning, 297–298
  olfactory impairment and, 43
  overeating, 209, 212, 296, 297–298
  physiological influences on, 247
  pre-eating phase, 74
  processed foods, 21

rates, food textures and, 194–195
  retronasal smell and, 70
  retronasal *vs.* orthonasal threshold, olfaction
    and, 67
  selective, physiological and social factors
    in, 223
  senses on, 159
  sensory-specific satiety and, 209–215
    olfactory and gustatory sensations,
      212–213
    termination, 212
    varied sensory experience, 210
  signal to stop, 74
  social relationships and, 3
  speed, 75
  sugary food, 283
Eight-cup technique, 106
Elderly population, 7
  age-related hearing impairment, waist
    circumference and, 205
  breast and lung cancer patients, 312
  cancer and, 74
  chemosensory disorders and, 30–36, 31t–35t
  cognitively impaired normosmic, 212
  food consumption, enhanced flavor and, 302
  glutamate/added aroma on appetite in, 284
  greater nutrition, need, 294
  with low blood urea nitrogen, 267
  non-obese, 194
  olfactory deficits, 30–31, 35, 36, 50, 298
  overweight, hedonically positive food odors
    and, 298–299
  sensory-specific satiety in, 212
  weight gain, antidepressants in, 75
Electrogustometry, 107–108
Elemente der Psychophysik, 104
Endocrine disorders, 36–37
Enduring changes, in taste, 88–89
Energy intakes, words for, 248–249
Environment, effect on taste and flavor, 151
Epidemiology, chemosensory disorders, 26–27
Epilepsy, temporal lobe, 38
Essence, 12
Essential tremor, 33t
Ethyl acetoacetate, 270–271, 271f
Ethyl mercaptan, 36
Etiologies, chemosensory disorders, 30–43
  aging, 30–36, 31t–35t
  Alzheimer's disease, 39–40
  diagnoses with olfactory impairment, 42–43
  endocrine disorders, 36–37
  meningiomas, 37
  nasal obstruction, 36
  nutritional deficiencies, 41–42
  Parkinson's disease, 38–39
  temporal lobe lesions, 37–38
  thalamic and hypothalamic lesions, 38

toxic agents, 40
trauma, 41
viral hepatitis, 36
European Organization for Research and
        Treatment of Cancer Quality of Life
        Questionnaire, 313
Excitation of ingestion, sweetness level, 224–230
    conditioned taste aversion, 229
    conditioned taste preference, 229–230
    learnt preferences for, 227–229, 228f
    reflex-ingestive movements to taste, 227
    saccharin preference as appetite model,
        224–225
    sensory motivation without pleasure/reward,
        227
    solutions, ingestive responses to, 225–226,
        226f
Expectations, judgments of food and, 167–169
Experiences, enduring changes in taste and,
        88–89

F

Family paradox, missing IP and, 245–246
Farm Bill, 21
Fat, dietary, tactile sensations from, 124
Fat taste, food preferences and obesity, 244–245
Feel, of food, 193–198. *See also* Food, look and
        feel
    burn and sting, 197
    physical texture, 194–195, 240
    pleasantness *vs.* pleasure, 250–251
Fifth taste, 268
Filter paper testing, 120–121
Flavor(s), 68–69
    colors cues to
        flavor-aroma identity, 144
        flavor-aroma intensity, 144–146
    enhancers, 35t
    identification, color and, 160–161
    intensity, color and, 161–162
    olfactory configurations in ingestion,
        276–278, 278f, 279f, 280f
    cuisines, not nutrients, 278, 279, 281
FMRI (functional magnetic resonance imaging),
        18, 213
Foliate papillae, 83
Food
    acceptance
        BMI and, 117
        long-term impairment of, 211–212
    amount of tastes, 254
    appetite for, hunger, 247–248
    aversion, cancer patients and, 317–319
    bitter, preference development for, 236, 237,
        238
    chemosensation and, 74–75

colors, 143–147. *See also* Color
        correspondences
    cues to flavor–aroma identity, 144
    cues to flavor–aroma intensity, 144–146
    cues to other sensations, 146–147
combinations of tastes, roles, 254
delivery modifications, for managing
        chemosensory alterations, 312–315,
        314t
different taste, 253
identification, color and, 160–161
judgments, expectations and, 167–169
look and feel, 193–198
    astringency, 197
    bite size, 195–196
    burn/sting, 197–198
    overview, 193–194
    texture, 194–195
    viscosity, 196–197
odors, 73–74
preferences
    obesity and, 241–245. *See also* Obesity,
        food preferences and
    PROP and, 238–239, 241
    responses, ingestive appetite and, 246
    words for, 250
presentation, 165–167, 210
quality
    direct route to, 269
    MSG quantity and, 269, 270f
value, freshness and, 203
visual cues on sensory and hedonic
        evaluation, 159–171. *See also* Visual
        cues
On Food, 5
Food choice, taste and, 81–96
    gustatory control of eating, 87–94
        enduring changes, 88–89
        momentary changes, 90–94, 92f, 94f
        taste system, organization, 87–88
        transient changes, 90
    gustatory functional anatomy, 83–86
        central taste system, 84–86. *See also*
            Central taste system
        peripheral nerves, 84
        receptors, 83–84. *See also* Receptors,
            taste
    overview, 81–83
Food Quality and Preference, 16–17
Fox, A. L., 109
Fragrances, 68–69, 73–74
Freshness
    colors and, 140, 146–147
    food value and, 203
    fruits and vegetables, 21, 50
    strawberries, aroma, 270, 271–272
    visual cues for, 164

Functional magnetic resonance imaging (fMRI), 18, 213
Fungiform papillae, 30, 121

G

Galen's concepts of bitterness, 3–10
Gastric distension, 91
General labeled magnitude scale (gLMS), 116–119, 118f
Genetics, PROP
food preferences and, 241
Georgians, taste preferences, 2
GLMS (general labeled magnitude scale), 116–119, 118f
Global intensity scales (GIS), 117, 119
Glomeruli, 27
Glossopharyngeal neuralgia, columella variant, 34t
Glucose, 229–230, 231–234, 232f, 233f
acceptance, NST and, 91, 92f, 94f
Glutamates
effect on appetite in older people, 284
MSG, 11, 13–15, 16, 265–267, 266f
amino acid detectors in mouth and brain, 267
quantity, quality of food and, 269, 270f
savory complex/fifth simple taste, 268
sensory vocabularies, 268–269
taste and flavor, 10–18
GMP (guanosine monophosphate), 11
GMP (guanylic acid), 16, 18
Gold standard technique, 112
Gonadotrophin, 37
Gonadotrophin-associated hypogonadism, 37
Grant, Mark, 8
Green peppers, 36
Group-averaged scores, for preference, 240–241
Guanosine monophosphate (GMP), 11
Guanylic acid (GMP), 16, 18
Gustatory adaptation, sensory-specific satiety and, 213–214
Gustatory configurations, in ingestion, 261–270
amino acid detectors in mouth and brain, 267
direct route to food quality, 269
direct stimulation of preference, 262–263, 262f
MSG
complex savory taste, 265–267, 266f
quantity, quality of food and, 269, 270f
savory complex/fifth simple taste, 268
sensations *vs.* thoughts controlling preference, 263–265, 264f
sensory vocabularies, 268–269
sweet and sour in oranges, balances, 261–262

Gustatory control, of eating, 87–94
tastes and
enduring changes in, 88–89
momentary changes, 90–94, 92f, 94f
system, organization, 87–88
transient changes in, 90
Gustatory functional anatomy, 83–86
central taste system, 84–86
NST, 84, 85f
primary taste cortex, 84–86, 85f
thalamic taste area, 84
peripheral nerves, 84
receptors, 83–84
papillae, 83
receptor cells, 84
taste buds, 83
Gustatory intensities, words for, 250

H

Half-discriminated fraction/disparity (HDF), 253, 254
Headache, 33t
Head injury, 41
Head trauma, 31t
Hearing impairment, age-related
waist circumference and, 205
Hedonic(s)
evaluation of food, visual cues on, 159–171. *See also* Visual cues
gLMS, 116–117, 118f
hedonically aversive odors and tastes, 295–298
hedonically positive odors, 298–300
hedonically positive tastes, 300–305
pairing of sound, 205–206
positive/negative beverage, 167–168
scale, 251
sensory-specific satiety and, 210, 211
Heinz, H. J., 21
Henderson, L. F., 14
Hue, defined, 143
Human oral experience, psychophysical measurement, 103–126
overview, 103–104
sensory evaluation, methods, 119–126
retronasal olfaction, 125–126
spatial taste testing, 122–125. *See also* Spatial taste testing
videomicroscopy of tongue, 121
whole mouth sensation, 120–121
thresholds *vs.* intensity, 104–119
direct scaling of suprathreshold intensity, 108–119. *See also* Suprathreshold intensity
procedures, threshold, 104–108. *See also* Thresholds, procedures

Human-oriented color spaces, 143
Human sensory preferences, learnt, 234
Humoral concepts of bitterness, of Galen, 3–10
Hunger, appetite for food, 247–248
Hunger levels, momentary changes in taste,
   90–94, 92f, 94f
Hunger pangs, 209
Huntington's chorea, 32t
Hydrogen sulfide, 297
   on overweight subjects, 297
Hyperphagia, 204
Hypocupria, 42
Hypogeusia, 37, 41, 48
Hyposmia, 37, 38, 41, 42, 48
Hypothalamic lesions, 38
Hypovitaminosis A, 41

I

Ideal point (IP)
   for bitterness of caffeine, 236, 237f–238f
   configured, 257–261
      identical/configured influences,
         260–261
      mixture statistics, 257–258
      scientific measurement of context,
         258–260
   missing, 240–249
      energy intakes and appetite ratings, words
        for, 248–249
      family paradox, 245–246
      food preferences and obesity, 241–245.
        See also Obesity, food preferences and
      food preferences and PROP genetics,
        241
      group-averaged scores for preference,
        240–241
      hunger, appetite for food, 247–248
      ingestive appetite and food preference
        responses, 246
      preference/appetite, 246–247
      sensations/sensed characteristics, 246
Identical influences, 260–261
Identification, food
   color and, 160–161
Ikeda, Kikunae, 10–20
Illness, bad taste and, 5–6
Illumination, on taste and flavor, 151
IMP (inosine monophosphate), 11, 13
Impaired olfactory acuity, 37
Impaired sensory-specific satiety, 212
Individual differences, in color correspondences,
   151–152
Infants, varied diet for, 211
Influences, in configured IP
   identical/configured, 260–261
   separate, interactions among, 260

Ingesting, convert sensing into, 255–261
   chemical stimulation to ingestive movement,
      processes, 255–256
   configured IP, 257–261
      identical/configured influences,
        260–261
      mixture statistics, 257–258
      scientific measurement of context,
        258–260
   mixing, 256–257
Ingestion
   excitation and inhibition, by sweetness level,
      224–230
      conditioned taste aversion, 229
      conditioned taste preference, 229–230
      learnt preferences for, 227–229, 228f
      reflex-ingestive movements to taste, 227
      saccharin preference as appetite model,
        224–225
      sensory motivation without pleasure/
        reward, 227
      solutions, ingestive responses to,
        225–226, 226f
   gustatory configurations, 261–270
      amino acid detectors in mouth and brain,
        267
      direct route to food quality, 269
      direct stimulation of preference, 262–263,
        262f
      MSG, complex savory taste, 265–267,
        266f
      MSG quantity, quality of food and, 269,
        270f
      savory complex/fifth simple taste, 268
      sensations *vs.* thoughts controlling
        preference, 263–265, 264f
      sensory vocabularies, 268–269
      sweet and sour in oranges, balances,
        261–262
   olfactory configurations, 270–281
      analytical and configured norms,
        275–276
      aroma of fresh strawberries, 271–272
      balances among components, 270–271,
        271f
      cognitive analysis of concentrations and
        ratings, 272, 273f–274f
      flavor of cuisines, not nutrients, 278, 279,
        281
      flavors, 276–278, 278f, 279f, 280f
Ingestive appetite, food preference responses
   and, 246
Ingestive behavior, basic theory, 223–224
Ingestive cortex, 85
Ingestive responses, to sweet solutions, 225–226,
   226f
Inhalation, dirhinous, 27

Inhibition of ingestion, sweetness level, 224–230
    conditioned taste aversion, 229
    conditioned taste preference, 229–230
    learnt preferences for, 227–229, 228f
    reflex-ingestive movements to taste, 227
    saccharin preference as appetite model, 224–225
    sensory motivation without pleasure/reward, 227
    solutions, ingestive responses to, 225–226, 226f
Inosine monophosphate (IMP), 11, 13
Inosinic acid, 13
Insular cortex, 84–85, 85f, 86
Insular neurons, 86
Intensity(ies)
    direct scaling of suprathreshold intensity, 108–119
    GIS, 117, 119
    labels, properties, 113–115
    magnitude estimation, 108–109
    oral sensory differences, measuring, 109–113. *See also* Oral sensory differences, measuring
    flavor, color and, 161–162
    gustatory and olfactory, words for, 250
    oral experience measurement, 104–119
International Congress of Applied Chemistry, 10, 12
Interventions, chemosensory alterations in cancer patients
    pharmacological, 316–317
    psychosocial, 317–319
Intranasal calcium inhibitors, for chemosensory disorder, 48–49
IP. *See* Ideal point (IP)
Irritation (mild pain), 240

J

Japanese Chemical Society, 19
Jelly beans, in retronasal smell, 71–72
Jelly Belly jelly beans, 71, 72
Journal of Tokyo Chemical Society, 10

K

Kallmann syndrome, 37
Katsuobushi, 11, 12, 13
Koadamada, Shintaro, 13
Konbu, 11, 12
Korsakoff's psychosis, 38
Kuninaka, Akira, 16

L

Labeled hedonic scale, 116–117, 118f
Labeled magnitude scale (LMS), 116–117, 118f

Labeled scales, measuring oral sensory differences, 113–119, 114f
    GIS, 117, 119
    gLMS, 116–119, 118f
    intensity labels, properties, 113–115
    invalid comparisons, consequences, 115–116, 115f
Laminaria japonica, 12
Lateral hypothalamic area (LHA), 86
Late twentieth-century diet, 20–22
Learnt peak of preference, for sweetness level, 230–240
    conditioned appetite for caffeine, 236
    development for bitter foods and drinks, 236, 237, 238
    evidence, human sensory preferences, 234
    facilitation by sensory factor, 234–235, 235f
    human preference for salt taste, 239–240
    IP for bitterness of caffeine, 236, 237f–238f
    likings for bitterness levels, 235–236
    most preferred strength, 230–231
    PROP and, 238–239
    somatic contexts, 231–234, 232f, 233f
    strengths of taste, 230
    tastes, smells, colors, and textures, 240
Learnt preferences, for sweetness level, 227–229, 228f
Leibig's meat extract, 12
Lettuce, humoral balance and, 7
Levodopa, on olfaction, 39
LHA (lateral hypothalamic area), 86
L-histidine, 42
Lighting, on taste and flavor, 151
Lightness, defined, 143
Likert scale, 113
Likings
    color and, 161
    learnt, for bitterness levels, 235–236
LMS (labeled magnitude scale), 116–117, 118f
Localized taste loss, clinical correlates, 122–125
    anesthesia in evaluation, 124–125
    oral disinhibition, 123–124

M

Maga, Joseph A., 15
Magnitude estimation, 108–109
Magnitude matching, 110–111
Magnitude scale, general labeled, 116–117, 118f
Malingering, 34t
Malnutrition
    cancer patients and
        risks, 310–311, 312, 319
        screening tool, 311
    chemosensory disorders and, 41–42
    elderly and, 36
    risks, 91

Malnutrition Screening Tool, 311
Maltodextrin, 230, 231, 232–233
Maltodextrin-averted taste-distension
        acceptance, 233f
Maltol, 270–271, 271f, 272
Mandibulation, symphony, 203
Manducation, sounds of, 203
Marinol, 316
Masking, 257–258
Measurement
    psychophysical, human oral experience, 103–
        126. *See also* Human oral experience
    scientific measurement, configured IP and,
        258–260
Medication effect, 34t
Megestrol, 75
Meningiomas, olfactory, 37
Menthone, 276–277, 278f, 279f, 280f
Messy presentations, food, 165–167
3-Methoxy-4-hydroxy-phenylethylene glycol
        (MHPG), 38
1-Methyl-4-phenyl-1,2,3,6-tetrahydropyridine
        (MPTP), 42
Migraine, 33t–34t
Mini Nutrition Assessment tool, 313
Minty smell, 276–277, 278f, 279f, 280f
Miracle fruit, 313
Miso soup, 11
Missing IP, 240–249
    energy intakes and appetite ratings, words
        for, 248–249
    family paradox, 245–246
    food preferences
        obesity and, 241–245. *See also* Obesity,
            food preferences and
        PROP genetics and, 241
    group-averaged scores for preference, 240–241
    hunger, appetite for food, 247–248
    ingestive appetite and food preference
        responses, 246
    preference/appetite, 246–247
    sensations/sensed characteristics, 246
Mitral cells, 27–28, 29
Mixing, sense of taste, 256–257
Mixture statistics, taste, 257–258
Mizushima, Sanishiro, 15
Momentary changes, in taste, 90–94, 92f, 94f
Monosodium glutamate (MSG), 11, 13–15, 16,
        265–267, 266f
    amino acid detectors in mouth and brain, 267
    quantity, quality of food and, 269, 270f
    savory complex/fifth simple taste, 268
    sensory vocabularies, 268–269
Motivating stimulus, words for, 252
Mouth
    amino acid detectors in, 267
    oral sensation, whole, 120–121

Movement disorders, 32t–33t
MPTP (1-methyl-4-phenyl-1,2,3,6-
        tetrahydropyridine), 42
MSG. *See* Monosodium glutamate (MSG)
Multiple sclerosis, 33t
Music-induced enhanced consumption, 204–205
Mustard, 176, 182

N

Nasal obstruction, chemosensory disorder, 36
Nasal polyposis, 31t
Nasogastric (NG) tube, 176, 182
Natick 9-point scale, 113
Nausea, in cancer patients, 318
Neat presentations, food, 165–167
Neophobia, 167
Nerve-stimulation phantom, 124
Neurotransmitters, smell mediators, 29
"New Seasonings," 11
New York Times, 20
NG (nasogastric) tube, 176, 182
Nippon kagaku zasshi, 10
Nitrogen, source, 267
Norephinephrine metabolite, 38
Norms, analytical and configured, 275–276
Nucleus of solitary tract (NST), 84, 85f, 91
    glucose acceptance and, 91, 92f, 94f
Nutrition
    auditory system and, 203–206
    intake in cancer patients, chemosensation for,
        309–319
        alterations, 309–319. *See also*
            Chemosensory alterations
    music on, 204–205
    sensory-specific satiety and, 209–215. *See
        also* Sensory-specific satiety
    taste on, long-term effects, 281–283
        salt and strokes, 281–283, 282f
        sugar and teeth, 283
    thermogenesis and, 175–189. *See also*
            Thermogenesis
Nutritional deficiencies, 41–42

O

Obesity
    aversion therapy and, 296
    benzocaine and, 300
    capsaicin and, 183–184
    children, flavor for satiety and, 302
    food preferences and, 241–245
        fat taste, 244–245
        sweet taste, 242–244, 243f
    hedonically positive food odors and, 298–299
    hedonically positive tastes, 302, 304
    high-viscosity foods/drinks, 197

music-induced enhanced consumption and,
    204–205
rates, 20–22
sensory-specific satiety for, 212, 214
sweetness and, 283
Odorants, 65, 68–69
    detecting, 67
Odors/smell, 73–74, 161–162
    anatomy of smell, 27–29, 28f
    blindness, 35t
    in cross-modal interaction, 196–197
    hedonically aversive, 295–298
    hedonically positive, 298–300
    mediators, neurotransmitters, 29
    minty, 276–277
    neurotransmitters, 29
    pairing with tastes, 170
    preferences for specific level of sweetness, 240
    retronasal, clinical testing, 70–73, 70f
OFC (orbitofrontal cortex), 83, 86, 91, 93, 213
Olfaction
    alcohol on, 40
    anatomy, 66–67
    assessing, 44–46, 45f
    in balladromic fashion, 26
    deficits, implications, 35
    impairment, diagnoses with, 42–43
    retronasal, 65–75. See also Retronasal
        olfaction
    retronasal vs. orthonasal threshold, during
        eating, 67
    sensory-specific satiety and, 212
    trigeminal sensation on, 198
Olfactory adaptation, sensory-specific satiety
    and, 213–214
Olfactory configurations, in ingestion, 270–281
    analytical and configured norms, 275–276
    aroma of fresh strawberries, 271–272
    balances among components, 270–271, 271f
    cognitive analysis of concentrations and
        ratings, 272, 273f–274f
    flavors, 276–278, 278f, 279f, 280f
    cuisines, not nutrients, 278, 279, 281
Olfactory deficits, elderly population and, 30–31,
    35, 36, 50, 298
Olfactory dysmorphophobia, 32t
Olfactory groove meningioma, 32t
Olfactory hallucination, 32t
Olfactory intensities, words for, 250
Olfactory receptor damage, 31t
Olfactory reference syndrome, 32t
Olfactory sensitivity
    in AD, 39
    with adrenal cortical insufficiency, 37
    prednisone and, 37
    temporal lobectomy, 37–38
    in viral hepatitis, 36

Olive oil, 10
Opsa, 7
Oral disinhibition, 123–124
Oral experience, human
    psychophysical measurement, 103–126. See
        also Human oral experience
Oral sensory differences, measuring, 109–119
    labeled scales, 113–119, 114f
        GIS, 117, 119
        gLMS, 116–119, 118f
        intensity labels, properties, 113–115
        invalid comparisons, consequences,
            115–116, 115f
    magnitude matching, 109–113
        genetic factors in variation, 111–112
        individual differences, 109–110
        overview, 110–111
        taster status classification, 112–113
Oral sensory evaluation, methods, 119–126
    retronasal olfaction, 125–126
    spatial taste testing, 122–125. See also Spatial
        taste testing
    videomicroscopy of tongue, 121
    whole mouth sensation, 120–121
Oral sensory variation, genetic factors, 111–112
Oranges, balance of sweet and sour in, 261–262
Orbitofrontal cortex (OFC), 83, 86, 91, 93, 213
Orthonasal olfaction, 125
    retronasal vs., 69
Orthonasal threshold
    olfaction, during eating, 67
Otitis media, recurrent, 205
Overeating, 209, 212, 296, 297–298
Overweight
    adults, hedonically positive food odors and,
        298–299
    aversion therapy and, 296
    benzocaine and, 300
    children, flavor for satiety and, 302
    high-viscosity foods/drinks, 197
    hydrogen sulfide and, 297
    music-induced enhanced consumption and,
        204–205
Overweight people
    capsaicin and, 183
    hedonically positive tastes and, 302, 304

P

Packaging
    color, 140, 141, 142
    of potato crisps, 193
Packaging color, 147–148, 148f, 193
Pairing
    hedonic, of sound, 205–206
    odors with tastes, 170–171
Papillae, 83

Parabrachial nucleus (PBN), 89, 95, 96
Parkinson–dementia complex of Guam, 32t
Parkinson's disease, 29, 32t, 38–39
Pathophysiology, chemosensory disorders, 29–43
  etiologies, 30–43
    aging, 30–36, 31t–35t
    Alzheimer's disease, 39–40
    diagnoses with olfactory impairment,
      42–43
    endocrine disorders, 36–37
    meningiomas, 37
    nasal obstruction, 36
    nutritional deficiencies, 41–42
    Parkinson's disease, 38–39
    temporal lobe lesions, 37–38
    thalamic and hypothalamic lesions, 38
    toxic agents, 40
    trauma, 41
    viral hepatitis, 36
  neurotransmitters, smell mediators, 29
  taste, physiology, 30
Patient evaluation, chemosensory disorders,
  43–46
  assessing olfaction, 44–46, 45f
Patients awareness, of altered eating habits, 50,
  51t
Pavlovian conditioning, 317–318
PBN (parabrachial nucleus), 89, 95, 96
Peanut oil, 210
Pentoxifylline, for chemosensory disorders, 48
Pepper, red hot, 176, 182–184
Peppermint candy, 277
PepsiCo, 21
Perception, color, 142–143
Perceptual learning, 169–171
Peripheral nerves, 84
  sodium in, 90
PET (positron emission tomography) study, 213
Phantoms, 123–125
Phantosmia, 39
Pharmacological interventions, chemosensory
  alterations in cancer patients, 316–317
Phenylthiocarbamide (PTC), 109, 111
Phosphatidylcholine, for chemosensory disorders,
  46–47
Physiological needs, transient changes in taste
  and, 90
Physiological signal, sensation and, 248–249
Physiological synesthesia, of smell, 301–302
Physiology
  changes to oral epithelium, astringency and,
    197
  influences on eating, 247
  pathophysiology, chemosensory disorders,
    29–43. *See also* Pathophysiology
  taste, 16, 17, 18, 19, 30
Pick's disease, 32t

Piperine, burn, 198
Plateware, color, 149–151
Plating, 165–167
Pleasure
  pleasantness *vs.*, 250–251
  sensory motivation without, 227
Polio virus, 47
Positron emission tomography (PET) study, 213
Post-ingestive negative alliesthesia, 210
Post's pseudodementia, 42
Postviral infection, 31t
Potato crisps, packaging, 193
On the Power of Foods, 8, 9
Prednisone, 37
  for chemosensory disorders, 49
Preferences
  acceptance and, 250–251
  conditioned taste, 229–230
  defined, 250
  direct stimulation, 262–263, 262f
  family paradox, 245–246
  for fats in foods, 244–245
  group-averaged scores for, 240–241
  learnt peak, for sweetness level, 230–240
    conditioned appetite for caffeine, 236
    development for bitter foods and drinks,
      236, 237, 238
    evidence, human sensory preferences,
      234
    facilitation by sensory factor, 234–235,
      235f
    food, PROP and, 238–239
    human preference for salt taste, 239–240
    IP for bitterness of caffeine, 236,
      237f–238f
    likings for bitterness levels, 235–236
    most preferred strength, 230–231
    somatic contexts, 231–234, 232f, 233f
    strengths of taste, 230
    tastes, smells, colors, and textures, 240
  missing IP, 246–247
  obesity and, 241–245. *See also* Obesity, food
    preferences and
  PROP genetics and, 241
  responses, ingestive appetite and, 246
  sensory, 250
  for tastes, 88–89
  thoughts controlling, sensations *vs.*, 263–265,
    264f
  words for, 250
Presentation, food, 165–167, 210
Primary taste cortex, 84–86, 85f
Pringles®, 203
Procedures, threshold, 104–108
  chemical taste, 106–107
  electrogustometry, 107–108
Progressive supranuclear palsy, 33t

PROP (6-*n*-propyl-thiouracil), 17, 43, 109,
110–111, 112, 120, 197
food preferences and, 238–239
genetics, 241
Propranolol, 182
6-*n*-propyl-thiouracil (PROP), 17, 43, 109,
110–111, 112, 120, 197
food preferences and, 238–239
genetics, 241
Pseudohypoparathyroidism, 37
Psychophysical measurement, of human oral
experience, 103–126. *See also* Human
oral experience
Psychosocial distress
on food intake and weight, 312
instruments for screening, 312
Psychosocial interventions, chemosensory
alterations in cancer patients, 317–319
PTC (phenylthiocarbamide), 109, 111
Pythagoras theorem, 260

Q

Quick Smell Identification Test (QSIT), 73
Quinine, 88, 167–168
Quintessence, 13

R

Ratings, cognitive analysis, 272, 273f–274f
Rats, diet-induced thermogenesis in, 176
Receptors, taste, 83–84. *See also* Taste
papillae, 83
receptor cells, 84
taste buds, 83
Recognition thresholds, for taste, 106
Recurrent otitis media, 205
Reduced acceptance, 249. *See also* Acceptance
Reflex-ingestive movements, to sweet taste, 227
Reflexive acceptance, 86. *See also* Acceptance
Refreshing appearance, 146, 164
Refreshment, colors and, 146–147, 163–164
Registered dietitians, 311, 312, 319
Rejection behavior, acceptance *vs.*, 87, 88, 223
Relaxation, olfaction role, 75
Release-of-inhibition phantoms, 123
Retronasal olfaction, 65–75
chemical signal, 67–68
chemosensation, response to, 73–74
clinical testing retronasal smell, 70–73, 70f
food and chemosensation, 74–75
function, 66
odorants and flavors, 68–69
olfactory anatomy, 66–67
oral sensory evaluation, 125–126
orthonasal *vs.*, 69
other behavioral realms, 75

overview, 65–66
sensory adaptation, role, 69
Retronasal smell, clinical testing, 70–73, 70f
Retronasal threshold
olfaction, during eating, 67
Reversal artifact, 116
Rewards
associative, words for, 252
food, 252
sensory motivation without, 227
Rice Krispies®, 203, 206
Rolls, B. J., 211–212
Rolls, Edmond T., 18–19
Room service method, 315

S

Saccharin, 88
preference as appetite model, 224–225
Salivation, 74
Salts
human preference for, 239–240
strokes and, 281–283, 282f
Satiety, 300, 301
chemosensory, 74–75
induction, 301, 302, 303
sensory-generalized, 303, 304
sensory-related, 299–300
sensory-specific, 301, 302, 303
nutrition and, 209–215. *See also* Sensory-
specific satiety
Saturation, defined, 143
Scammony, 6
Schizophrenia, 32t
Scientific measurement, of contexts, 258–260
separate influences, interactions, 260
Scopolamine, 46
Seiyakusho, Suzuki, 13
Senescence, 34t
Senile dementia of Alzheimer's type, 32t, 46
Sensations, 246, 248
thoughts controlling preference *vs.*, 263–265,
264f
Sensed characteristics, 246
Sensing into ingesting, converting, 255–261
chemical stimulation to ingestive movement,
processes, 255–256
configured IP, 257–261
identical/configured influences, 260–261
mixture statistics, 257–258
scientific measurement of context,
258–260
mixing, 256–257
Sensory adaptation, role, 69
Sensory evaluation
of food, visual cues on, 159–171. *See also*
Visual cues

oral, methods, 119–126
   retronasal olfaction, 125–126
   spatial taste testing, 122–125. *See also*
      Spatial taste testing
   videomicroscopy of tongue, 121
   whole mouth sensation, 120–121
Sensory factor, peak of learnt facilitation by,
   234–235, 235f
Sensory motivation, without pleasure/reward, 227
Sensory preferences, 250
Sensory-related satiation, 299–300
Sensory-specific satiety, nutrition and, 209–215,
   301, 302, 303
   anorexia and, 214
   of beverages, 214
   on changes in visual sensation, 211
   chewing gum on, 214
   defined, 210
   in elderly population, 212
   hedonics on, 210, 211
   impaired, 212
   localize to brain, 213
   mechanisms, 209
   for obesity, 212, 214
   OFC in, 213
   olfaction and, 212
   olfactory or gustatory adaptation and, 213–214
   post-ingestive negative alliesthesia, 210
   VMH syndrome, 210
Sensory vocabularies, social names, 268–269
Sensual pleasure, sweetness and, 227
7UP, 167–168, 171
Shininess, 164
Sinusitis, 33t
Size, of bite, 195–196
Smell. *See* Odors/smell
SNAP (supplemental nutrition and assistance
   plan), 21
Sniff therapy, for chemosensory disorders, 49
Social names, sensory vocabularies, 268–269
Sodium
   acceptance curve for, 90
   dietary restriction, 90
   in peripheral taste nerves, 90
Sodium glutamate, 12
Solutions, sweet
   ingestive responses, 225–226, 226f
Somatic contexts, of sweet preference, 231–234,
   232f, 233f
Sour taste, balance in oranges, 261–262
Southerners, taste preferences, 2
Soy sauce, 11
Spatial taste testing, 122–125
   localized taste loss, clinical correlates,
      122–125
      anesthesia in evaluation, 124–125
      oral disinhibition, 123–124

Spurge, 6
St. Louis encephalitis, 39–40
Steroid-dependent anosmia, 36
Stevens, S. S., 108, 109
Stimulation
   chemical, to ingestive movement, 255–256
   from citric acid, 263
   direct, of preferences, 262–263, 262f
   nerve-stimulation phantom, 124
Sting, 197–198
Strawberries, aroma, 271–272
   analytical and configured norms, 275–276
   cognitive analysis of concentrations and
      ratings, 272, 273f–274f
Strengths
   of influence, stimulus, 252–253
   preferred, of sweet taste, 230
      most preferred, 230–231
Strokes, salt and, 281–283, 282f
Strychnine, 87
Sucrose, 257, 276–277, 278f, 279f, 280f
Sugar
   in diet, 20–22
   sweetened gum, 214, 276–277
   sweet taste
      balances in oranges, 261–262
      food preferences and obesity, 242–244,
         243f
      level. *See* Sweetness level
   teeth and, 283
Supertasters, 17
   defined, 110
   PROP, 197
Supplemental nutrition and assistance plan
   (SNAP), 21
Suprathreshold intensity, direct scaling, 108–119
   magnitude estimation, 108–109
   oral sensory differences, labeled scales,
      113–119, 114f
      GIS, 117, 119
      gLMS, 116–119, 118f
      intensity labels, properties, 113–115
      invalid comparisons, consequences,
         115–116, 115f
   oral sensory differences, magnitude
      matching, 109–113
      genetic factors in variation, 111–112
      overview, 110–111
      taster status classification, 112–113
Surroundings, color, 151
Sweetness level
   excitation and inhibition of ingestion,
      224–230
      conditioned taste aversion, 229
      conditioned taste preference, 229–230
      learnt preferences for, 227–229, 228f
      reflex-ingestive movements to taste, 227

saccharin preference as appetite model,
   224–225
sensory motivation without pleasure/
   reward, 227
solutions, ingestive responses to,
   225–226, 226f
learnt peak of preference for, 230–240
   conditioned appetite for caffeine, 236
   development for bitter foods and drinks,
      236, 237, 238
   evidence, human sensory preferences, 234
   facilitation by sensory factor, 234–235,
      235f
   human preference for salt taste, 239–240
   IP for bitterness of caffeine, 236,
      237f–238f
   likings for bitterness levels, 235–236
   most preferred strength, 230–231
   PROP and, 238–239
   somatic contexts of, 231–234, 232f, 233f
   strengths of taste, 230
   tastes, smells, colors, and textures, 240
Sweet taste
   acceptance, 228, 228f, 230
   balances in oranges, 261–262
   food preferences and obesity, 242–244, 243f
Sweet tooth, 244
Synsepalum dulcificum, 313
Synthroid, 48

T

Tableware, color, 149–151
Tactile referrals, 122
Taste and Smell Survey, 311
Taste and tasting
   amount, 254
   combinations of tastes, roles, 254
   conditioned taste aversion, 229
   conditioned taste preference, 229–230
   different taste, 253
   enduring changes, 88–89
   fat, food preferences and obesity, 244–245
   food choice and, 81–96. *See also* Food choice
   hedonically aversive, 295–298
   hedonically positive, 300–305
   history, 1–22
      basic tastes, 2–3
      biological aspects, 1, 3
      Galen's concepts of bitterness, 3–10
      overview, 1–3
      umami, 10–20
   mixing, sense of taste, 256–257
   mixture statistics, 257–258
   on nutrition, long-term effects, 281–283
      salt and strokes, 281–283, 282f
      sugar and teeth, 283

pairing odors, 170
physiology, 16, 17, 18, 19, 30
preferences for specific level of sweetness,
   240
salt, human preference for, 239–240
savory complex/fifth simple taste, 268
spatial taste testing, 122–125. *See also* Spatial
   taste testing
stimulus levels, 254–255
sweet
   acceptance of, 228, 228f, 230
   food preferences and obesity, 242–244,
      243f
   most preferred strength, 230–231
   preferred strengths of, 230
   reflex-ingestive movements to, 227
system, organization, 87–88
transient changes, 90
Taste buds, 83
Taste cortex, primary, 84–86, 85f
Taste receptor gene (T2R38), 111–112
Taster status classification, 112–113
Tea, black, 214
Teeth, sugar and, 283
Temporal lobe lesions, 37–38
Testosterone, 37
Texture, food, 194–195, 240
Thalamic lesions, 38
Thalamic taste area, 84
Theophylline, for chemosensory disorders, 49
Thermogenesis, 175–189
   capsaicin on, 176, 177t–181t, 182–184, 188t,
      189
   capsiate on, 185t–187t, 188t
   concept, 175
   diet-induced, in rats, 176
   ingestion, 175–176
   nonchemosensory origins, 176
   sensory mechanisms in, 189
Thiamine, for chemosensory disorders, 47
Thiamine deficiency, alcohol and, 42
Thiourea bitterness, 113
Thirst, 81, 247
Thirst-quenching beverage, 147, 163
Thoughts controlling preference, sensations *vs.*,
   263–265, 264f
Three-drop technique, 106
Thresholds
   retronasal *vs.* orthonasal, olfaction and, 67
Thresholds, oral experience measurement,
   104–119
   direct scaling of suprathreshold intensity,
      108–119
      magnitude estimation, 108–109
      oral sensory differences, measuring,
         109–113. *See also* Oral sensory
         differences

procedures, 104–108
  chemical taste, 106–107
  electrogustometry, 107–108
Threshold testing, 311
Tofu, 11
Tongue, videomicroscopy of, 121
Toothpastes, refreshing properties, 146
Toxic agents, 40
T2R38 (taste receptor gene), 111–112
Traditional method, defined, 314
Transient changes, in taste, 90
Transient receptor potential vanilloid 1 (TRPV1), 176
Trauma, 41
Trigeminal sensation, on olfaction, 198
TRPV1 (transient receptor potential vanilloid 1), 176
Tufted cells, 27, 28, 29
Turner's syndrome, 37

U

Umami, 10–20
Umami Research Association, 17
Uncinate fits, 29
Unconscious sensation, 248
On Uneven Bad Temperament, 7–8
University of Pennsylvania Smell Identification Test (UPSIT), 45

V

Valeric acid, 297
VAS (visual analog scale), 113
Ventromedial hypothalamic (VMH) syndrome, 210
Videomicroscopy, of tongue, 121
Viral hepatitis, chemosensory disorder, 36
Viscosity, food, 196–197
Visual analog scale (VAS), 113
Visual cues, on sensory and hedonic evaluation of food, 159–171
  color(s) and
    flavor intensity, 161–162
    food identification, 160–161
    liking, 161
    refreshment, 163–164
  expectations, 167–169
  food presentation, 165–167
  for freshness, 164
  mechanisms by effects occur, 167

overview, 159–160
perceptual learning, 169–171
Visual sensation, changes
  sensory-specific satiety on, 211
Vitamin A, for chemosensory disorders, 47
VMH (ventromedial hypothalamic) syndrome, 210

W

Wakame, 11
Weber, E. H., 252–253, 254–255
Weight loss, chemosensation for, 295–305
  hedonically aversive odors and tastes, 295–298
  hedonically positive odors, 298–300
  hedonically positive tastes, 300–305
  overview, 295
Wernicke–Korsakoff syndrome, 32t, 42
Western diet, capsaicin in, 184, 189
Whole mouth oral sensation, 120–121
Wild leeks, 7
Wine, 70, 144, 151, 168
  astringent beverages, 197
  background music, 204, 205
  white, 170
Wolpe, Joseph, 295–296, 318–319
Words
  for energy intakes and appetite ratings, 248–249
  for intensities and preferences, 250–255
    amount of tastes, 254
    combinations of tastes, roles, 254
    different taste, food, 253
    food preferences, 250
    intensities, gustatory and olfactory, 250
    motivating stimulus/associative reward, 252
    pleasant *vs.* pleasurable, 250–251
    stimulus levels, 254–255
    strength of influence, 252–253

Y

Yamaguchi, Shizuko, 18
Yamasa Shoyu Company, 16

Z

Zinc, for chemosensory disorders, 47–48
Zinc sulfate, 316

Printed in the United States
by Baker & Taylor Publisher Services